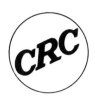

Cocaine: Chemical, Biological, Clinical, Social and Treatment Aspects

A CRC Drug Dependence Series Title

Editor-in-Chief
Drug Dependence Series

S. J. Mulé

Assistant Commissioner and Director
New York State ODAS Testing and Research Laboratory
Brooklyn, New York

Published by

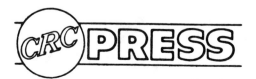

CRC PRESS, Inc.
18901 Cranwood Parkway · Cleveland, Ohio 44128

Library of Congress Cataloging in Publication Data

Main entry under title:

Cocaine.

   Includes bibliographical references and indexes.
   1. Cocaine. I. Mulé, S. J.
QP921.C7C6   362.2'93   76-25486
ISBN 0-87819-082-1

International Standard Book Number 0-8493-5057-3

Library of Congress Card Number 76-25486

Printed in the United States

CONTRIBUTORS (continued)

Ronald R. Hutchinson, Ph.D.
Research Director
Foundation for Behavioral Research
600 South Cherry Street
Augusta, Michigan

Darryl S. Inaba, Pharm. D.
Director of Pharmaceutical Services
Haight-Ashbury Free Medical Clinics
San Francisco, California
and
Assistant Clinical Professor
University of California
School of Pharmacy
San Francisco, California

Peter Jatlow, M.D.
Professor of Laboratory Medicine
Yale University School of Medicine
New Haven, Connecticut

Norman A. Krasnegor, Ph.D.
Assistant Chief, Clinical Behavior Branch
Division of Research
National Institute on Drug Abuse
11400 Rockville Pike
Rockville, Maryland

Masaji Matsuzaki, M.D., Ph.D.
Associate Research Scientist
New York State Office of Drug Abuse Services
Testing and Research Laboratory
80 Hanson Place
Brooklyn, New York

Anand L. Misra, Ph.D.
Associate Research Scientist
New York State Office of Drug Abuse Services
Testing and Research Laboratory
80 Hanson Place
Brooklyn, New York

Joel L. Phillips, B.A.
Research Associate
Wynne Associates
3804 Legation Street, N.W.
Washington, D.C.

Roy Pickens, Ph.D.
Psychiatry Research Unit
Mayo Memorial Building
University of Minnesota Medical School
Minneapolis, Minnesota

Robert M. Post, M.D.
Chief, 3-West Clinical Research Unit
Section on Psychobiology
Adult Psychiatry Branch
National Institute of Mental Health
9000 Rockville Pike
Bethesda, Maryland

Elaine S. Resnick, M.S.W.
Research Associate
Division of Drug Abuse Research and Treatment
Psychiatric Social Worker
Department of Psychiatry
New York Medical College
New York, New York

Richard B. Resnick, M.D.
Director, Division of Drug Abuse Research and Treatment
Associate Professor
Department of Psychiatry
New York Medical College
New York, New York

Jeffrey S. Stripling, Ph.D.
Post-Doctoral Fellow
Behavioral Neuropharmacology Section
Department of Psychiatry
Duke University Medical Center
Durham, North Carolina

Ronald D. Wynne, Ph.D.
Co-director
Wynne Associates
3804 Legation Street, N.W.
Washington, D.C.

CONTRIBUTORS

Michael R. Aldrich, Ph.D.
Executive Curator
Fitz Hugh Ludlow Memorial Library
1445 Stockton
San Francisco, California

Harold L. Altshuler, Ph.D.
Chief, Neuropsychopharmacology
Texas Research Institute of Mental Sciences
Houston, Texas

Sydney Archer, Ph.D.
Research Professor of Medicinal Chemistry
Department of Chemistry
Rensselaer Polytechnic Institute
Troy, New York

Robert Barker
Director
Fitz Hugh Ludlow Memorial Library
1445 Stockton
San Francisco, California

Milton L. Bastos, Full Professor
Department of Forensic Medicine
New York University School of Medicine
520 First Avenue
New York, New York

Neil R. Burch, M.D.
Research Division Head
Chief, Psychophysiology Section
Texas Research Institute of Mental Sciences
Texas Medical Center
Houston, Texas

John Caldwell, Ph.D.
Lecturer in Biochemical Pharmacology
Department of Biochemical and Experimental
    Pharmacology
St. Mary's Hospital Medical School
London W2 1PG
England

**Anna Maria Di Giulio, Doctor in Biological
Sciences**
Assistant Professor
2nd Chair, Department of Pharmacology
School of Medicine
University of Milan
Italy

John Dougherty, Ph.D.
Drug Abuse Research Laboratory (116-CDD)
Veterans Administration Hospital
Lexington, Kentucky

Everett H. Ellinwood, Jr., M.D.
Professor of Psychiatry
Director, Behavioral Neuropharmacology
    Section
Department of Psychiatry
Duke University Medical Center
Durham, North Carolina

Grace S. Emley, M.A.
Research Associate
Foundation for Behavioral Research
600 South Cherry Street
Augusta, Michigan

George R. Gay, M.D.
Family Practice, Toxicology and
    Anesthesiology
Mendocino, California
        Formerly
Director of Clinical Services
Haight-Ashbury Free Medical Clinics
San Francisco, California

Antonio Groppetti, Doctor in Pharmacy
Libera Docenza in Pharmacology
Associate Professor
2nd Chair, Department of Pharmacology
School of Medicine
University of Milan
Italy

Richard L. Hawks, Ph.D.
Research Technology Branch
Division of Research
National Institute on Drug Abuse
11400 Rockville Pike
Rockville, Maryland

Donald B. Hoffman, Ph.D.
Senior Chemist
Toxicological Laboratories
Office of the Medical Examiner
New York, New York

THE EDITOR

S. J. Mulé, Ph.D., is Assistant Commissioner and Director of the New York State Office of Drug Abuse Services Testing and Research Laboratory, New York.

Dr. Mulé received his B.A. degree in Chemistry in 1954 from College of Wooster, Wooster, Ohio; the M.S. degree in Biochemistry and Physiology in 1955 from Rutgers University, New Brunswick, New Jersey; and the Ph.D. degree in Pharmacology in 1961 from the University of Michigan, Ann Arbor, Michigan. Dr. Mulé subsequently received postdoctoral training in the Departments of Physiological Chemistry and Pharmacology at the University of Wisconsin. He continued his research at the Addiction Research Center of the National Institute of Mental Health, Lexington, Kentucky. His present research concerns the pharmacokinetics and biotransformation of narcotic analgesics, the detection and identification of drugs subject to abuse, and the biochemical mechanisms of drug dependence.

Dr. Mulé, who has published extensively in the scientific literature and is a member of pharmacological, chemical, clinical, and forensic societies, is editor-in-chief of the CRC Drug Dependence Series.

PREFACE

Cocaine, "The Champagne of Drugs of Abuse," has periodically enjoyed "center stage" in the drama of drug misuse for more than ten centuries. Once again, "La Dama Blanca" (The White Lady) flies high especially among the opiate dependent, the affluent, and the creative and innovative. The need for more knowledge and information concerning this heavily abused drug is thus self-evident. Therefore, the purpose of this text is to provide the scientist (chemical, pharmacological, physiological, psychological, clinical, behavioral, and social) with currently available data (state of the art) on cocaine's use and abuse in our society. The sophisticated laymen may also find interest in this material. Logically, the text was organized by first reviewing the historical evolution of cocaine, followed by a thorough study of the chemistry including physical and chemical properties, stereochemistry, and synthetic mechanisms of not only cocaine, but also many of its derivatives and congeners. The detection of cocaine has advanced considerably over the years both in regards to identification in biological materials and the analysis of "street" derived substances. The recent synthesis of radioactive cocaine and derivatives coupled with the development of methods and techniques for the identification of cocaine and metabolites have allowed complete studies on the pharmacokinetics and biotransformation in animals. The neurotransmitter mechanisms whereby cocaine may exert some of its pharmacological actions are presented. Psychic dependence, the essential driving force behind "drug seeking behavior," is viewed from a neurophysiological and self-administration perspective. Furthermore, the effects of cocaine (acute and chronic) on the electrical activity of the brain and the subsequent development of tolerance to these effects are thoroughly explored. Behavioral correlates of cocaine use, especially as it applies to aggression are delightfully discussed. The physiological effects of cocaine following acute and chronic administration are reviewed in depth. Clinical assessments of acute and chronic use of cocaine in man in relation to physiological effects and behavior are scientifically presented. The sociological implications and treatment of the toxic effects of cocaine overdose and rehabilitation of the chronic user are vividly reviewed.

The highly technical nature of this monograph required the efforts of many authors who brought their special expertise to a given chapter. In a text of this nature, it is almost impossible to eliminate all duplication of data and information as well as to be absolutely certain that all the essential available research data are presented. However, a serious effort was exerted to reduce duplication and to see that all the critical available data on a given subject were presented. Furthermore, diverse viewpoints unsupported by data and impinging upon biases were hopefully eliminated.

Special thanks is given to Virginia Sebastiano for her marvelous efficiency in handling the innumerable daily tasks required in order to complete this monograph for publication.

S. J. Mulé, Ph.D.
New York, New York

TABLE OF CONTENTS

Historical Aspects

Historical Aspects of Cocaine Use and Abuse

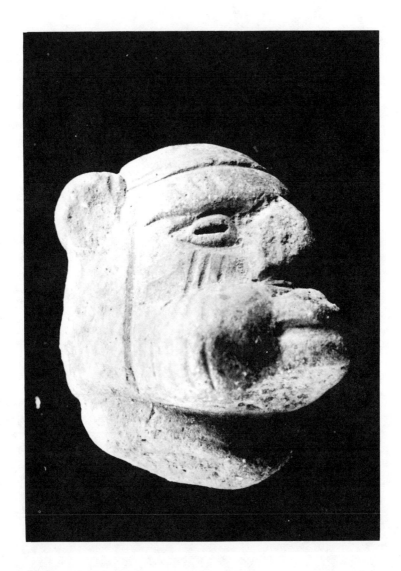

FIGURE 1. Head of coca-chewer, terracotta whistle, Colombia, ca. 1300 A.D. (Courtesy of The Fitz Hugh Ludlow Memorial Library, San Francisco. Photo by Jeremy Bigwood.)

HISTORICAL ASPECTS OF COCAINE USE AND ABUSE

Michael R. Aldrich and Robert W. Barker

Amerigo Vespucci was the first European to describe coca-chewing in the New World which now bears his name. Disembarking at Isla de Margarita off the coast of Venezuela in 1499, he was greeted by "the most bestial and brutal race ever seen," (Figure 1) as he recalled in a letter about his voyages:[1]

> They were very brutish in appearance and behavior, and their cheeks bulged with the leaves of a certain green herb which they chewed like cattle, so that they could hardly speak. Each had around his neck two dried gourds, one full of that herb in their mouths, the other filled with a white flour like powdered chalk. From time to time, each put a small stick (which had been moistened in his mouth) into the gourd full of flour. Then they would draw it forth and put it in both sides of their cheeks, mixing the powder with the herb in their mouths. They did this frequently, a little at a time; and the thing seemed wonderful for we could not understand the secret, or with what object they did it.

After asking for drinking water and being offered coca instead, Vespucci surmised that "they kept this herb in their mouths to stave off thirst." Fifty years later the youthful Conquistador Pedro Cieza de Leon gave a more informed, though equally disdainful, explanation:[2 A]

> When I asked some of these Indians why they carried these leaves in their mouth, which they do not eat, but merely hold between their teeth, they replied that it prevents them from feeling hungry, and gives them great vigor and strength. I believe that it has some such effect, although perhaps it is a custom only suitable for people like these Indians.

Coca has been cultivated for these purposes since the dawn of agriculture in South America. Cord bags containing leaves, flowers, and even a chewed quid of coca have been unearthed in burial middens dating back to c. 2500 B.C. at Huaca Prieta on the north coast of Peru.[3] Such finds point to aboriginal shamanistic rites in which coca was deposited in graves to facilitate the departed spirit's journey through death, as it had in life. Voluminous evidence of trephined skulls (Figure 2), coca quids, obsidian knives, and cotton bandages in ancient Peruvian graves leads to the conclusion that "cocaine-filled saliva of the chewed coca leaves was used as a local anesthetic in early, yet highly sophisticated, trephining operations."[4]

From these prehistoric beginnings, the multiple uses of coca became known to every pre-Colombian civilization in western South America. To appreciate the reverence with which coca was regarded, one needs only to glimpse the desolate and inhospitable conditions of life in the high Andes, where even now food will not grow without a farmer's utmost efforts. Yet for millenia before the Spanish conquest, without horses, cattle, or even the wheel, with simple digging tools and clod breakers, the highlanders not only survived but built irrigation aqueducts for terrace farming, magnificent stone temples and buildings, and a road network that was a wonder of the ancient world. Artifacts from many cultures attest the inextricable link between coca and the advancement of civilization in these regions. In Colombia, the mysterious San Agustín monolithic idols (500 B.C. to 300 A.D.) display the characteristic distended cheek of the coca-chewer,[5] while exquisite Quimbaya gold vessels for powdered lime, and Tairona gold priests' bells cast as human faces with prominent lip-bulges bespeak the awe in which coca was held by artists and priests.[6] In Peru, certain elements of the Inca religion appear to derive, ultimately, from Mochica clan rituals of the Classic Period (200 to 800 A.D.), judging by a huge gold coca bag in the shape of a puma with a human head on its tongue, as well as numerous stirrup-jars depicting warriors and shamans in ecstatic poses blessing their weapons, praising sky gods, or nursing their wounds while clutching coca bags and lime gourds.[7-9] Very precious ceremonial containers and delicate gold, silver, and bronze lime spoons from Post Classic cultures reveal a continuous progression of sacramental coca use right up to the time of Pizarro's entry in 1532.[3,10]

The Incas, however, made coca the center of a religion and social system distinctly their own. Inca legend has it that the plant was divine, brought from heaven by the first emperor Manco Capac. The Inca (Quechua) word *coca*, cognate with Aymara *khoka*, meant simply "the tree."[2 B] The bright star Spica was "Mama Coca," a name

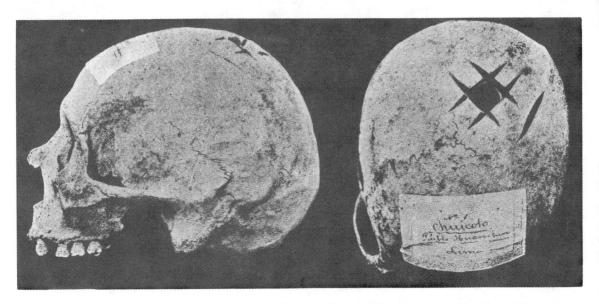

FIGURE 2. Peruvian trephining. (From Mortimer, W. G., *Peru: History of Coca,* Vail & Co., New York, 1901, reprinted as *History of Coca,* And/Or Press, San Francisco, 1974. With permission.)

also taken by an early empress symbolizing her role, and coca's role, as "mother" of the expanding Inca empire.[2C] Throughout the empire, from Ecuador to Chile, use of coca was restricted to the conquering Inca aristocracy, though it could be given to chiefs (*curacas*) of conquered tribes assimilated into the empire, and to other persons designated by royalty.[2D,7] Among these were priests, doctors, youths selected for initiation into warrier or priestly clans, the fabled relay runners who conveyed messages 150 miles a day along the stupendous Inca road system, and the scholars who kept the empire's accounts on intricately knotted strings called *quipus.*[2E,7] The sovereign gift of the right to chew coca thus signified acceptance into the aristocracy and into the Inca religion. Solid gold models of coca sprigs adorned the gold-plated Temples of the Sun, whose altars could be approached only by the elite with coca in their mouths.[2F,11] This strict control over who could use coca may have been a form of protection against abuse of the plant; it was also perhaps the social mechanism which gave the aristocracy their divine powers.

Precisely because coca was an integral part of native religion, the Spanish first forbade it as satanic idolatry. The roots of anti-coca sentiment, which still pervades South American officialdom, may be found in the Spanish Inquisition, which regarded coca use as devil worship; racism, which in its mildest form may be seen in Cieza's statement quoted above; and genocide, which in a few years exterminated the Incas and curacas along with their centralized social system. Yet another aspect of Spanish imperialism, commercial exploitation of the subjugated natives, overcame the first impulse to prohibit coca. The Conquistadores recognized that coca enabled their slaves to endure forced labor, and thus encouraged its use and cultivation. By Spanish decree, workers were both paid and taxed in coca, and great plantations sprang up as close to the mines as possible, i.e., at altitudes of up to 6,000 feet. By 1590, traffic in coca at Potosi, the rich silver mines 17,000 feet high in southern Bolivia, was valued at over half a million dollars a year.[2G] Further regulations stipulated that a portion of each worker's income had to be given to the Church. Father Blas Valera, a 16th-century chronicler, says flatly that "the greater part of the revenue of the bishops and canons of the cathedrals of Cuzco is derived from the tithes of Coca leaves."[2H] Only then, after living for decades in the Andes, did the Conquistadores glimpse coca's medical value. Valera continues:

Cuca preserves the body from many infirmities, and our doctors use it pounded for applications to sores and broken bones, to remove cold from the body or to prevent it from entering, as well as to cure sores that are full of maggots. It is so beneficial and has such singular virtue in the cure of outward sores, it will surely have even more virtue and efficacy in the entrails of those who eat it!

Despite such reports, coca did not attract much attention in Europe except as a contemptible form of native intoxication. Nicolas Monardes of Seville in 1565 attempted a technical description of coca's characteristic leaf-within-a-leaf pattern, and related what appears to be a sailor's story in a curious passage which surely confuses "Tabaco" with one of the hallucinogenic snuffs:[12]

When thei will make them selves dronke, and bee out of judgements, thei mingle with the Coca the leaves of the Tabaco, and thei doe chewe them alltogether, and thei goe as thei were out of their wittes, like as if thei were dronke which is a thynge that dooeth geve them greate contentement . . .

With such descriptions of "Tabaco" circulating, it is no wonder that King James and other monarchs later tried to outlaw tobacco; the wonder is that no one except botanists took much interest in coca. Perhaps the leaves deteriorated during the long voyage from America; then, too, the practice of sucking a mouthful of leaves did not exactly commend itself to the world of fashion. The earliest "taxonomic" classification of the plant, if it may be called that, was given by Plukenet in 1692, who described "Mamacoca" as the divine name in Peru. Then in 1749 Joseph de Jussieu sent carefully collected specimens of Bolivian coca to his brother Antoine in Paris, who placed them in the family *Malpighiaceae*. This classification was changed by Linnaeus, who put coca in its own family, *Erythroxyleae,* and genus, *Erythroxylon.*[21,11] (The generic name sometimes seen, *Erythroxylum,* from the plant's "red wood," was that used by Browne in a 1756 report on Jamaican flora.) Lamarck gave the most important species the name *Erythroxylon coca* in 1786.

European interest in coca's legendary efficacy as a stimulant perked up in the early 19th century, inspired by the fascinating accounts of the great naturalists Unanue (1794), Humboldt, Poeppig, Tschudi, Bibra, Martius, Weddell, Spruce, Herndon, and Markham (1862).[2J] Most of these writers penned glowing descriptions of coca's virtues, often including accounts of their own use of the leaves. None was more extravagant, however, than Dr. Paolo Mantegazza, an eminent Italian neurologist who wrote in 1859, after chewing more than an ounce of fresh leaves: "Borne on the wings of two coca leaves, I flew about in the spaces of 77,438 worlds, each one more splendid than the others . . . I prefer a life of

ten years with coca to one of a hundred thousand without it."[4,13]

At about the same time, the search for medically useful alkaloids, begun in 1806 with Sertürner's isolation of morphine from opium, began to awaken scientific interest in coca. Interestingly, perhaps because of European disdain for the plant inevitably associated with the downtrodden natives of South America, cocaine was the last of the major 19th-century drug plant alkaloids to be isolated. A substance called "erythroxyline," probably cocaine, was extracted by Gaedecke about 1855, while "cocaine," so named, was isolated independently by Albert Niemann of Göttingen (Figure 3) 4 or 5 years later.[14] As investigation of cocaine began, some of Europe's and America's finest scientists — as well as one of history's greatest entrepreneurs — began experimenting with coca in earnest.

Angelo Mariani (Figure 4), a young Corsican chemist living in Paris, manufactured a coca-based wine, instantly acclaimed by opera singers and musicians as a tonic to soothe their sore throats and stimulate their often prodigiously long performances.[2K,15] Sir Robert Christison, the 78-year-old President of the British Medical Association, astonished colleagues in 1876 by describing how coca chewing enabled him to take 16-mile hikes and climb mountains with "youthful vigour."[14,2L] American physicians, including the noted throat specialist Dr. Louis Elsberg, began using coca, *Vin Mariani*, and cocaine in their practice; the leaves became official in the U.S. Pharmacopia in 1880, cocaine in 1890.[2K,11] The *Detroit Therapeutic Gazette* ran a series of articles touting cocaine as a cure for morphine addiction, while in Germany an army doctor, Theodor Aschenbrandt, dosed his fatigued troops with cocaine and noted a marvelous increase in their energy and endurance.[16A] A distinguished pharmacologist, Dr. August Vogl, regaled the academicians of Vienna with the beneficial effects of a coca tea he brewed himself; Vogl is significant because one of his students was Carl Koller, and Sigmund Freud researched his papers on cocaine in Vogl's library.[16B]

The year 1884 was the watershed in cocaine history. That year young Freud published the first of five papers on cocaine which have recently been revived in an exhaustively annotated edition by Dr. Robert Byck.[16] *Über Coca* was, as Dr. Byck observes, "a brilliantly written review of the

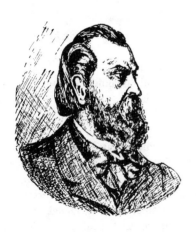

FIGURE 3. Albert Niemann. (From Mortimer, W. G., *Peru: History of Coca,* Vail & Co., New York, 1901, reprinted as *History of Coca,* And/Or Press, San Francisco, 1974. With permission.)

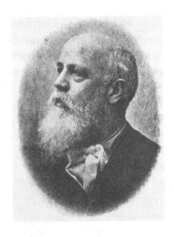

FIGURE 4. Angelo Mariani. (From Mortimer, W. G., *Peru: History of Coca,* Vail & Co., New York, 1901, reprinted as *History of Coca,* And/Or Press, San Francisco, 1974. With permission.)

knowledge of cocaine up to that time and one of the finest reviews of cocaine ever done. Much of it is still authoritative."[17] Freud recommended the "magical drug" for a variety of therapeutic purposes, not the least of which was curing his own severe depressions; for treating nervous exhaustion, hysteria, hypochondria, neurasthenia, digestive disorders; for "all diseases which involve degeneration of the tissues, such as severe anemia, phthisis, long-lasting febrile diseases, etc.;" as a possible aphrodisiac and cure for syphilis, asthma, and altitude sickness; as "a local anesthetic, especially in connection with affections of the mucous membrane;" to "suppress the craving for morphine in habitual addicts," and similarly to treat alcoholism.[16C] Freud particularly hoped that cocaine might cure the morphine addiction of his friend Dr. Ernst von Fleischl-Marxow — which it did; but Fleischl soon developed an irresistible craving for hypodermic injections of cocaine, and Freud came to blame himself for hastening his friend's death 7 years later.[16D] The prominent pharmacologists Louis Lewin and A. Erlenmeyer soon denounced Freud's advocacy of cocaine, Erlenmeyer calling it "the third scourge of mankind" after alcohol and morphine.[18] Freud stopped proselytizing the drug after his fifth essay on the subject in 1887, but continued taking it intermittently himself through at least 1895, when beginning his seminal work on dream interpretation. It may be argued that cocaine contributed, perhaps substantially, to the origins of psychoanalytic theory, for the first of Freud's own dreams submitted to detailed analysis occurred when he was, by his own admission, "making frequent use" of cocaine.[16E]

And when Carl Koller, a young Viennese intern who experimented with cocaine at Freud's request, noticed its numbing effect on the tongue, he suddenly realized it might be the anesthetic for eye surgery which he had been seeking for some time. As early as 1862, Schraff had remarked on this numbing effect, while in 1868 Moreno y Maiz had suggested the possibility of local anesthesia while studying cocaine acetate on frogs;[11] but Koller designed a series of experiments to prove the theory. Too poverty-stricken himself to attend an ophthalmological conference in Heidelberg, Koller had a friend there demonstrate his experiments and read his paper on September 15, 1884, announcing the discovery of local anesthesia.[16B]

Koller's discovery had stunning world-wide impact. Newspapers reported it regularly for months; the pharmaceutical companies were swamped with orders for cocaine hydrochloride, which suddenly skyrocketed in price; doctors vied with each other to invent new applications for the revolutionary anesthetic. But as cocaine's therapeutic usefulness became apparent, so did its potential for abuse. The pioneer American surgeon Dr. William Halsted demonstrated cocaine's nerve-blocking effects which rendered it useful for dozens of surgical procedures, and became so dependent on the drug that his associates had to put him aboard an ocean-bound schooner to kick the habit. This he accomplished, but at the expense of becoming a morphine addict — the reverse of what had happened to Freud's friend Fleischl. For a very long time thereafter, one of Johns Hopkins University's most closely-guarded secrets was that one of its founders was a junkie.[16 F,19] Dr. J. L. Corning, Halsted's student, was the first to use cocaine in spinal anesthesia.[20]

Two classmates at City University of New York who heard about Koller's discovery were destined to play important roles in the history of coca. One was Henry H. Rusby, who immediately upon graduation departed for Bolivia to study coca for Parke-Davis & Co. He made the best early taxonomic field studies of the plant and became the first to insist that "the properties of cocaine, remarkable as they are, lie in an altogether different direction from those of coca."[2 M,21] Rusby became Dean of Pharmacy at Columbia, one of the most distinguished ethnopharmacologists of his time. His classmate, W. Golden Mortimer, became editor of the *Pharmaceutical Journal* in New York and the author of the best book about coca in any language, *Peru: History of Coca* (1901). In this definitive 576-page work, Mortimer constantly reiterated the key distinction between coca and cocaine:[2 M]

Since 1885, most of the writings and the experiments of physiologists upon Coca seem to have been based upon the idea of a single active principle which should represent the potency of the leaf. As is clearly indicated in the history which has been traced through nearly four centuries, this is a false supposition. The qualities of Coca are not fully represented by any one of its alkaloids so far isolated.

Contemporary research is beginning to show that Rusby and Mortimer were correct. Coca is a natural powerpack of energy sources — not only cocaine, which is present in proportions varying from 0.25 to 1.0%[22,23] — but also other alkaloids, notably ecgonine and cuskohygrine, which also may be active,[10] and a rich complement of vitamins A, B_1, C, E, riboflavin, calcium, phosphorus, and iron.[7,24,36]

The explosive controversy over cocaine's therapeutic value, and growing abuse, naturally found expression in the flourishing literature of the time. Dr. Myron G. Schultz has suggested that Robert Louis Stevenson's *Dr. Jekyll and Mr. Hyde*, in which a newly-discovered powder transforms a respectable physician into "the grotesque embodi-

ment of the basest part of his nature," may have been written under the stimulus of cocaine prescribed, as Freud recommended, for his tuberculosis.[25] Dr. Arthur Conan Doyle, an eye specialist, would not have missed the news of Koller's great discovery, and began inserting references to Sherlock Holmes's use of cocaine in stories as early as 1886.[14,26] The great detective, depicted elegantly injecting cocaine in *The Sign of Four*, is the perfect prototype of the gentlemanly intellectual cocaine user (as opposed to the later stereotype of the depraved cocainist), and was so portrayed by the celebrated actor William Gillette on the New York stage in 1901 (Figure 5). This image was soon debunked by no less an actor than Douglas Fairbanks, Sr., whose self-produced *The Mystery of the Leaping Fish* (1916) featured a detective named "Coke Ennyday" snorting and shooting great handfuls of cocaine to subdue an opium smuggling ring operating near "Short Beach," California. This was perhaps the first screen

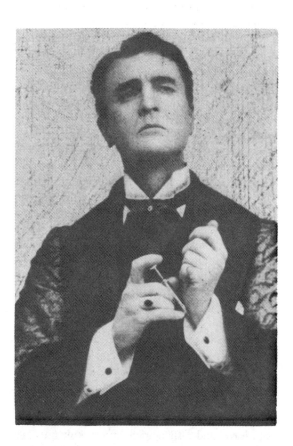

FIGURE 5. William Gillette as Sherlock Holmes, 1901. (Courtesy of The Fitz Hugh Ludlow Memorial Library, San Francisco.)

portrayal of the drug user as a "hop-head," with Fairbanks literally hopping up and down every time he takes either cocaine or opium. More recently, novelist Nicholas Meyer has climbed the best-seller lists with *The Seven-Per-Cent Solution* (1975), which proposes that Holmes had his cocainomania cured by none other than Dr. Sigmund Freud.

The chief beneficiary of the *fin de siècle* cocaine explosion, however, was not Freud, Koller, Stevenson, or Doyle. It was Angelo Mariani, whose coca-leaf Bordeaux became the most avidly endorsed tonic in the world. Among the luminaries who graced the pages of Mariani's testimonial albums[27] were the Czar and Czarina of Russia, the Prince and Princess of Wales, the King of Norway and Sweden, King Norodom of Cambodia, the Commander of the French Forces in Indochina, the Commanding General of the British Army, and Pope Leo XIII, who awarded Mariani a special gold medal for the wine. Over 8,000 doctors, including physicians to all the royal houses of Europe, testified to the elixir's virtues, along with the greatest authors, performers, and artists of the era: Dumas *fils*, H. G. Wells, Verne, Rostand, Zola, France, Ibsen; Bernhardt, Duse, Gounod, Massenet; and Rodin, Robida, Chéret, Mucha. August Bartholdi, sculptor of the Statue of Liberty, wrote that this "precious wine will give me strength to carry out certain other projects already formed." In America, President McKinley's secretary wrote that a case of *Vin Mariani* had been received enthusiastically, while physicians of former President U. S. Grant said that Mariani's coca tea enabled the failing general to work several hours a day. Even Thomas Alva Edison sent in a note and picture for Mariani's endorsement albums; interestingly, his biographers are fond of noting that the busy inventor slept only a few hours a night when absorbed in some particularly thorny problem.

It was not long before American entrepreneurs leaped into this booming market. In 1885 John S. Pemberton, a patent-medicine maker in Atlanta, brought out *French Wine Coca – Ideal Nerve and Tonic Stimulant*. Alcohol-prohibitionist sentiment ran high at the time, however, so a year later Pemberton launched a nonalcoholic extract of coca leaves and caffeine-rich African kola nuts in a sweet carbonated syrup.[19] *Coca-Cola®*, advertised as the "intellectual beverage and temperance drink," soon inspired a horde of imitators.

But the commercial explosion was getting out of hand. Reports of medical and nonmedical cocaine abuse, often from police sources, poured in to the authorities, and several states moved to make it illegal except by prescription. What was it that in a decade or two turned public sentiment against this drug? Most succinctly put, it was the transition from use of a green plant (and its leaf extracts) to use of a white powder. First, there were few complaints of harm resulting from widespread use of coca leaves, wines, teas, soft drinks, and patent medicines, arising from their consumers; rather, physicians and public health officials led a campaign against patent medicines not being labeled with their ingredients. Investigations of fraud culminated in the Pure Food and Drug Act of 1906 and forced the makers of Coca-Cola to remove cocaine from their product. D. W. Griffith, in a scathing short film called *For His Son* (1912), looked back on the early days of soft drinks with a tale of how the son of one of these manufacturers became "addicted" to cocaine by downing great quantities of daddy's soda pop. Even Mariani was forced to advertise that *Vin Mariani* was not a cocaine wine[16G] — which was, strictly speaking true, for he'd always insisted that his wine be made from an extract of the whole leaf, not the alkaloid — but the suddenly drug-conscious public would no longer support such niceties. The distinction between coca and cocaine was ignored, and both were misclassified as "narcotics" and banned by the Harrison Narcotic Act in 1914. That was the year Mariani died, leaving a museum of artifacts and books as the only memory of an era of coca commerce, an empire that was never to be rebuilt, a green magnificence scuttled in the outcry against white powder.

Secondly, racism played an important part in the formation of anti-cocaine legislation, as it was to do some years later with anti-marijuana laws. At the turn of the century, black laborers in New Orleans discovered that cocaine enabled them to load and unload steamboats more easily, and soon plantation owners were issuing regular rations of cocaine to their field hands.[11] The original "dope fiends" of American folklore were black cocaine-using workers and prostitutes.[28] As Dr. David Musto has observed,[29]

The fear of the cocainized black coincided with the peak of lynchings, legal segregation, and voting laws all designed to remove political and social power from him ... So far, evidence does not suggest that cocaine caused a crime wave but rather that anticipation of black rebellion inspired white alarm.

Up the river from New Orleans with jazz and marijuana, cocaine spread to the northern urban ghettoes and became a target for fear-stricken white lawmakers. Here it merged with the image of the white working-class drug abuser whose craving for "dope" is uncontrollable, as in Pendleton King's popular one-act play *Cocaine* (1917) which portrays an ex-boxer and his prostitute girlfriend in suicidal depression when they can no longer afford to buy the drug.[30]

Thirdly, beginning in the 1880's, pharmaceutical companies made cocaine hydrochloride widely available and it could be snorted as well as intravenously injected. Sniffing cocaine was preferred since it left no needle marks, required no special equipment, and allowed the habit to be continued discreetly. This mode of administration contributed greatly to the expansion of cocaine use as it suffused from the cultured and professional classes down to less wealthy economic levels. In Europe, the descent of the depraved cocainist (Figure 6) was brilliantly presented in Pitigrilli's 1921 novel *Cocaine,*[31] a mordantly witty satire on the cocaine-crazed demimonde of Montmartre, and in Aleister Crowley's *Diary of a Drug Fiend* 2 years later. American tabloids boosted their circulation with lurid articles on the drug underworld, which were later collected into books like Fred V. Williams's *The Hop-Heads* (1920) and Winifred Black's *Dope* (1928).

Medicinal use of cocaine tarried well into the Roaring Twenties. Sajous's *Analytic Cyclopedia of Practical Medicine* (1924) lists both internal uses for the drug (in seasickness, vomiting, shock, narcotics poisoning, gastritis, fatigue, neurasthenia, melancholia, etc.) and dozens of analgetic or anesthetic uses, but devotes as much space to grave warnings about cocainism, "the most insidious of all drug habits." Yet diagnosis of the "cocainomaniac" was difficult, Sajous declares, because he "quite often shows no symptom of bodily or mental disturbance." In other words, a stereotyped image is difficult to treat.[32] Sajous's tome signaled the culmination and end of cocaine therapy; other -caine derivatives without psychoactivity soon replaced cocaine even in anesthesia.

So strong were the dope-fiend images of cocaine use in the Twenties that they were sometimes used to denigrate any daring experimental writer. In 1921 James Joyce had to fend off his detractors' rumors that he was a "cocaine victim." Nevertheless it is true that Joyce

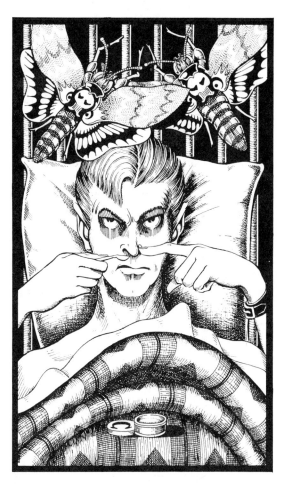

FIGURE 6. "What boredom, life!" (Drawing by Jim Osborne illustrating Pitigrilli's *Cocaine,* © Jim Osborne, 1974. From Segre, D. "Pitigrilli," *Cocaine,* Milano, 1921, English translation [1933] reprinted by And/Or Press, San Francisco, 1974. With permission.)

revised the penultimate chapters of *Ulysses* and began the most celebrated soliloquy in modern literature, Molly Bloom's interminable sentence at the end of the book, "with the aid of repeated doses of cocaine to relieve the pain" of an iritis attack in July, 1921.[33] Other authors —Herman Hesse, for instance, in *Steppenwolf* (1927) — made fictional use of cocaine in recreating the decadent ambiance of between-war Europe. Several passages in Marcel Proust's *À La Recherche du Temps Perdu* reflect widespread social cocaine use and abuse.[14] With stunning power, for example, Proust portrays a once-elegant lady

. . . whose features were so chipped away that the lines of her face could no longer be reconstructed . . . She had been taking cocaine and other drugs for three years past. Her eyes, circled with deep black rings, wore almost a haunted look . . . Time has in this way express trains and special trains to carry people to a premature old age.

World War II ground the decadent cabaret atmosphere of Europe into the dust beneath the clanking of panzers and the roar of the blitzkrieg. It has long been held that various members of the Nazi High Command – particularly Luftwaffe chief Hermann Goering – were cocainists,[34] but here it is difficult to separate truth from anti-Nazi propaganda. Amphetamines and synthetic narcotics replaced medical use of cocaine in many countries when supplies of coca were cut off during the war. Certainly social use of cocaine continued underground among entertainers, musicians, wealthy jet-setters, and *littérateurs* in post-war Europe and America, suddenly and dramatically reemerging from the drug culture of the Sixties into the "glitter crowd" of the Seventies.[35] Today it is the darling of discotheques around the world, as it once was in the dance halls of Vienna, Paris, and London, and the cabarets of Berlin and Buenos Aires.

In the fifty eventful years between Freud's paper and Proust's masterpiece, cocaine plunged from the bright hopes of medical science to the twilight of the underworld. Yet for centuries before and after that sunny Caribbean morning when Amerigo Vespucci wondered at "the secret" of the plant, coca and cocaine have intrigued some of the greatest writers, artists, and scientists of all time. Elixir of youth, revolutionary anesthetic, choice of aristocracy and slaves, lauded and maligned, the drug's fascination continues to this day.

REFERENCES

1. **Vespucci, A.,** Letter to a magnificent lord, 1504. Translation based on: (A) Markham, C., *The Letters of Amerigo Vespucci,* Hakluyt Society, London, 1894, 25; (B) Brooks, J., *Tobacco,* Rosenbach, New York, 1937, 189, cited in Wassen, S. H., Anthropological survey of the use of South American snuffs, in *Ethnopharmacologic Search for Psychoactive Drugs,* Efron, D., Holmstedt, B., and Kline, N., Eds., U.S. Govt. Printing Office, Washington, D.C., 1967, 234.
2. **Mortimer, W. G.,** *Peru: History of Coca,* Vail & Co., New York, 1901, reprinted as *History of Coca,* And/Or Press, San Francisco, 1974, (A) Cieza (1550), 151; (B) Weddell (1853), 7; (C) Hagar (1899), 66 – see also 152, 230; (D) 37, 152; (E) 37–50; (F) 63–4; (G) Acosta (1590), 155; (H) Valera (in Garcilasso, 1609), 159–60; (I) 165–6, 228–31, 531; (J) 167–77; (K) 412, 460; (L) Christison (1876), 362–6; (M) Rusby (1888), 17–19, (1898), 182–3.
3. **Bushnell, G. H. S.,** *Peru,* Praeger, New York, 1957, 28.
4. **Gay, G. R., Sheppard, C. W., Inaba, D. S., and Newmeyer, J. A.,** Cocaine in perspective: 'gift from the sun god' to 'the rich man's drug,' *Drug Forum,* 2(4), 409, 1973.
6. **Anon.,** *Gold Museum* (Catalogue), 3rd ed., Bank of the Republic, Bogotá, Colombia, 1972, 5–21.
7. **Martin, R.,** The role of coca in the history, religion, and medicine of South American Indians, *Econ. Bot.,* 24, 422, 1970.
8. **Benson, E.,** *The Mochica: A Culture of Peru,* Praeger, New York, 1972, 59–62.
9. **Grimal, P., Ed.,** *Larousse World Mythology,* 3rd ed., Paul Hamlyn, London and New York, 1971, 484.
10. **Nieschulz, O.,** Cocaism and cocainism, (1969), in *The Coca Leaf and Cocaine Papers,* Andrews, G. and Solomon, D., Eds., Harcourt Brace Jovanovich, New York and London, 1975, 269.
11. **Woods, J. H. and Downs, D. A.,** The psychopharmacology of cocaine, in *Drug Use in America: Problem in Perspective, The Technical Papers of the Second Report of the National Commission on Marihuana and Drug Abuse,* Appendix, Vol. 1, U.S. Govt. Printing Office, Washington, D.C., 1973, 116.
12. **Guerra, F.,** Sex and drugs in the 16th century, *Br. J. Addict.,* 69, 269, 1974.
13. **Mantegazza, P.,** *Sulle virtio igieniche e medicinale della Coca, a sugli alimenti nervosi in generale,* Milan, 1859, cited in Gay, et al. (see Reference 4), 423.
14. **Ashley, R.,** *Cocaine: Its History, Uses and Effects,* St. Martin's Press, New York, 1975.
15. **Mariani, A.,** *Coca and its Therapeutic Application,* Jaros, New York, 1890.
16. **Byck, R., Ed.,** *Cocaine Papers by Sigmund Freud,* Stonehill, New York, 1975, (A) Aschenbrandt (1883), 21; (B) Becker, H. K., 261, 276, 283–6; (C) Freud (1884), 47, 63–73; (D) Jones, E., 197–202; (E) Freud (1895), 205; (F) Byck, xxxi, Jones, 199; (G) Byck, xxviii.
17. **Byck, R.,** personal communication, 1975.

18. **Holmstedt, B.,** Historical survey, in *Ethnopharmacologic Search for Psychoactive Drugs,* Efron, D., Holmstedt, B., and Kline, N., Eds., U.S. Govt. Printing Office, Washington, D.C., 1967, 3.

19. **Brecher, E. and the Editors of Consumer Reports,** *Licit and Illicit Drugs,* Little, Brown & Co., Boston, 1972, 33–6, 270.

20. **Blejer-Prieto, H.,** Coca leaf and cocaine addiction – some historical notes, *Canad. Med. Assoc. J.,* 93, 700, 1965.

21. **Rusby, H. H., Bliss, A. R., and Ballard, C. W.,** *The Properties and Uses of Drugs,* Blakiston's Son & Co., Philadelphia, 1930, 125, 386, 407.

22. **Anon.,** The Commission of Enquiry on the Coca Leaf, *Bull. Narc.,* 1, 20, 1949.

23. Commission of Inquiry into the Non-Medical Use of Drugs, *Final Report,* Information Canada, Ottawa, 1973, 349.

24. **Alcalá, R. P.,** citing coca producers, in The coca question in Bolivia, *Bull. Narc.,* 4, 10, 1952.

25. **Schultz, M. G.,** The 'strange case' of Robert Louis Stevenson, *JAMA,* 216, 90, 1971.

26. **Musto, D.,** A study in cocaine: Sherlock Holmes and Sigmund Freud, *JAMA,* 204, 125, 1968.

27. **Mariani, A., Ed.,** *Album Mariani, Les Figures Contemporaines, Contemporary Celebrities from the Album Mariani,* etc., various publishers for Mariani & Co., 13 Vols., 1891–1913. See also Groff, J., The golden age of cocaine wine, *High Times,* #5, 31, 1975.

28. **Schatzman, M.,** Cocaine and the 'drug problem,' *J. Psychedelic Drugs,* 7, 7, 1975.

29. **Musto, D.,** *The American Disease: Origins of Narcotic Control,* Yale University Press, New York and London, 1973, 7.

30. **King, P.,** *Cocaine – A Play in One Act,* Frank Shay, New York, 1917.

31. **Segre, D. ("Pitigrilli"),** *Cocaine,* Milano, 1921, English translation (1933) reprinted by And/Or Press, San Francisco, 1974.

32. **Sajous, C.,** Coca, cocaine, and cocainomania, in *Sajous's Analytic Cyclopedia of Practical Medicine,* Vol. 3, 9th ed., Davis, Philadelphia, 1924, 506.

33. **Ellmann, R..** *James Joyce,* Oxford University Press, New York and London, 1959, 512, 524, 530.

34. **Andrews, G. and Solomon, D.,** Coca and cocaine: uses and abuses, in *The Coca Leaf and Cocaine Papers,* Andrews, G. and Solomon, D., Eds., Harcourt Brace Jovanovich, New York and London, 1975, 3.

35. **Hopkins, J.,** Cocaine consciousness: the gourmet trip, in *The Coca Leaf and Cocaine Papers,* Andrews, G. and Solomon, D., Eds., Harcourt Brace Jovanovich, New York and London, 1975, 277.

36. **Duke, J. A., Aulik, D., and Plowman, T.,** Nutritional value of coca, *Harv. Univ. Bot. Mus. Leaflets,* 24, 113, 1975.

Chemical Aspects

The Chemistry of Cocaine and Its Derivatives

THE CHEMISTRY OF COCAINE AND ITS DERIVATIVES

Sydney Archer and Richard L. Hawks

TABLE OF CONTENTS

INTRODUCTION

The chemistry of cocaine has a very long history which has been the subject of several reviews.[1-3] Cocaine was first isolated from coca leaves in 1862 by Wohler.[4] The gross structure was finally established in 1923 by the total synthesis achieved by Willstätter et al.[5] However the stereochemical problems remained and these were not resolved until the mid-1950s. The correct stereochemical formula of the compound is shown in Structure 1. It is a member of the tropane family of alkaloids

which includes the belladonna alkaloids such as atropine and scopolamine. These are esters of tropine (Structure 2) whereas cocaine is an ester of ψ-tropine (Structure 3).

The *Chemical Abstracts* name for tropine ($\underset{\sim}{2}$) is *endo*-8-methyl-8-azabicyclo[3.2.1]octane-3-ol. Fodor has used α and β to designate *endo* and *exo* respectively so that tropine becomes tropan-3α-ol and ψ-tropine is tropan-3β-ol. This is a much less cumbersome nomenclature and we will use it in this chapter to designate stereochemistry. The use of the Greek letter has been superseded by use of the prefix *pseudo* to designate the *exo* (or β) forms of this alkaloid family. For the sake of consistency, we will use the *pseudo* designation throughout this discussion when reference to the trivial name is necessary, keeping in mind that the ψ-designation was the commonly accepted prefix up to the mid-20th century. The entry for cocaine in *Chemical Abstracts* is 8-azabicyclo[3.2.1] octane-2-carboxylic acid, 3-benzoyloxy-8-methyl methyl ester [1R-(*exo-exo*)].

ISOLATION AND PHYSICAL PROPERTIES

Cocaine and its companions are found in coca leaves of *Erythroxylon coca* which occur in western South America and are cultivated in Java. The alkaloid content of South American coca leaves is about 0.5 to 1.5%, with cocaine representing about 75% of the total alkaloid content of Bolivian coca leaves. The total alkaloid content of Java coca leaves is somewhat higher (1.0 to 2.5%), but cocaine represents only 50% of the total alkaloid content.[6] Only trace amounts of cocaine can be detected in other species of the genus *Erythroxylum.*[7]

In South America the crude alkaloid was traditionally exported for refining[8] up to the middle of this century. Now clandestine laboratories on that continent perform the function either by extraction and crystallization or by methods of hydrolysis and reesterification similar to those traditionally used in Java.[9]

Cocaine crystallizes from ethanol as monoclinic prisms, mp 98°C, [α] -16.2°C (CHCl$_3$). It is used mainly as the hydrochloride which crystallizes from ethanol as prisms, mp 200 to 202°C, [α] -71.95 (H$_2$O). It forms a variety of salts including the bitartrate which is obtained as a hydrate, mp 114 to 115°C, [α] -41.2 (H$_2$O).[5] The companion alkaloids are discussed below (see Table 1).

STRUCTURAL STUDIES

Cocaine forms a quaternary ammonium salt when treated with methyl iodide,[10] and on treatment with cyanogen bromide affords cyano-norcocaine.[11] Thus the alkaloid is a monomethyl tertiary base, which on hydrolysis with dilute sulfuric acid yields (-)-ecgonine, benzoic acid, and methanol.[12] Partial hydrolysis can be effected by boiling with water, whereupon methanol and (-)-benzoylecgonine are obtained.[13] Further hydrolysis furnishes (-)-ecgonine and benzoic acid. Thus cocaine contains a carbomethoxy and benzoyloxy group.

Structures $\underset{\sim}{4}$, $\underset{\sim}{5}$, and $\underset{\sim}{6}$ are shown in Figure 1, and as can be seen, the structure of (-)-ecgonine ($\underset{\sim}{4}$) and thus cocaine itself was established by oxidation. Oxidation with chromic oxide in sulfuric acid converted (-)-ecgonine to 2-carboxytropinone ($\underset{\sim}{5}$), which lost carbon dioxide spontaneously to furnish tropinone ($\underset{\sim}{6}$).[14] These experiments demonstrated that the hydroxyl group of ecgonine is located at C-3. The spontaneous loss of carbon dioxide suggested that the intermediate was a β-keto acid, thereby locating the carboxyl function of ecgonine at C-2. Since it already had been established that cocaine is the *O*-benzoyl, methyl ester or ecgonine, the nonstereochemical aspects of the structure of cocaine were secured.

As shown in Figure 2, ecgonine ($\underset{\sim}{4}$) can be converted into an amide[15] and dehydrated to give anhydroecgonine ($\underset{\sim}{9}$).[16] The latter can be reduced to give two 2-carboxytropanes ($\underset{\sim}{10}$) depending on reaction conditions.[11,17] Oxidation of (-)-ecgonine with chromic acid yields (-)-tropinic ($\underset{\sim}{7}$) and (-)-ecgoninic acid ($\underset{\sim}{8}$).[18] The latter was used as a relay point to establish the absolute configuration of (-)-cocaine.[19] Upon treatment with hydrochloric acid at high temperature, anhydroecgonine ($\underset{\sim}{9}$) was decarboxylated to afford tropidine ($\underset{\sim}{11}$),[20] which was obtained independently by dehydration of tropine (see Structure $\underset{\sim}{2}$), thus establishing a structural link between cocaine and atropine, a belladonna alkaloid.

Like ecgonine, anhydroecgonine furnishes an amide ($\underset{\sim}{12}$) which undergoes the Hofmann reaction to yield optically active tropan-2-one ($\underset{\sim}{13}$).[21] Upon reduction the ketone gave (+)-tropan-2β-ol ($\underset{\sim}{14}$), which upon treatment with acetic anhydride in the presence of perchloric acid furnished

TABLE 1

Physical Properties of Cocaine and Selected Derivatives

	Molecular weight	Melting point* (°C)	R_f(TLC)**	Mass spectrum***	
				CI	EI
(–)-Cocaine	303	98°	0.98(A–E) 0.83(F) 0.75(G)	182(100) 304(92) 204(10)	182(100) 82(95) 83(41)
hydrochloride	339	197°		332(3) 272(6)	105(35) 94(33)
bitartrate	339	115°			77(31) 96(27) 303(25)
(–)-Ecgonine	185	205°	0.00(A) 0.03(B)		
hydrochloride	221	275° 241°	0.33(C) 0.11(D) 0.28(E) 0.48(F) 0.37(G)		
(–)-Benzoylecgonine	289	195° (dec)		290(100) 168(90)	
tetrahydrate	361	90°	0.00(A–B) 0.29(C)	291(17) 318(8)	
hydrochloride	325	200°	0.50(D) 0.73(E) 0.88(F)		
(–)-Norcocaine hydrochloride	325	116–117°	0.67(G)	168(100) 290(88) 318(14)	
(–)-Benzoylnorecgonine	275		0.00(A) 0.00(B)		
hydrochloride	311	200°(27)	0.12(C) 0.30(D) 0.46(E) 0.95(F) 0.47(G)		
(–)-Ecgonine methylester	199	oil at room temp	0.98(A) 0.64(B)	200(100) 182(52)	
hydrochloride	235	215°[27]	0.98(C) 0.98(D) 0.98(E) 0.66(F) 0.62(G)	201(11) 168(9)	
Pseudococaine (C-2α, C-3β)	303	217°[29]			
hydrochloride	339				

TABLE 1 (continued)

Physical Properties of Cocaine and Selected Derivatives

	Molecular weight	Melting point* (°C)	R_f(TLC)**	Mass spectrum*** CI	EI
(±)Allococaine (C-2β, C-3α)	303	95−97°[32],[35]			
picrate	532	161°[32],[35]			
(±)Allopseudococaine (C-2α, C-3α)	303	83−84°[32]			
hydrochloride	339	209−210°[32]			
picrate	532	179°[35]			

*From Reference 5 (Willstätter et al.) except where noted.
**Solvent-developing systems: (a) $CHCl_3$/acetone/NH_4OH (5/94/1);[64] (b) Benzene/EtOAc/MeOH/NH_4OH (80/20/1.2/.01);[64] (c) $CHCl_3$/acetone/Et_2NH (5/4/1);[64] (d) EtOAc/MeOH/NH_4OH (17/2/1);[64] (e) EtOAc/MeOH/NH_4OH (15/4/1);[64] (f) n-BuOH/AcOH/H_2O (35/3/10);[64] (g) MeOH/NH_4OH (99/1).[62]
***CI = Chemical Ionization (methane carrier gas); EI = Electron Impact (70 eV).

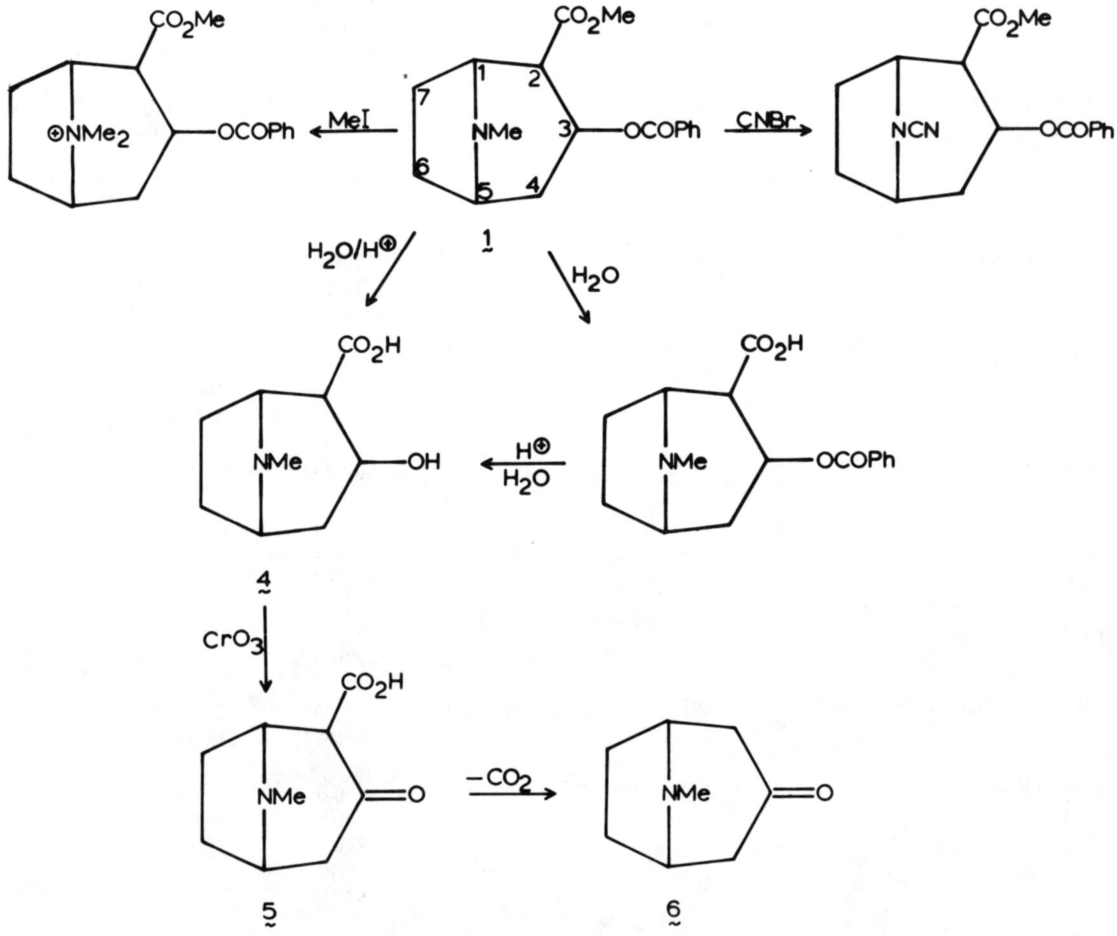

FIGURE 1.

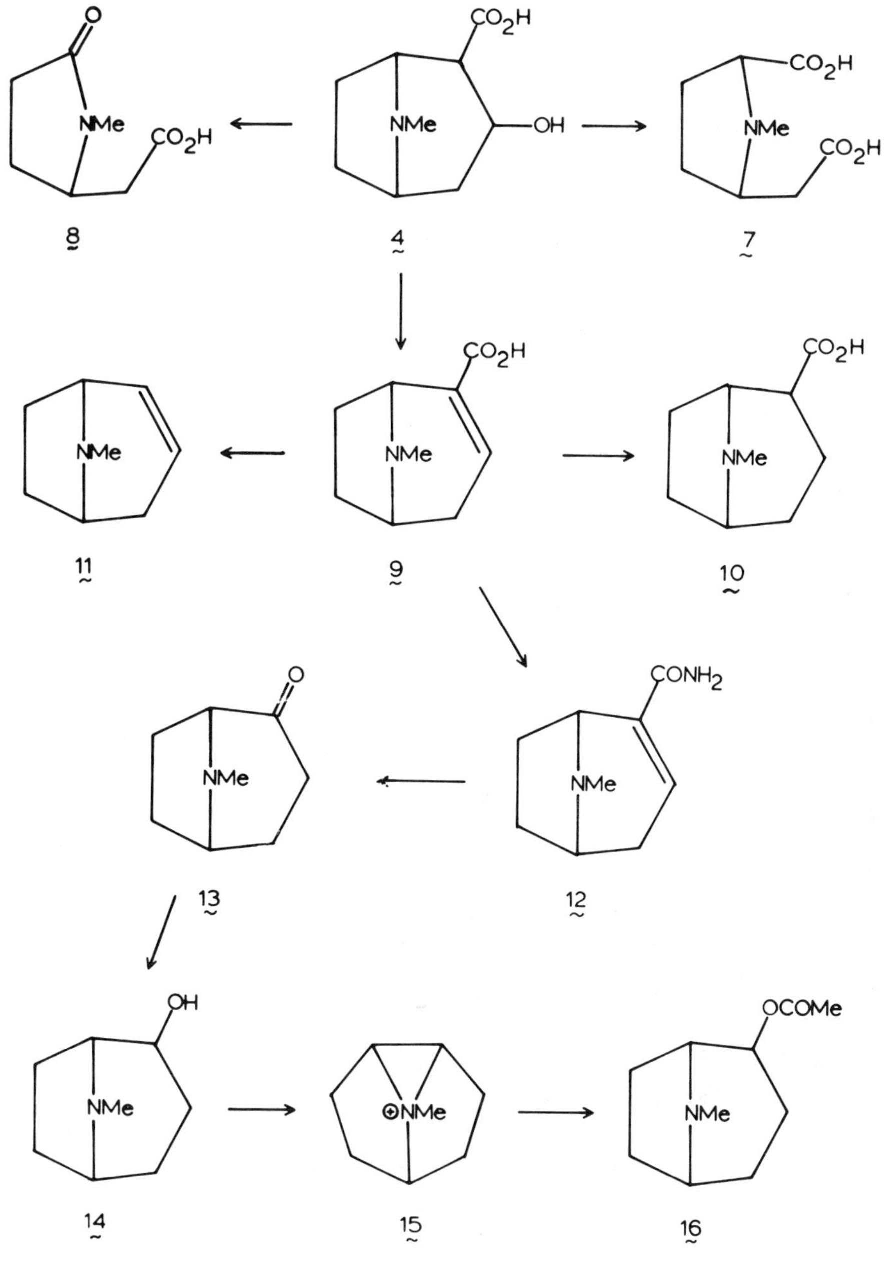

FIGURE 2.

(tropane-2β-acetate (16). This took place via the symmetrical ion (15).[22] The NMR spectral data are listed in Table 2.

SYNTHESIS OF COCAINE

Willstätter et al. completed the total synthesis of cocaine in 1923.[5] Succindialdehyde, methylamine, and monomethyl β-ketoglutarate (as the potassium salt) were condensed by a Robinson-type tropane synthesis to give methyl 2-carbomethoxytropinone (Structure 17-Figure 3). The keto-ester was reduced with sodium amalgam to give a mixture of diastereomeric methyl tropan-3-ol-2-carboxylates (18). These were converted to a mixture of their corresponding benzoates (19) which were separated by fractional crystallization. The more soluble benzoate proved to be (±)-cocaine, which was resolved as the bitartrate salt. The levo-isomer of the liberated base proved to be

TABLE 2

NMR Spectral Data of Cocaine and Selected Derivatives

Compound	Solvent	Chemical shifts, δ-values (ppm)									Reference
		C-1H	C-2H	C-3H	C-4H₂	C-5H	C-6H₂ C-7H₂	Arom.-H₅	N-CH₃	O-CH₃	
Cocaine Hydrochloride	CDCl₃	3.55(m)	3.03(m)	5.27(m)	2.30(m)	3.27(m)	2.45(m)	7.75(m)	2.21(s)	3.71(s)	32
	D₂O	4.28(m)	3.64(m)	5.58(m)		4.15(m)			2.93(s)	3.67(s)	62
Norcocaine Hydrochloride	CDCl₃	4.10(m)	3.25(m)	5.59(m)	2.22(m)	4.31(m)	2.36(m)	7.80(m)	–	3.74(s)	63
	D₂O	4.42(m)	3.60(m)	5.58(m)				7.75(m)		3.64(s)	62
Benzoylecgonine Hydrochloride	CDCl₃	3.62(m)	3.02(m)	5.30(m)	2.30(m)	3.55(m)	2.44(m)	7.75(m)	2.25(s)		63
	D₂O	4.28(m)	3.53(m)	5.55(m)		4.12(m)		7.75(m)	2.92(s)	–	62
Ecgonine Hydrochloride	D₂O	4.20(m)	3.19(m)	4.40(m)		3.93(m)		–	2.75(s)	–	62
Ecgonine methylester Hydrochloride	CDCl₃	3.60(m)	2.75(m)	3.85(m)	2.22	3.19(m)		–	2.20(s)	3.75(s)	32
	D₂O	4.16(m)	3.32(m)	4.46(m)		4.00(m)			2.82(s)	3.79(s)	62
Benzoylnorecgonine Hydrochloride	D₂O	4.37(m)	3.42(m)	5.53(m)	2.20(m)	4.29(m)	2.35(m)	7.75(m)	–	–	62
Pseudococaine (C-2α, C-3β)	CDCl₃	3.50(m)	3.15(m)	5.58(m)		3.25(m)			2.41(s)	3.63(s)	32
Allococaine (C-2β, C-3α)	CDCl₃	3.65(m)	2.82(m)	5.67(m)		3.17(m)			2.25(s)	3.76(s)	32
Allopseudococaine (C-2α, C-3α)	CDCl₃	3.50(m)	3.15(m)	5.65(m)		3.15(m)			2.33(s)	3.53(s)	32

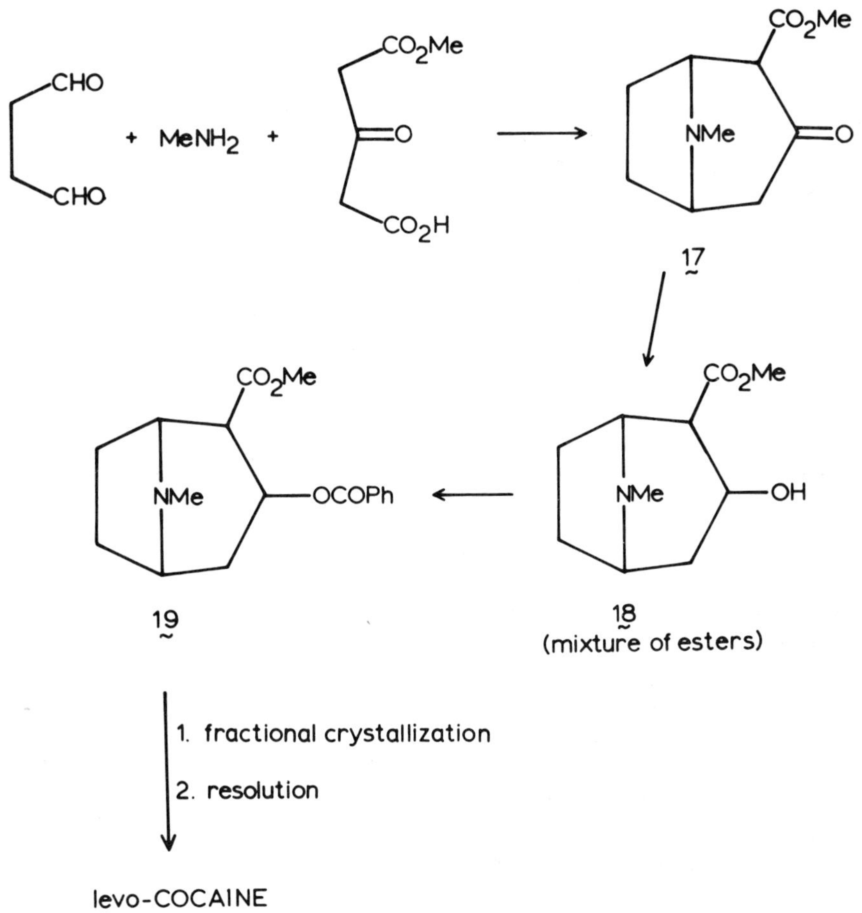

FIGURE 3.

identical in all respects with the natural alkaloid. The synthesis shown in Figure 3 has not been improved upon in subsequent years except for the development of a better preparation of the monomethyl β-ketoglutarate salt, which gives an improvement in overall yield from 30 to 60%.[23] Preobrashenski et al.[24] reported the synthesis of the tropinone (17) using the β-ketoglutaric acid (19) rather than the monomethyl ester to give tropinone (6) as the intermediate product, which was subsequently treated with sodium or potassium and dimethyl carbonate in refluxing benzene or xylene to yield 2-carbomethoxytropinone (17). Although the yield of Structure 17 was reported to be 75% and would thus significantly improve the overall yield of cocaine using this approach, subsequent investigation[23] indicated the yield to be 35%; thus no overall improvement could be realized in the yield of cocaine. This reaction is significant, however, since it affords a potential means of conveniently introducing a ^{14}C-carbon

at the C-2 carboxy position at a late stage in synthesis.[26]

STEREOCHEMISTRY

Even though Willstätter et al.[5] reported the synthesis of (−)-cocaine in 1923, the absolute stereochemistry remained unresolved until 1955. In order to appreciate the chemical transformation involved in the establishment of the relative configuration of cocaine and its isomers, the stereochemistry of tropine (see Structure 2) and ψ-tropine (pseudotropine [see Structure 3]) are considered first.

Pseudotropine was converted (see below) to norpseudotropine (20), which upon acetylation gives N-acetylnorpseudotropine (21). When the hydrochloride of Structure 21 was heated at 150°C it rearranged quantitatively to give O-acetylnorpseudotropine hydrochloride (22).[27]

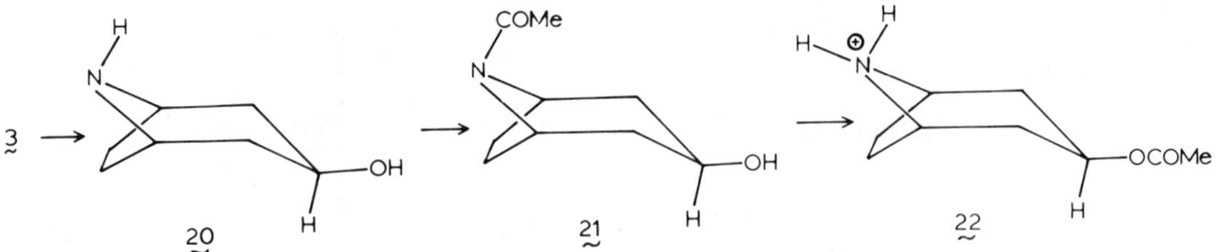

3 → 20 → 21 → 22

On the other hand, when N-acetylnortropine hydrochloride (23) derived from tropine was heated at 150°C, it did not rearrange to give O-acetylnortropine (24).

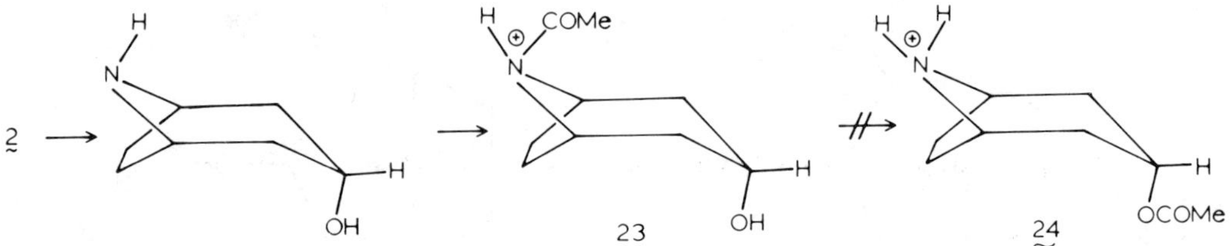

2 → 23 → 24

This series of experiments established that the hydroxyl in pseudotropine (3) was β (exo) and in tropine was α (endo), since acetyl transfer takes place via an intermediate such as Structure 25.

The same type of experiments was used to establish the configuration of the 3-hydroxyl group in ecgonine obtained from cocaine and the isomeric pseudoecgonine, which was derived from pseudococaine. N-Acetylnorpseudoecgonine ethyl ester (26) was converted to the O-acetate (27) under acid conditions. Under alkaline conditions the reverse reaction occurred.[26]

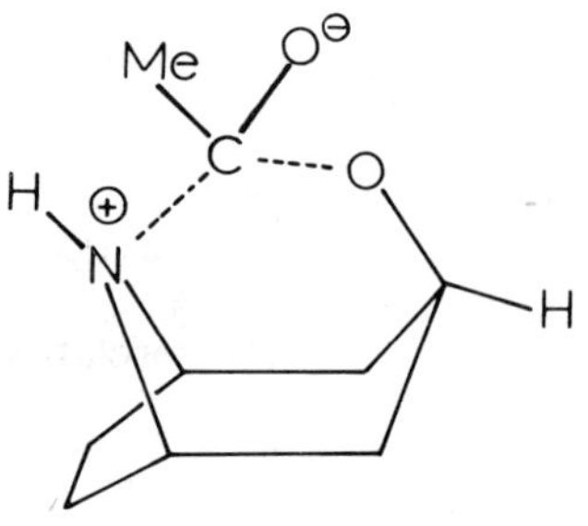

25

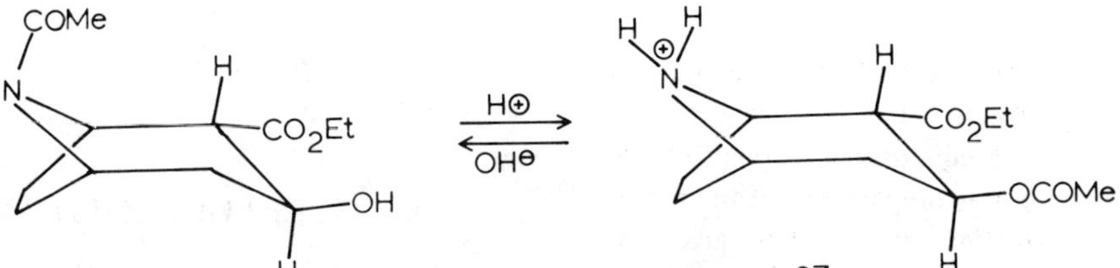

26 $\xrightarrow[\text{OH}^\ominus]{\text{H}^\oplus}$ 27

Similarly, Findlay[27] found that O-benzoylnorecgonine (28) underwent an O → N migration at pH 11. Kovacs et al.[28] found the reverse to occur in acid.

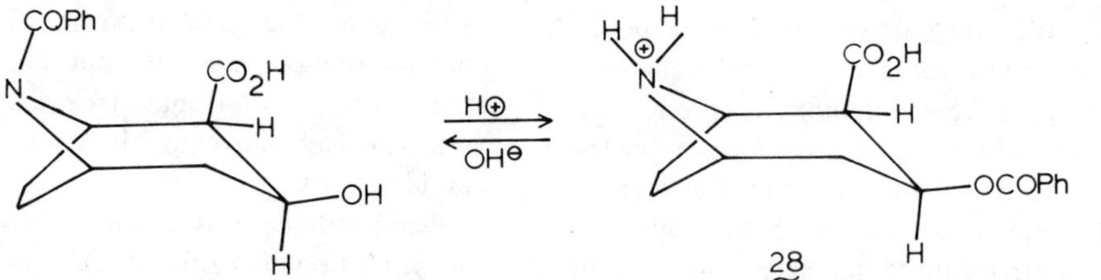

28

Findlay[27] showed that ecgonine methyl ester (29) epimerizes in alkaline methanol solution to pseudoecgonine methyl ester (30).

This result suggests that the carbomethoxy group in cocaine is in the less stable β (axial) conformation. Fodor et al.[29] and Kovacs et al.[30] carried out a series of transformations (Figure 4) which supported this suggestion. Cocaine and pseudococaine (Structure 31 – Figure 4) were converted to two isomeric 2-methyl-tropan-3-ones (40 and 41), which formed the same oxime when the oxidation was carried out in alkaline medium. This compound was later determined to have C-2 configuration. Clearly the difference between the two was the conformation at C-2, but the series of reactions shown do not allow unequivocal assignment of Structures to 1 and 31.

However, the hydroxymethyl-tropan-3-ol (32) derived from cocaine gave the acetal (34) when treated with benazaldehyde,[25] whereas the epimeric glycol (33) did not form an acetal. The 2-chloromethyltropan-3-ol (35) from cocaine gave the cyclic ether (36),[28] whereas the isomeric chloride (37) did not undergo such a reaction.[30] These experiments showed that the functionalites at C-2 and C-3 in cocaine were cis, whereas in pseudococaine they were trans. Since it had been shown that the benzoyloxy group in cocaine is β, it follows that the group at C-2 must also be β.

N → O Migration experiments were used to establish the relative configuration of cocaine and pseudococaine (see below).[26] O-Benzoylecgonine (42) and O-benzoylpseudoecgonine (45) were converted to the corresponding 2-benzamido-tropan-3β-ols (43 and 46).

Upon treatment with acid, alcohol (43) rearranged to give the amino ester (44), whereas in the pseudo-series, 2α-benzamido-tropan-3β-ol (46) did not give Structure 47 under comparable conditions. Since the Curtius reaction proceeds with retention of configuration, these experiments show that in ecgonine the hydroxyl and carboxyl groups are cis, whereas in pseudoecgonine they are trans. It follows that cocaine is methyl 3β-benzoyloxy-tropan-2β-carboxylate (1) and pseudococaine is methyl 3-benzoyloxy-tropan-2α-carboxylate (48).

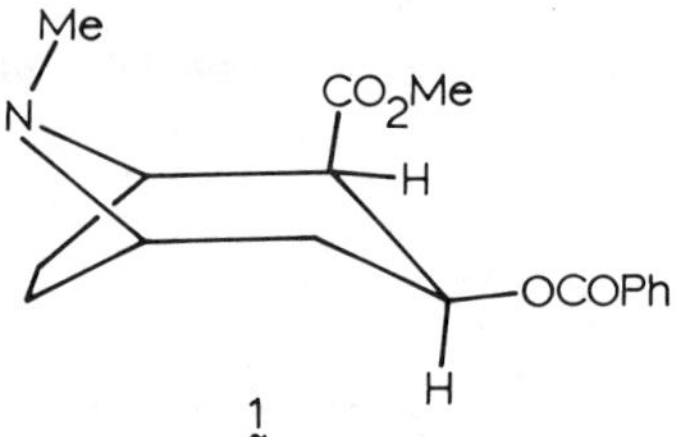

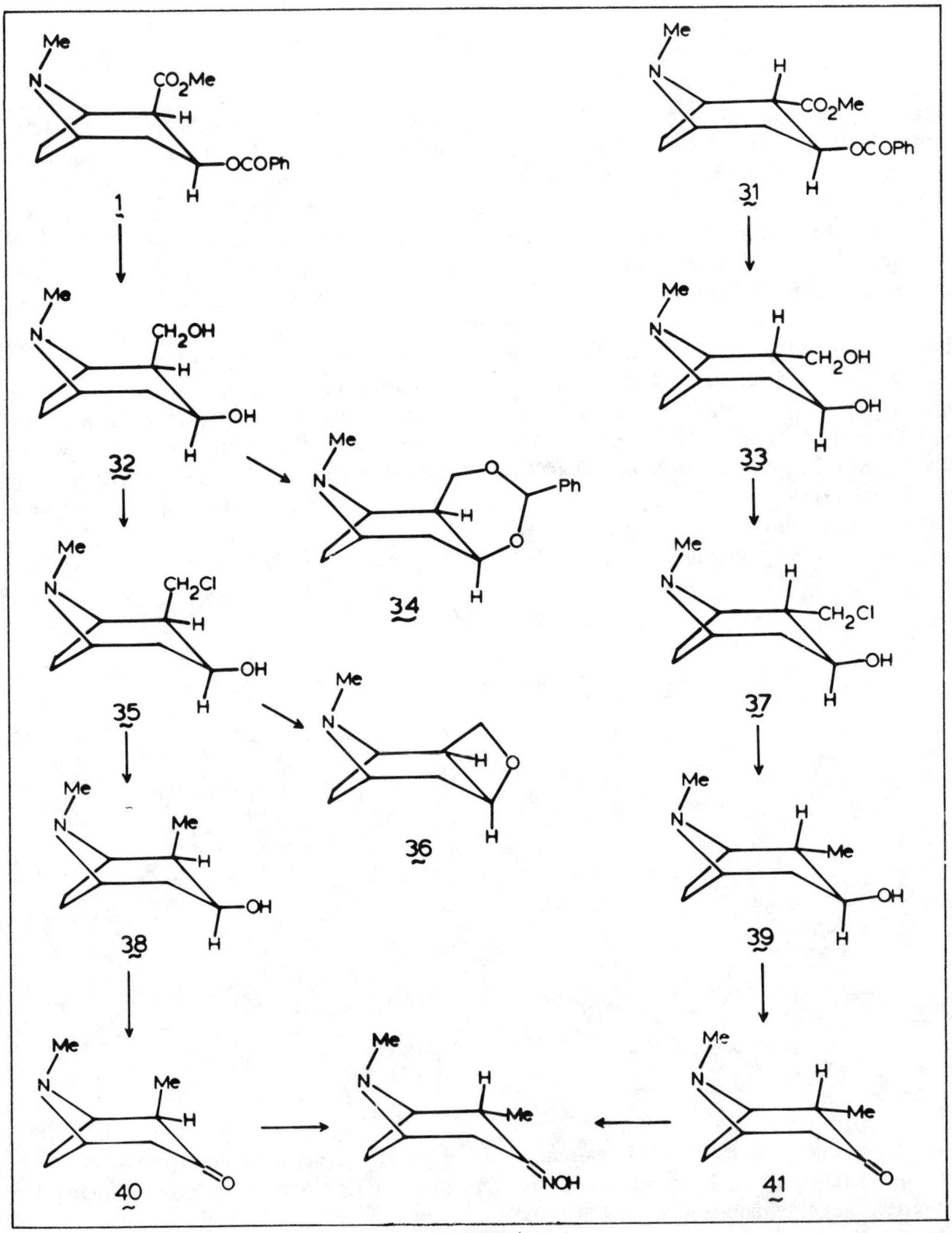

FIGURE 4.

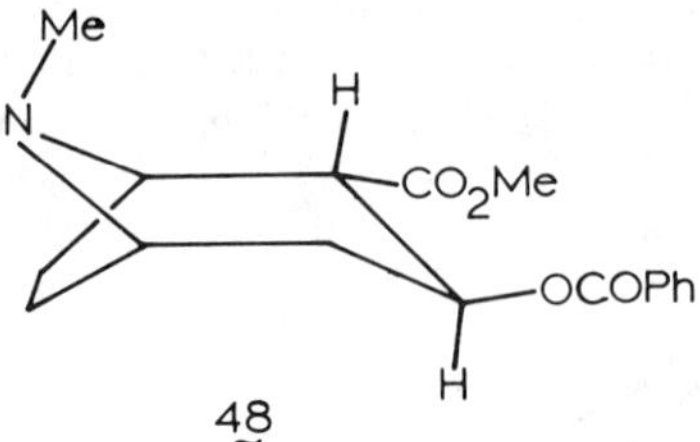

An infrared analysis of hydrogen bonding in the isomeric ecgonines by Bainova et al.[31] supported the assignments for ecgonine, pseudoecgonine, alloecgonine, and allopseudoecgonine as determined by the chemical methods discussed above. These authors, as well as those applying chemical methods, assumed a chair conformation of the piperidine ring in making their assignments of configuration. The chair form was determined to be in fact the preferred conformation by analysis of proton magnetic resonance spectra of the four racemic cocaines.[39]

Hardegger and Ott[19] established the absolute stereochemistry of cocaine by relating it to L-glutamic acid by means of the transformations shown in Figure 5. L-Glutamic acid (Structure 49 – Figure 5) was converted to pyroglutamic acid, which upon esterification with diazomethane afforded the methyl ester (50). Reduction with lithium aluminum hydride gave the carbinol (51) which upon tosylation gave Structure 52. Treatment with potassium cyanide gave the nitrite (53) which was methylated without racemization to give Structure 54. Partial hydrolysis of Structure 54 gave the amide (55) which was obtained from

ecgoninic acid (8), derived from (−)-cocaine, by conversion to the methyl ester followed by ammonolysis.

This stereochemical configuration was further substantiated by Gabe and Barnes in 1963 by their report of the X-ray crystal structure of cocaine hydrochloride.[33] They found that the piperidine ring of the tropane nucleus has the chair form, with the carbomethoxy function at C-2 occupying an axial position and the benzoyloxy at C-3 the equatorial position. This conformation was postulated in 1953 by Fodor and Kovacs,[26] based on their observation of the ease of elimination of water from ecgonine but not from pseudo-ecgonine. The chair conformation would allow a *trans* elimination in the former but not the latter. The conformational disposition of the molecule is only slightly different in the case of cocaine methiodide, whose crystal structure was recently reported.[34] This unequivocally establishes (−)-cocaine as (−)-3R-methoxycarbonyl-2S-benzoyloxytropane.

The other isomers of cocaine, allococaine (56) and allopseudococaine (57), are derived from tropan-3α-ol.

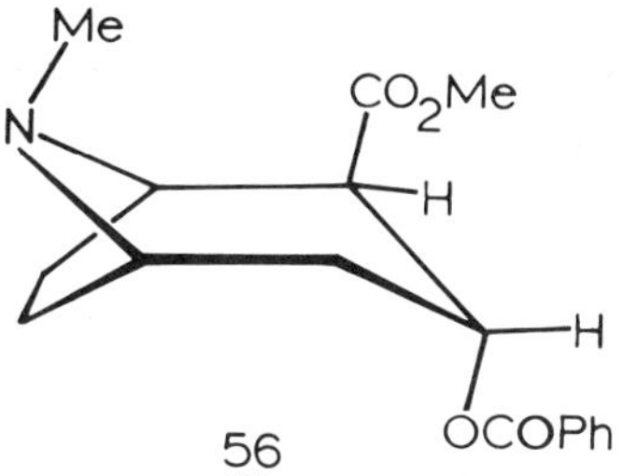

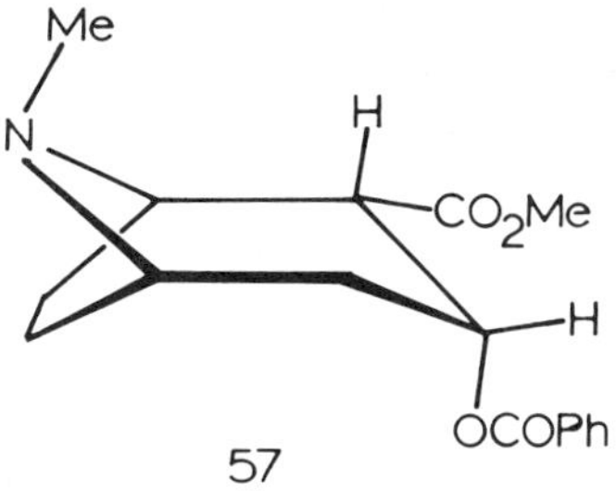

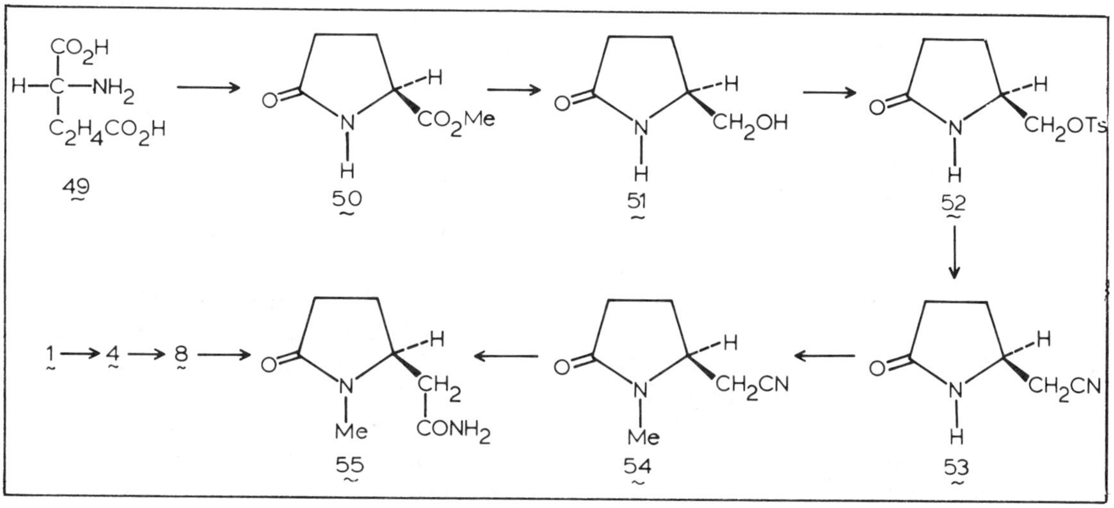

FIGURE 5.

Findlay[35] reduced α-carbomethoxytropinone (17) over a platinum catalyst and obtained the carbinol (58), which upon benzoylation furnished allococaine (56).

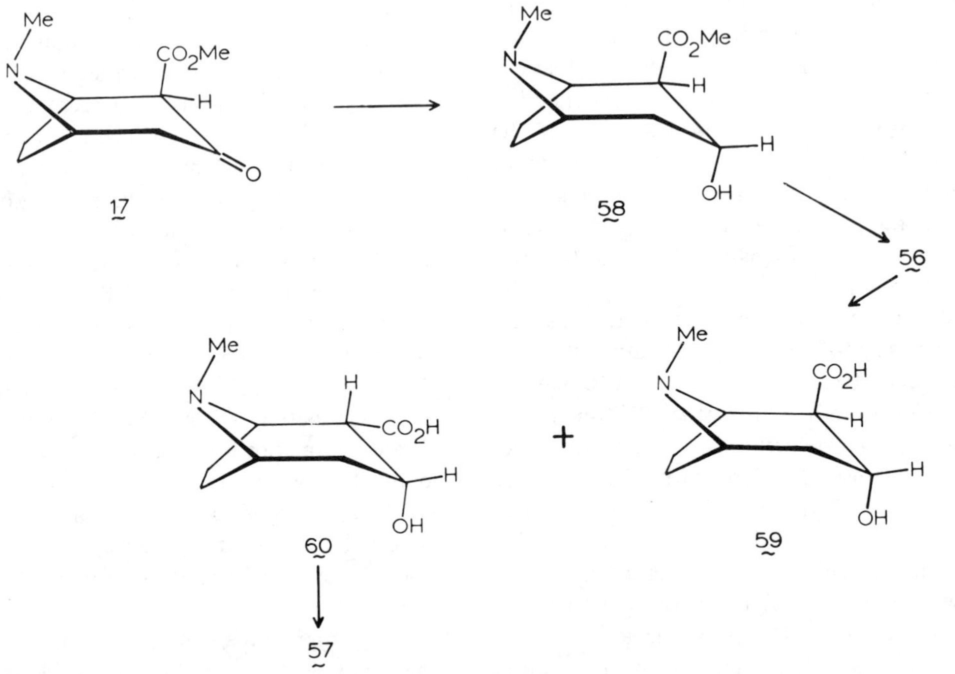

17

58

56

60

57

+

59

Saponification of Structure 56 gave a mixture of hydroxy acids, alloecgonine (59) and allopseudoecgonine (60). The latter, upon methylation followed by benzoylation, gave the remaining isomer, allopseudococaine (57).

It should be noted at this point that the nomenclature convention chosen for allococaine and allopseudococaine is that recommended by Simmema et al.,[32] which designated the 2β-benzoyloxytropan-3α-carboxylate isomer as allococaine (56) and 2α-benzoyloxytropan-3α-carboxylate as allopseudococaine (57). This convention is the opposite to that used by Findlay,[35] who designated the 2β-, 3α-isomer as allopseudococaine and the 2α-, 3α-isomer as allococaine.

COMPANIONS OF COCAINE IN COCA LEAVES

Pseudococaine (31) was isolated from coca leaves by Liebermann and Giesel.[36] It is probably an artifact of the isolation procedure, arising from the action of alkali on cocaine itself.

Cinnamoylcocaine (61) was isolated from Java coca leaves and proved to be identical with a substance obtained by treatment of ecgonine with cinnamic anhydride, followed by esterification with methanol.[37]

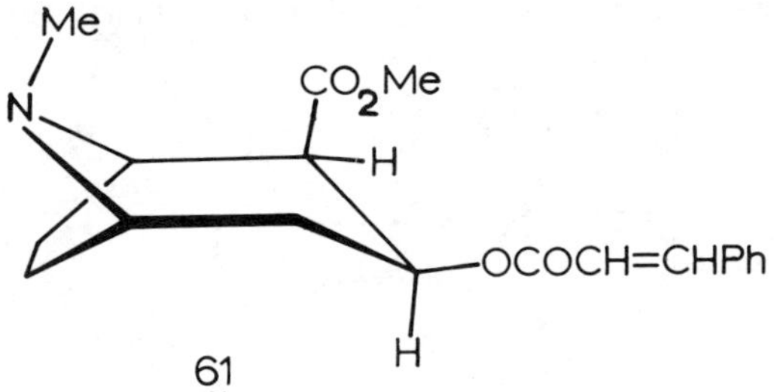

61

Benzoylecgonine was isolated from Peruvian coca leaves, but not from the variety obtained from Java.[38] It may be an artifact arising by hydrolysis of cocaine. The same author found that ecgonine methyl ester occurs naturally in Java coca leaves. Tropacocaine, the benzoate ester of tropan-3β-ol, occurs in Java coca leaves[39] and in Peruvian coca leaves.[40]

METABOLITES OF COCAINE

The biotransformation, disposition, and excretion of cocaine have been the subjects of numerous investigations. Figure 6 outlines the observed metabolic pathways. Cocaine's principle metabolites in man and animals appear to be O-benzoylecgonine (42) and ecgonine (4),[41-45] compounds resulting from esterase enzyme activity.[46-50] Liver N-demethylase enzymes convert cocaine to norcocaine (62).[45,47,51-53] Norcocaine can in turn be converted to O-benzoylnorecgonone (28)[43] and finally to norecgonine (63).[53] Enzymatic hydrolysis of the benzoate function of cocaine in an initial step leads to ecgonine methyl ester (29).[43,53] Suggestive evidence exists for a minor hydroxylated metabolite, where the hydroxy function presumably resides on the *para* position of the aromatic ring of the benzoate moiety (64).[43]

The syntheses of most of these metabolites were carried out as part of the studies previously discussed in the section on "Structual Studies," with the exception of the N-demethylated compounds. Ecgonine methyl ester (29) may be prepared by treatment of cocaine (1)[54] or ecgonine (4)[27] with refluxing methanolic hydrochloric acid. When refluxed in water cocaine is converted to O-benzoylecgonine (42).[27] Refluxing in aqueous hydrochloric acid gives ecgonine (4).[21] Norcocaine (62) results from the treatment of cocaine with alkaline potassium permanganate.[54,55] An improved synthesis of norcocaine from cocaine has recently been achieved,[56] which provides the N-demethylation by formation of the norcocaine carbamate derivative with trichloro-ethylchloroformate followed by hydrolysis. Benzoylnorecgonine (28) is prepared by the action of alkaline potassium permanganate on benzoylecgonine (42).[27,55]

ISOTOPIC LABELING OF COCAINE AND ITS METABOLITES

Interest in the metabolism, disposition, and excretion characteristics of cocaine has generated a need for isotopically labeled material. Schmidt and Werner[54] prepared the ^{14}C-labeled derivatives of cocaine (1), O-benzoylecgonine (47), ecgonine methyl ester (29), and ecgonine (4). Norcocaine (62) was treated with ^{14}C-methyl iodide to yield cocaine-(N-methyl-^{14}C) (65), specific activity 4.5 mCi/mmol. Hydrolysis of Structure 65 in hydrochloric acid yielded ecgonine-(N-methyl-^{14}C) (66), specific activity 0.17 mCi/mmol. Treatment of Structure 66 in methanolic hydrochloric acid provided ecgonine methyl ester-(N-methyl-^{14}C) (67), specific activity 0.17 mCi/mmol. Alternatively, Structure 66 was treated with benzoic anhydride to give O-benzoylecgonine-(N-methyl-^{14}C) (68), specific activity 0.17 mCi/mmol.

Cocaine-(benzoyl carbonyl-^{14}C) (69), specific activity 0.64 mCi/mmol, was prepared by treatment of ecgonine methyl ester (29) with benzoyl chloride-(carbonyl-^{14}C). The label was placed in the methyl ester moiety by treatment of O-benzoylecgonine (42) with ^{14}C-diazomethane to provide cocaine of specific activity 0.62 mCi/mmol (70).

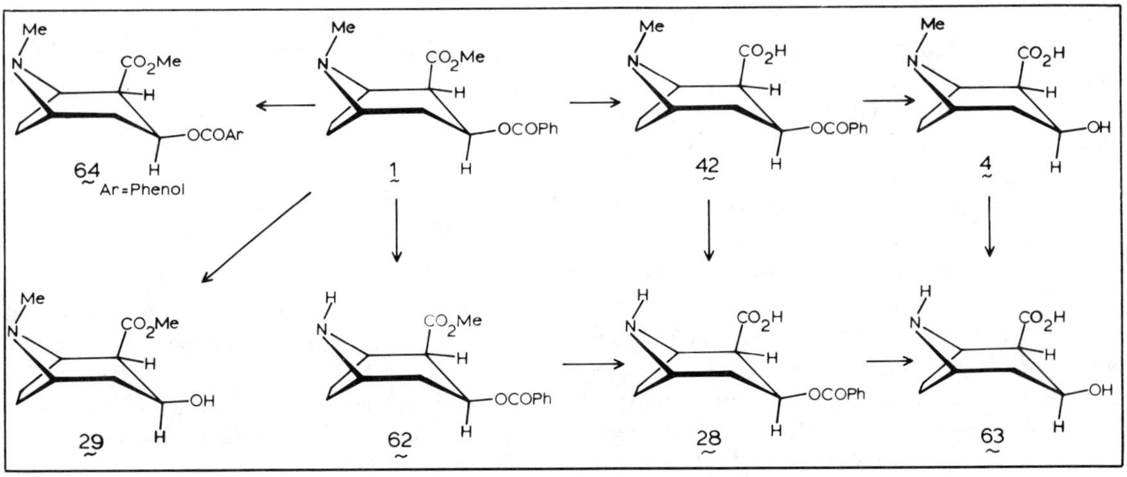

FIGURE 6.

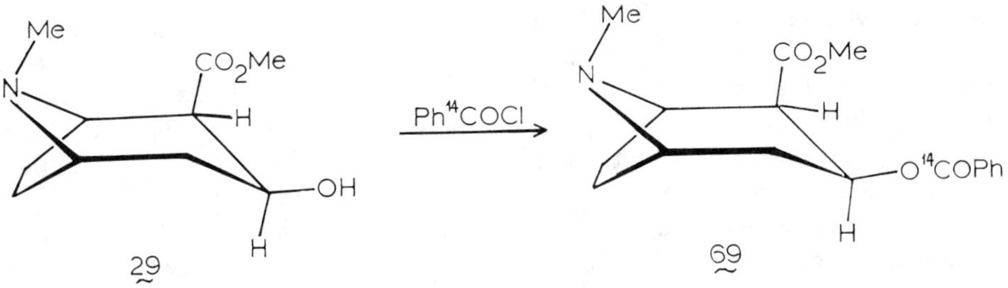

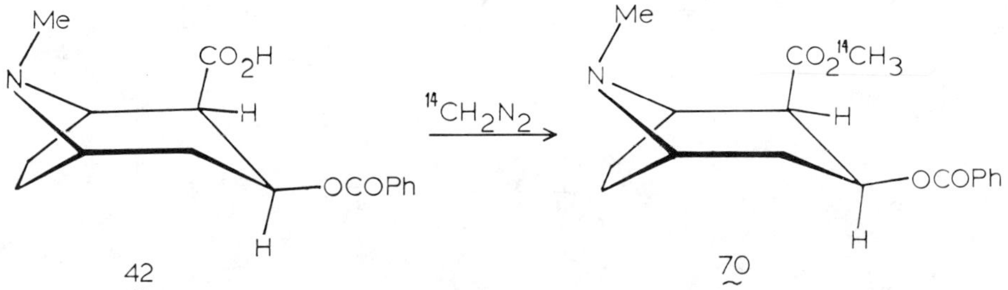

There have been several reports of the general labeling of cocaine and derivatives with tritium gas. Schmidt and Werner[55] prepared norcocaine (specific activity 2.5 mCi/mmol) by exposing that compound to tritium gas and removing the labile tritium with a methanol wash. The same authors prepared cocaine (specific activity 1.2 mCi/mmol) by absorbing it on activated charcoal and treating it with tritium gas.[57] A higher specific activity generally labeled cocaine was prepared by Gosztonyi and Walde[58] by subjecting the compound to a microwave discharge while in the presence of tritium gas. This technique allowed the

uptake of 12% of the available tritium gas and provided material of 29 mCi/mmol. Nayak et al.[59] achieved even higher levels of activity by treating cocaine dissolved in acetic acid tritium gas while in the presence of a platinum catalyst. This catalyzed treatment yielded material of 189 mCi/mmol. Werner and Mohammad[60] prepared cocaine-(N-methyl-^{3}H), specific activity 36 mCi/mmol, by treatment of norcocaine (62) with tritium-labeled methyl iodide. Pseudococaine (31) of similar activity was prepared in an analogous fashion from norpseudococaine.

All the compounds mentioned in the foregoing

paragraphs involved radiolabels which are situated, at least in part, on metabolically labile positions and are therefore not ideal compounds to use for studies of metabolism. Ideally, the label should be located in a position not prone to enzymatic attack. In the case of cocaine, this would be in the nortropane nucleus. Nayak et al.[59] used the method of tritiation in the presence of platinum to generally label ecgonine and then replace the methyl ester and benzoyl functions to prepare cocaine (specific activity 14.5 mCi/mmol) containing the general label in the tropane nucleus. This material was subsequently hydrolyzed in water to provide O-benzoylecgonine with the labeled tropane nucleus. This approach does not unequivocally rule out label in the labile N-methyl position. As yet, there have been no reports of labeling confined strictly to the nortropane nucleus.

Cocaine and two of its metabolites have been prepared which incorporate the heavy isotope, deuterium. Deuterated compounds are employed as internal standards for quantitative analysis by gas chromatography-mass spectrometry, a technique which provides high sensitivity as well as high specificity. Since the mass spectrometer can distinguish between the compound and its deuterated derivative, and these deuterium-labeled compounds are essentially chemically equivalent to their unlabeled counterparts, they provide the ideal internal standard. The label chosen for incorporation is not limited of course to deuterium, but could be nitrogen-15, oxygen-18, or carbon-13. Deuterium is the most commonly used isotope because it is usually the easiest isotope to synthetically incorporate in the molecule.

Deuterium-labeled compounds prepared for use in quantitative GC-MS usually contain a minimum of three deuterium atoms. This is to minimize overlap problems with the naturally occurring isotopes in the compound to be measured, although corrections can be made for isotopically labeled compounds containing fewer deuteriums. Bosin et al.[61] have prepared cocaine (72) and O-benzoylecgonine (73) containing one and two deuterium atoms in the aromatic ring of the benzoyl moiety. The incorporation was achieved by synthesis of the aryl chloride analog of cocaine (71) followed by reduction with sodium borodeuteride. Hydrolysis with water provides O-benzoylecgonine (aryl-^{2}H).

Hawks et al. have prepared cocaine containing six deuteriums (74) by treatment of O-benzoylnorecgonine with deuterated methyl iodide in the presence of potassium carbonate.[51]

$$75 \qquad 28 \qquad 74$$

Treatment of the same compound with deuterated methanol saturated with deuterated hydrochloric acid yields norcocaine-(methoxy-$^2H_3$) (75).[62] Jeffs and Baldwin have prepared benzoylecgonine-(benzoyl-$^2H_5$) by the treatment of ecgonine methyl ester with $^2H_5$-benzoyl chloride.[63]

Table 1 lists some of the physical properties of cocaine and a selection of some of its derivatives. Table 2 contains NMR data pertinent to structural studies within the cocaine series.

REFERENCES

1. **Holmes, H. L.,** The chemistry of the tropane alkaloids, in *The Alkaloids,* Vol. I, Manske, R. H. F. and Holmes, H. L., Eds., Academic Press, New York, 1950, 272.
2. **Fodor, G.,** The tropane alkaloids, in *The Alkaloids,* Vol. VI, Manske, R. H. F., Ed., Academic Press, New York, 1960, 151.
3. **Fodor, G.,** Tropane alkaloids, in *Chemistry of the Alkaloids,* Pelletier, S. W., Ed., Van Nostrand Reinhold, New York, 1970, 440.
4. **Wohler, F.,** Fortsetzung der Untersuchungen über Coca und das Cocain, *Ann. Chem. (Justus Liebigs),* 121, 372, 1862.
5. **Willstätter, R., Wolfes, O., and Mader, H.,** Synthese des naturlichen cocaines, *Ann. Chem. (Justus Liebigs),* 434, 111, 1923.
6. **DeJong, A. W. K.,** The alkaloids of coca, *Recl. Trav. Chim. Pays-Bas,* 25, 233, 1906.
7. **Aynilian, G. H., Duke, J. A., Gentner, W. A., and Farnsworth, N. R.,** Cocaine content of *Erythroxylum* species, *J. Pharm. Sci.,* 63, 1938, 1974.
8. **Luzio, F.,** Manufacture of cocaine in huanuco, *Agronomie,* 3, 44, 1938; *Chem. Abstr..* 33, 3075, 1939; Binda, D., Cocaine, an industrial problem in Peru, *Actas Trabajos Congr. Peruano Quim.,* 2, 375, 1943; *Chem. Abstr.,* 39, 3629, 1945.
9. **DeJong, A. W. K.,** The extraction of coca leaves, *Recl. Trav. Chim. Pays-Bas,* 25, 311, 1906; DeJong, A. W. K., Research on the coca leaf of Java and its alkaloids, *Recl. Trav. Chim. Pays-Bas,* 42, 980, 1923; Duilius, Cocaine, *Chem. Ztg.,* 54, 31, 1930.
10. **Einhorn, A.,** Weitere untersuchungen über das Cocain, *Ber. Dtsch. Chem. Ges.,* 21, 3029, 1888.
11. **Braun, J. and Muller, E.,** Umwandlung des Cocains in neue, physiologisch wirksame Substanzen, *Ber. Dtsch. Chem. Ges.,* 51, 235, 1918.
12. **Lossen, W.,** *Ann. Chem. (Justus Liebigs),* 133, 351, 1865.
13. **Einhorn, A.,** Beitrage zur Kenntniss des Cocains, *Ber. Dtsch. Chem. Ges.,* 21, 47, 1888.
14. **Willstätter, R. and Muller, W.,** Ueber die Constitution des Ecgonins, *Ber. Dtsch. Chem. Ges.,* 31, 2655, 1898.
15. **Einhorn, A. and de Norwall, F. K.,** Uber die Amide der Ecgonin, *Ber. Dtsch. Chem. Ges.,* 26, 962, 1893.
16. **Einhorn, A.,** Ueber Ecgonin, *Ber. Dtsch. Chem. Ges.,* 20, 1221, 1887.
17. **Gadamer, J. and John, C.,** Ecgonine, *Arch. Pharm.,* 259, 227, 1921; Willstätter, R., Ueber Hydroecgonidin, *Ber. Dtsch. Chem. Ges.,* 30, 702, 1897.
18. **Liebermann, C.,** Ueber die Oxydation von Ecgonin, *Ber. Dtsch. Chem. Ges.,* 23, 2518, 1890; Liebermann, C., Ueber Tropinsaure und die Oxydation des Linksecgonins, Rechtsecgonins und Tropins, *Ber. Dtsch. Chem. Ges.,* 24, 606, 1891; Willstätter, R. and Bode, A., Zur Kenntnis der Ecgoninsaure, *Ber. Dtsch. Chem. Ges.,* 34, 519, 1901.
19. **Hardegger, E. and Ott, H.,** Konfiguration des Cocains und Derivate der Ecgoninsaure, *Helv. Chim. Acta,* 38, 312, 1955.
20. **Ladenburg, A.,** Die Constitution des Atropins, *Ann. Chem. (Justus Liebigs),* 217, 74, 1883.
21. **Bell, M. R. and Archer, S.,** L(+)-2-Tropinone, *J. Am. Chem. Soc.,* 82, 4642, 1960.
22. **Archer, S., Lands, A. M., and Lewis, T. H.,** Isomeric 2-acetoxytropine methiodides, *J. Med. Chem.,* 5, 423, 1962.

23. **Findlay, S. P.,** Concerning 2-carbomethoxytropinone, *J. Org. Chem.,* 22, 1385, 1957.
24. **Preobrashenski, N. A., Schtschukina, M. N., and Lapina, R. A.,** Cocain-Synthese aus Hyoscyamin. I. Mitteil: Darstellung von Tropinon-carbonsaure-estern, *Ber. Dtsch. Chem. Ges.,* 69, 1615, 1936.
25. **Fodor, G. and Nador, K.,** The stereochemistry of the tropane alkaloids. I. The configuration of tropine and pseudotropine, *J. Chem. Soc.,* 721, 1953.
26. **Fodor, G. and Kovacs, O.,** The stereochemistry of the tropane alkaloids. Part II. The configurations of the cocaines, *J. Chem. Soc.,* 724, 1953.
27. **Findlay, S. P.,** The three-dimensional structure of cocaine, *J. Am. Chem. Soc.,* 75, 4626, 1953; Findlay, S. P., The three-dimensional structure of the cocaines. Part I. Cocaine and pseudococaine, *J. Am. Chem. Soc.,* 76, 2855, 1954.
28. **Kovacs, O., Fodor, G., and Weisz, I.,** Konfigurationsbeweis des Cocains, *Hel. Chim. Acta,* 37, 892, 1954.
29. **Fodor, G., Kovacs, O., and Weisz, I.,** Stereochemistry of cocaine, *Nature,* 174, 131, 1954.
30. **Kovacs, O., Weisz, I., Zoller, P., and Fodor, G.,** Konstitutionsbeweis eines Tropan-Vierringathers. Darstellung von zwei neuen epimeren Ecgoninolen, *Helv. Chim. Acta,* 39, 99, 1956.
31. **Bainova, M. S., Bazilevskaya, G. I., Miroshnichenko, L. D., and Prebrazhenski, N. A.,** Conformational investigation in the cocaine series, *Dokl. Akad. Nauk. SSSR,* 157, 599, 1964.
32. **Simmema, A., Matt, L., Van Der Gugten, A. J., and Beyerman, H. C.,** Configuration and Conformation of all four cocaines from NMR spectra, *Recl. Trav. Chim. Pays-Bas,* 87, 1027, 1968.
33. **Gabe, E. J. and Barnes, W. H.,** The crystal and molecular structure of l-cocaine hydrochloride, *Acta Crystallogr.,* 16, 796, 1963.
34. **Shen, M., Ruble, J. R., and Hite, G.,** Stereochemical aspects of local anesthetic action. II. The crystal structure of cocaine methiodide, *Acta Crystallogr.,* in press, 1976.
35. **Findlay, S. P.,** Synthesis of racemic allocaine and racemic allopseudococaine, *J. Org. Chem.,* 21, 711, 1956.
36. **Liebermann, C. and Giesel, F.,** Ueber ein Nebenproduct der technischen cocainsynthese, *Ber. Dtsch. Chem. Ges.,* 23, 508, 1890.
37. **Liebermann, C.,** Ueber Cinnamylocacain, *Ber. Dtsch. Chem. Ges.,* 21, 3372, 1888; Liebermann, C., Ueber das Cinnamylcocain der Cocablatter, *Ber. Dtsch. Chem. Ges.,* 22, 2661, 1889.
38. **DeJong, A. W. K.,** The absence of l-benzoylecgonine and the presence of an ester very probably the methylester of l-ecgonine in Java coca leaves, *Recl. Trav. Chim. Pays-Bas,* 58, 107, 1939; DeJong, A. W. K., The determination of ecgonine alkaloids in coca leaves, *Recl. Trav. Chim. Pays-Bas,* 59, 687, 1940.
39. **Willstätter, R.,** Über ein Isomers des Cocains, *Ber. Dtsch. Chem. Ges.,* 29, 2216, 1896.
40. **Hesse, O.,** Zur Kenntniss der Cocablatter, *J. Pract. Chem.,* 66, 401, 1902.
41. **Fish, F. and Wilson, W. D. C.,** Excretion of cocaine and its metabolites in man, *J. Pharm. Pharmacol.,* 21, 1355, 1969.
42. **Montesinos, A. F.,** Metabolism of cocaine, *Bull. Narc.,* 17, 11, 1965.
43. **Nayak, P. K., Misra, A. L., and Mulé, S. J.,** Physiological disposition and biotransformation of [^{3}H] cocaine in acute and chronically treated rats, *J. Pharmacol. Exp. Ther.,* 196, 556, 1976.
44. **Werner, G.,** Investigations of the transformations of tropane alkaloids in mammalian species, *Planta Med.,* 9, 293, 1961.
45. **Misra, A. L., Nayak, P. K., Bloch, R., and Mulé, S. J.,** Estimation and disposition of ^{3}H-benzoylecgonine and pharmacological properties of some cocaine metabolites, *J. Pharm. Pharmacol.,* 27, 784, 1974.
46. **Blaschko, H., Himms, J. M., and Stromblad, B. C.,** The enzymatic hydrolysis of cocaine and alpha-cocaine, *Br. J. Pharmacol. Chemother.,* 10, 442, 1955.
47. **Leighty, E. C. and Fentiman, A. F.,** Metabolism of cocaine to norcocaine and benzoylecgonine by an *in vitro,* microsomal enzyme system, *Res. Commun. Chem. Pathol. Pharmacol.,* 8, 65, 1974.
48. **Stormont, C. and Suzuki, Y.,** Atropinesterase and cocainesterase of rabbit serum: Localization of the enzyme activity in isozymes, *Science,* 167, 200, 1970.
49. **Werner, G.,** Studies on the metabolism of tropane alkaloids 3. On the mode of action of rabbit "(–)-cocaine-3-acylhydrolase," *Hoppe Seyler's Z. Physiol. Chem.,* 348, 1151, 1967.
50. **Yamamoto, I., Mikami, K., and Kurogochi, Y.,** The enzymatic break-down of cocaine by the rabbit liver, *Jpn. J. Pharmacol.,* 3, 39, 1953.
51. **Hawks, R. L., Kopin, I. J., Colburn, R. W., and Thoa, N. B.,** Norcocaine: A pharmacologically active metabolite of cocaine found in brain, *Life Sci.,* 15, 2189, 1974.
52. **Misra, A. L., Nayak, P. K., Patel, M. N., Vadlamani, N. L., and Mulé, S. L.,** Identification of norcocaine as a metabolite of [^{3}H]-cocaine in rat brain, *Experimentia,* 30, 1312, 1974.
53. **Misra, A. L., Patel, M. N., Alluri, V. R., Mulé, S. J., and Nayak, P. K.,** Disposition, metabolism and regional brain distribution of [^{3}H]-cocaine in acute and chronically-treated dogs, submitted for publication, 1976.
54. **Schmidt, H. L., and Werner, G.,** Synthetic incorporation of ^{14}C- in (–)cocaine, (–)ecgonine and derivatives, *Ann. Chem. (Justus Liebigs),* 653, 184, 1962.
55. **Schmidt, H. L. and Werner, G.,** Preparation of ^{3}H-atropine and ^{3}H-nor(–)cocaine, *Ann. Chem. (Justus Liebigs),* 656, 149, 1962.
56. **Baldwin, S. W. and Jeffs, P. W.,** Preparation of norcocaine, submitted for publication, 1976.
57. **Werner, G. and Schmidt, H. L.,** The general labeling of (–)-cocaine with tritium, *J. Labelled Compds.,* 5, 200, 1969.

58. **Gosztonyi, T. and Walde, N.,** Studies on the tritium labeling of some local anaesthetics and amino acids by the microwave, discharge modification of the Wilzbach technique, *J. Labelled Compds.,* 2, 155, 1966.

59. **Nayak, P. K., Misra, A. L., Patel, M. N., and Mulé, S. J.,** Preparation of radiochemically pure randomly labeled and ring labeled ³H-cocaine, *Radiochem. Radioanal. Lett.,* 16, 167, 1974.

60. **Werner, G. and Mohammad, N.,** Radioactive tagging of tropane alkaloids. V. Synthetic incorporation of tritium in (−)cocaine, (+)pseudocaine and (−)scopolamine, *Ann. Chem. (Justus Liebigs),* 694, 157, 1966.

61. **Bosin, T. R., Garbrecht, F. C., and Raymond, M. G.,** Preparation of deuterium-labeled cocaine and benzoylecgonine, *Res. Commun. Chem. Pathol. Pharmacol.,* 11, 405, 1975.

62. **Hawks, R. L.,** unpublished results.

63. **Jeffs, P. W. and Baldwin, S. W.,** unpublished results.

64. **Misra, A. L., Pontani, R. B., and Mulé, S. J.,** Separation of cocaine, some of its metabolites and congeners on glass fibre sheets, *J. Chromatogr.,* 81, 167, 1973.

Detection and Identification

Detection and Identification of Cocaine, Its Metabolites, and Its Derivatives

DETECTION AND IDENTIFICATION OF COCAINE, ITS METABOLITES, AND ITS DERIVATIVES

TABLE OF CONTENTS

Milton L. Bastos and Donald B. Hoffman

INTRODUCTION

Cocaine is a natural component of coca leaves (*Erythroxylum coca*) and other species, occurring together with other alkaloids such as *cis-* and *trans*-cinnamoylcocaine, truxilline, tropacocaine, and their amino acid derivatives, methylecgonine, benzoylecgonine, cinnamoylecgonine, and ecgonine.[1] Some of them are known to arise from the hydrolysis of the methyl ester group of the original alkaloid, and are also believed to be produced during the manufacture of cocaine together with pseudococaine and cocaethyline.[2]

GENERAL PROPERTIES

Cocaine crystallizes as large, colorless, monoclinic prisms (mp 96 to 98°C[3]); its solutions are levo-rotatory (-29.46°, 2% solution in alcohol); and it has a faintly bitter taste and causes temporary anesthesia on the tongue. Cocaine is only very slightly soluble in water (1 g/1300 ml), but it readily dissolves in ethanol (1 g/7 ml), ether (1 g/4 ml), and chloroform (1 g/0.5 ml).[3] Cocaine hydrochloride (mp > 197°C) dissolves easily in water (1 g/0.5 ml), ethanol (1 g/4.5 ml), and chloroform (1 g/18 ml).[3] A 2% aqueous solution has a specific rotation of 70° to 72°.

Benzoylecgonine (tetrahydrate, mp 86 to 92°C)[4] and ecgonine (mp 98°C with decomposition) are very soluble in hot water, ethanol, and in acid and basic media, owing to their amphoteric nature (both contain amino and carboxyl groups). They are insoluble in ether, chloroform, and other organic solvents.

Ecgonine loses water when heated in the presence of $POCl_3$, becoming transformed to anhydroecgonine, a β unsaturated acid with characteristic UV absorption maxima at 213 nm.[5]

The hydrolysis of cocaine to benzoylecgonine may be accomplished by heating under reflux for 10 hr a suspension of 28 g cocaine in 300 ml of water. The benzoylecgonine tetrahydrate so formed (21 g) is recovered by cooling the 100 ml concentrate obtained by vacuum evaporation of the original suspension, from which any nonhydrolyzed cocaine has been removed by extraction with 2 × 150 ml of ethyl ether.[6]

Ecgonine results from further hydrolysis of the ester group present in benzoyl- and cinnamoylecgonine. It may be found among the cocaine metabolites or artifacts formed upon heating aqueous acidic or alkaline solutions of cocaine.

METHODS OF ANALYSIS

Spectrophotometry

Although cocaine, benzoylecgonine, and ecgonine may be detected and quantitated by spectrophotometric methods,[7] these methods are neither specific nor sufficiently sensitive for use in most cases involving the analysis of these drugs.

The ultraviolet spectrophotometry of cocaine utilizes the absorption peaks at 233, 275, and 281 nm (E $_{1\,cm}^{1\%}$ = 470, 38, and inflection, respectively) of the alkaloid dissolved in 0.1 N sulfuric acid,[3] or those of 230, 274, and 281 nm of the free base dissolved in ethanol.[3,8] The peak at 274 nm may be used for quantitating concentrations above 5 mg%.[9-11] The UV spectra of cocaine (Figure 1) are similar to those given by amydricaine, amylocaine, benzoic acid, benzoylecgonine, eucaine, di-*n*-butyl phthalate, dipiperocaine, hexylcaine, hippuric acid, phthalate esters, piperocaine, meprilcaine, tropacocaine,[12] and cinnamoylcocaine.[8] The ultraviolet spectra of cinnamoylcocaine in dilute acid solution reveal an absorption maximum at 280 nm which interferes with the quantitation of cocaine, when assayed using its absorption at 275 nm, but which does not interfere with the absorption at 232 nm.[1] The ultraviolet spectra of cocaine solutions containing cinnamoylcocaine show an inflection around 300 nm which is not present in pure cocaine solutions.[1]

The UV spectra of benzoylecgonine are similar to that of cocaine, showing absorption peaks at 234 nm and 275 nm (E$_{1\,cm}^{1\%}$ 392 and 26.4, respectively). Ecgonine, however, has considerably different spectra with peaks at 218 and 274 nm (E$_{1\,cm}^{1\%}$ 329 and 151, respectively, in ethanol).[7,13] The spectral region is not suitable for analytical purposes despite its having been used for quantitation of anhydroecgonine (213 nm).[10]

Visible range spectrophotometry can be used only with chromophoric compounds obtained from the reaction of cocaine with dyes[14,15] such as bromocresol purple[16] and bromophenol blue,[17] or with chromophores derived from other color reactions.

Infrared spectrophotometry is useful for the

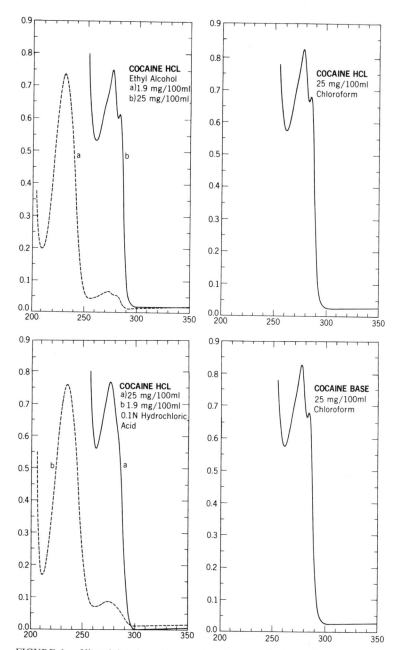

FIGURE 1. Ultraviolet absorption spectra of cocaine hydrochloride and cocaine base. (Courtesy of John W. Gunn, Jr., Analytical Manual, Laboratory Division, Bureau of Narcotics and Dangerous Drugs, Drug Enforcement Administration, U. S. Department of Justice.)

identification of pure samples of cocaine, utilizing the peaks at wave numbers 1275, 1700 and 1728, or 1106 cm^{-1} (KBr pellet). Two milligram quantities are required for production of a suitable spectra (Figure 2). *cis-* and *trans-*Cinnamoylecgonine are also easily identifiable by their infrared spectra.[1]

Chemical Reactions

Functional Group Analysis

The presence of a benzoyl group in cocaine and benzoylecgonine may be utilized for the determination of these drugs via formation of chromophoric derivatives. However other natural ester alkaloids of coca can interfere.

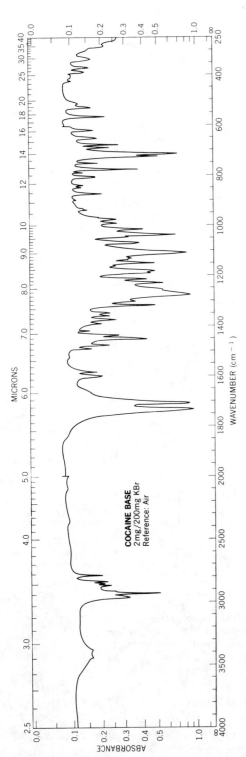

FIGURE 2. Infrared spectra of cocaine base (KBr pellet) showing the characteristic peaks 1275, 1700, 1728, and 1106 cm^{-1}. (Courtesy of John W. Gunn, Jr., Analytical Manual, Laboratory Division, Bureau of Narcotics and Dangerous Drugs, Drug Enforcement Administration, U. S. Department of Justice.)

A stable red-purple color (ferric hydroxymate derivative, 520 nm absorption) is obtained from the reaction sequence of 50 to 250 μg of cocaine first with hydroxylammonium chloride and NaOH followed by Fe (ClO$_4$)$_3$ reagent.[18] Tropic acid esters of atropa alkaloids require heating and any other ester-type alkaloids may interfere.[18]

The benzoyl group of cocaine and benzoylecgonine may further be identified after transesterification which may be effected by heating these alkaloids with sulfuric acid to obtain the volatile methyl ester of benzoic acid. This compound may be recognized by its characteristic odor.[19] The formation of methylbenzoate (using a methanolic KOH reagent) and its subsequent sensory detection have recently been made the basis of a sensitive, specific field test for cocaine.[20]

Higher sensitivity may be achieved with a procedure involving the nitration of the aromatic nucleus of the benzoyl ester alkaloids. This step is followed by alkalinization of the reaction products and is carried out as Vitali reaction for tropane alkaloids.[21] The application of this reaction was extended to cocaine by improvement of the nitration conditions so as to increase the yield of the m-dinitro derivatives.[22] These react with acetone and KOH to form blue derivatives[23] or purple derivatives,[24,25] depending on the conditions of the nitration which is carried out in the presence of sulfuric acid. This reaction was used for atropine, amphetamine, procaine, and homatropine,[24,25] and for the colorimetric determination of between 4 to 10 mg of cocaine.[26]

Color Tests

Cocaine forms precipitates with both Reinecke salts and thiocyanate, which are soluble in organic solvents, forming colored solutions that may be used for colorimetric determinations.[26,27]

Cobalt thiocyanate is the best known color reagent for the detection of cocaine and other alkaloids. It can form two types of complexes:[27] the more common blue, in which the cobalt forms a complex anion with [SCN$^-$], and a red-brown or violet type in which the cobalt forms a complex cation with the organic base.[27] By suitable control of the reaction media, it is possible to increase the selectivity of the test for cocaine, an attribute of great importance in field tests. An evaluation of the use of cobalt thiocyanate for this purpose has recently been given.[28] It should be noted that all such tests involving the use of this reagent must be backed up by additional confirmatory procedures.

Precipitation Reactions

Cocaine is precipitated, as are other alkaloids, by the general alkaloid precipitants which are still in use for screening purposes[29] or for locating alkaloids in paper and thin-layer chromatography.

Spray reagents – Platinum iodide has been widely used as a general chromophoric locating agent for alkaloids and other basic compounds. However, acidified bismuth polyiodide reagents, e.g., Dragendorff[30] or Ludy Tenger,* appear to be more sensitive for these compounds, and hence, are more suitable for the differentiation of ecgonine and norecgonine. These compounds give a brown color with Ludy Tenger reagent, whereas other coca alkaloids show characteristic orange colors.[31]

Copper chloride (5% solution) is recommended as a spray reagent for the detection of the thiocarbamates formed from the interaction of NH$_3$ and CS$_2$ vapors with secondary amines. This special reaction is useful for the differentiation of the demethylated metabolites of coca alkaloids from the other present, without however interfering with their detection by the iodoplatinate or Ludy Tenger reagents which may be applied in succession on the same chromatogram.[32]

Microcrystal reagents – When the precipitates derived from the reactions of coca alkaloids and various microcrystal reagents are examined under a microscope, their observed forms and optical properties provide the best chemical identification method for these compounds.

The cocaine picrates have specific characteristics, but because picric acid precipitates itself and many other drugs (for which it has been a microcrystal reagent), it is no longer employed for cocaine.[22]

Potassium permanganate forms very characteristic crystals with cocaine,[33,34] but this technique becomes very tedious and complicated if reproducible results are to be insured,[34] and in addition, cocaine concentrations as high as 10 μg/μl are

---

*Ludy Tenger Spray Reagent: dissolve 0.5 g bismuth carbonate in 1.5 ml concentrated hydrochloric acid. Add 3 g KI and adjust the volume to 50 ml.

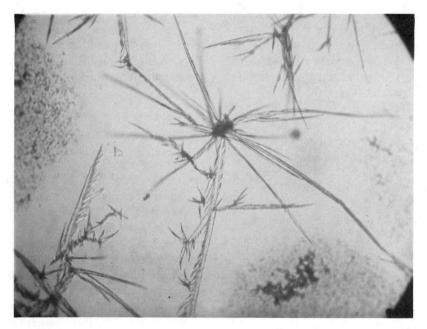

FIGURE 3. Crystals of cocaine with 5% gold chloride reagent, as seen under microscope, 90 × magnification. Crystals are strongly birefringent with a 9° extension.

required. Benzoylecgonine, 2.5 $\mu g/\mu l$, forms branched needles with acidified 2% $KMnO_4$ solution.[35]

Both silver iodide[36] and lead iodide[35,37] yield very characteristic crystals (Figure 3) with cocaine solutions of 2 $\mu g/\mu l$[36] and 0.33 $\mu g/\mu l$,[3] respectively, for the two reagents. Fulton[38] described the successful use of a modified PbI_2 reagent* which was applied to a cover glass that in turn was placed over the dried residue contained on a glass slide. This technique afforded a differentiation of cocaine (needles showing dendritic branching and positive elongation) from both benzoylecgonine (rosette shaped needles with weak birefringence and positive elongation after 15 min) and ecgonine (straight shaped individual needles).[39]

Gold chloride is the best microcrystal reagent for the identification of cocaine (0.33 $\mu g/\mu l$).[3,22,34,35,40] The crystals formed (Figure 4) exhibit perpendicular branching, are strongly birefringent, and have an extension angle of 9° and a positive elongation. Benzoylecgonine (5 $\mu g/\mu l$) forms plates and needles of larger size with the same reagent,[3] but ecgonine requires a gold bromide precipitant.[38]

Platinic chloride (5% aqueous solution) reagent gives highly characteristic crystals with cocaine solutions containing more than 0.25 $\mu g/\mu l$[22] and is used frequently by forensic chemists.[38,41] Ecgonine (2.5 $\mu g/\mu l$) requires platinic iodide reagents to insure the precipitation of small rectangular plates.[3]

Ecgonine does not react well to form highly characteristic crystals with most of the previously discussed precipitant reagents. Potassium bismuth iodide solutions form hexagonal- or octagonal-shaped plates (depending upon the temperature)[38] with ecgonine concentrations greater than 1 $\mu g/\mu l$.[3] More stable forms are obtained with a special acidified reagent.**

A solution of 10 g phosphomolybdic acid in 100 ml dilute nitric acid (1:9 v/v) is an excellent reagent for ecgonine[38] since it gives amorphous precipitates with most other drugs.

The sensitivity of an aqueous microcrystal test for coca alkaloids may be calculated by multi-

*(a) Dissolve 0.24 g $Pb(OAc)_2 \cdot 3H_2O$ and 0.27 g KI in 1 ml of acetic acid, add 5 ml of a solution of Mg $(OAc)_2$ (40 g/100 ml).

**(a) Dissolve 50 g of bismuth subnitrate in 70 ml of diluted HNO_3 (1:1 v/v). (b) Dissolve 1.25 g of KI in 2 ml of H_2O. Add 2.5 ml of diluted sulfuric acid (1:3 v/v). (c) To solution (b) add 0.5 ml solution (a). (d) Add 0.1 g sodium hypophosphite to solution (c) Evaporation of the reagent should be avoided as KNO_3 may precipitate out.

plying the volume of the drop used by the concentration threshold of identification. Working with a 0.1 μl hanging drop inside a sealed cavity glass slide,[35] levels as low as 25 ng may be detected; however, working with the usual 50 μl drops, the sensitivity ranges from 7.5 to 500 μg, depending upon the particular reagent and alkaloid involved.

PREPARATIVE CHROMATOGRAPHY

Several paper[42-46] and thin-layer[31,47-61] chromatographic systems are available, and the most representative of these are presented in Table 1. Solvent S-1 (methanol:ammonium hydroxide; 100:1.5, v/v) used with silica gel systems is best for the separation of benzoylecgonine from ecgonine.[62]

The use of gas chromatography does not provide good separation with underivatized ecgonine compounds. Applications of liquid column chromatography for cocaine have been described.[8,54,63] The use of high performance liquid chromatography for the analysis of drugs of abuse is gaining increasing prominence as a tool for the forensic chemist.[64,65] As reported by these workers, cocaine may be readily separated from other drugs on a column of Corasil® II (Figure 5).

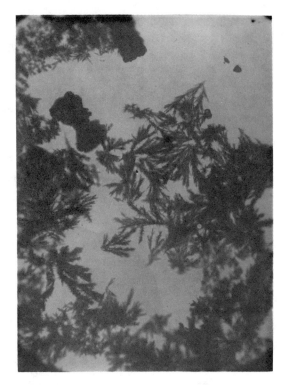

FIGURE 4. Crystals of cocaine with lead iodide (Wagenaar reagent), as seen under microscope, 90 × magnification. Crystals not birefringent. Reagent prepared by adjusting a 30% wt/v solution of potassium acetate to pH 6 with 2 N acetic acid and then saturating with lead iodide.

TABLE 1

R_f × 100 Values of Coca Alkaloids and Metabolites

	Silica Gel Plate		Gelman® I TLC		Paper, Whatman® No. 1		
	S-1[57]	S-2[46]	S-3[31]	S-4[31]	S-5[46]	S-6[43]	S-7[42]
Benzoylecgonine	78	80	29	73	60		53
Benzoylnorecgonine			12	46			
Cocaine	77	90	98	98	98	60	97
Ecgonine	32	60	33	28	35	–	0
Ecgonine methyl esther			98	98			
Norecgonine			12	15			
Tropacocaine						82	75

S-1 — methanol:ammonium hydroxide (99:1)
S-2 — ethyl ether:benzene:methanol (5:3:2) adjusted to pH 9.5 with ammonium hydroxide
S-3 — chloroform:acetone:diethylamine (5:4:1)
S-4 — ethyl acetate:methanol:ammonium hydroxide (15:4:1)
S-5 — ethyl acetate:pyridine:water (75:23:16.5)
S-6 — ethyl acetate:pyridine:water (75:23:16.5) adjusted to pH 6.8
S-7 — methyl acetate:water:pyridine:ethylene glycol:ligroin (bp 95°C) (30:0.5:1.5:3:5).

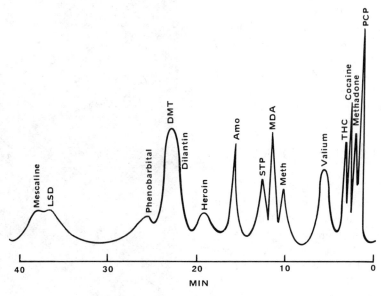

FIGURE 5. Use of high pressure liquid chromatography for the separation of drugs of abuse. Gradient elution of drugs. Column packing material: Corasil II. Column dimensions: 2.3 mm (I.D.) × 1 m. Solvent gradient: (a) 0.5% ethanol, 1.25% dioxane, and 0.2% cyclohexylamine in hexane; (b) 10% ethanol, 20% dioxane, and 1.2% cyclohexylamine in hexane. Flow rate: 1.45 ml/min. Temperature: 23°C. Sample size: 5 to 8 g each substance in total injection volume of 10 μl. (From Chan, M. L., Whetsell, C., and McChesney, J. D., *J. Chromatogr. Sci.*, 12, 512, 1974. With permission.)

Although this technique has not yet been applied to isolation of ecgonine derivatives, it would appear to be an excellent choice for this particular analysis judging by the successful results obtained on tropane alkaloids.

CHROMATOGRAPHIC SEPARATION

The difference in the physical properties of the basic compound cocaine and the amphoteric ecgonine derivatives is such that there are no suitable chromatographic systems available for effective separations of these compounds, either among themselves or from other interfering compounds. Thus, the chromatographic conditions that provide acceptable separation of cocaine from other interfering basic compounds do not resolve the amphoteric ecgonine derivatives and vice versa.

Masking of the acidic carboxyl group by derivatization of ecgonine will allow a general chromatographic separation of cocaine and its derivatives; however, the presence of other drugs will necessitate selection of operating conditions which will vary according to the particular type of

sample under investigation, i.e., pharmaceutical product, street sample, or biological material.

Thin-Layer Chromatography

The separation of cocaine from other drugs of abuse is not a simple matter. The special systems presented in Table 2 have been developed for use as screening systems in forensic toxicology; however, they do not separate cocaine from phencyclidine (PCP). The selection of a single thin-layer chromatographic system which allows the separation of all such drugs has been attempted.[3,47, 48,66] Although the general usefulness of different thin-layer systems may be readily ascertained by noting their respective resolving powers,[61] a more realistic judgment of the effectiveness of such systems must take into account the particular field of analysis involved and the recommendation that two or more systems be used to resolve the problems arising from the frequent conjunction of R_f values of members of a group of compounds.

Gas-Liquid Chromatography

Cocaine may be separated from other coca alkaloids on a coiled glass column (4′ × 1/4″ I.D.)

TABLE 2

R$_f$ × 100 Values of Cocaine and Other Drugs of Abuse Chromatographed on Silica Gel

	S-8[58,59]	S-9[11]	S-10[60]	S-11[32]
Amphetamine	0	58	49	26
Methamphetamine		50	37	21
Cocaine	84	94	79	80
Codeine	11	31	–	40
DMT	10	43	48	
LSD	34	85	69	65
Heroin	34	79	45	58
MMT			21	
Mescaline	5	28	27	
Methadone				32
Morphine	0	18		21
Nicotine				68
PCP (Phencyclidine)	89	97	79	
Propoxyphene				95
STP	13	42		

S-8 ethyl acetate:propanol:ammonium hydroxide (40:30:3), Merck® SG plates

S-9 – chloroform:ethyl acetate:ammonium hydroxide (40 ml:10 ml:10 drops) Eastman® sheets

S-10 – chloroform:ethyl ether:methanol:ammonium hydroxide (75:25:5:1) Merck SG plates

S-11 – chloroform:methanol (90:10) – a drop of ammonium hydroxide is spotted at the origin.

packed with 3% OV-1 on 100-200 mesh Chromosorb® W-HP; with a linear temperature program of 190° to 280°C, the retention times increase in the following order: tropacocaine, cocaine, cis-cinnamoylcocaine, and trans-cinnamoylcocaine.[1]

The relative retention times, expressed in Kovat units, of cocaine and other basic drugs on the commonly used SE-30 and OV-17 columns are shown in Table 3.[61,67]

The columns OV-1[68-71] or SE-30,[72] which are used instead of the OV-17 previously reported[73] in the laboratories of the Office of Chief Medical Examiner, New York City, for general screening of basic drugs in blood extracts, do not provide a separation of cocaine, dextropropoxyphene, and methaqualone (Table 3). In addition, tetracaine and amitriptyline are not well resolved from cocaine.[74] Columns of OV-17 allow better resolutions of cocaine and have been selected for analysis of this drug,[75-78] despite the fact that the retention time for cocaine is the same as that of methaqualone and is in close proximity to those of pentazocine, desipramine, nortriptyline, and atropine.[77]

Cocaine and its metabolites, which decompose in strongly alkaline media, are completely trapped

TABLE 3

Kovat Values of Some Drugs of Abuse with Retention Times in the Range of Cocaine[61,67]

	SE-30	OV-17
Methadone	2,170	2,445
Oxymetazoline	2,170	
Atropine	2,175	2,310
Fluopromazine	2,175	
Linolenic Acid	2,175	
Stearic Acid	2,175	
Codeine	2,180	2,625
Dextropropoxyphene	2,180	2,465
Cocaine	2,180	2,625
Metaxalone	2,180	
Methaqualone	2,180	2,553
Mefenamic Acid	2,180	
Adiphenine	2,190	
Amitriptyline	2,200	2,550
Chloroprocaine	2,200	
Perphenazine	2,200	

by columns of Apiezon® pretreated with potassium hydroxide.[57,75]

The development of polyamide liquid phases[79-81] has brought about the use of new stationary phases of particular interest for toxicological analysis,[82] but the importance of the Poly-A-103[®] columns now available has not yet been established for cocaine.[76]

OV-225 columns[83] and others such as OV-101 and OV-25 have been suggested for the separation of cocaine from the silyl derivatives of benzoylecgonine and ecgonine.[84] The derivatization of cocaine and GLC of the transformed product has also been proposed as a means of differentiating cocaine from other bases. As already noted, the most commonly used columns fail to provide good separation of cocaine from other drugs.

Derivatization Techniques

Cocaine does not require derivatization for gas chromatographic separation; however, certain derivatives have been used to confirm the presence of cocaine or to extend the threshold of detection by the use of electron-capture detection for halogenated derivatives.

Blake described the lithium aluminum hydride reduction of cocaine to 2-hydroxymethyltropine, followed by a pentafluoropropionic anhydride esterification of the two hydroxyl groups.[85] Benzoylecgonine, but not ecgonine, could also be determined by reduction and subsequent acylation, thereby allowing very sensitive determination with the electron-capture detector.[86]

The presence of cocaine may be confirmed by an on-column derivatization technique which produces a specific pattern of compounds with characteristic R_T values different from that of the parent compound. A combined aliquot containing cocaine and 2 M methanolic trimethylanilinium hydroxide is co-injected onto a column packed with 7% OV-17 on 80-100 mesh Chromosorb W (port temperature 275°C, column temperature 250°C, detector temperature 275°C).[87] An ecgonidine methyl ester is formed (R_T 12.5 min) together with ecgonine methyl ester (R_T 14.2 min) and three other decomposition products, all with R_T values much different from that of cocaine (R_T 23.3).

The mechanism of the decomposition reaction probably involves formation of a Hofmann degradation product.[87] Such is the case when benzphetamine, imipramine, and chlorpromazine undergo[88] alkylation of their tertiary amine groups with methyl iodide and subsequent treatment with moist silver oxide, with the resulting formation of a quaternary ammonium hydroxide derivative which, upon gas chromatographic injection, decomposes according to the Hofmann degradation mechanism to yield products with different retention times.

Derivatization of benzoylecgonine and ecgonine by esterification of their carboxylic acid groups is required prior to gas chromatography. The simplest reagent for this purpose is a mixture of sulphuric acid and methanol[78] or butanol.[89] This procedure allows for the differentiation of cocaine from the butyl ester of benzoylecgonine, but the conditions of esterification are critical,[78] presumably because of transesterification reactions involving benzoylecgonine. Milder conditions prevail with diazomethane,[75] dimethylacetal,[62] *N,N*-dicyclohexylcarbodiimide,[90] phenyltrimethylammonium hydroxide and iodobutane,[91] or *n*-butanol-boron trifluoride.[92] Alternately, derivatization may be achieved using 10% boron trichloride in 2-chloroethanol,[93] a method which has the advantage of introducing a halogenated substituent in the molecule for subsequent electron-capture detection.

For the same reason, *N,O*-bis(trimethylsilyl) trifluoroacetamide (BSTFA)[71,72] has been used in place of *N,O*-bis(trimethylsilyl) acetamide (BSA) as a derivatizing agent; however, Moore obtained the best results for the derivatization of ecgonine and benzoylecgonine with BSA.[84] The use of either a hexafluoroisopropanol-heptafluorobutyric anhydride (HFBA) mixture (1:2)[86] or that of ethanol, pyridine, and HFBA is the best approach[94] when the simultaneous esterification of both carboxyl and hydroxyl groups with alcohol-HFBA is required. When only hydroxyl groups are involved, as after the reduction of cocaine and benzoylecgonine, only acylation is required and pentafluorproprionic anhydride is the reagent of choice.[86]

Mass Spectrometry

Gas chromatography in conjunction with mass spectrometry has been considered the ideal screening procedure in forensic[68,95-98] and other fields of toxicology.[99-103] Cocaine metabolites subjected to GC-MS will, however, present many of the same problems and restrictions described in the preceding section on gas chromatography, unless they are detected only by mass spectrometry using either direct sample injection with chemical ionization[104] or direct multiple-mass fragmentography (ion monitoring).[105]

Other limitations of the GC-MS techniques are the small number of samples per day that can be effectively analyzed and the high investment cost of the equipment.

DETERMINATION IN PHARMACEUTICAL PREPARATIONS

The concentration of cocaine and other coca alkaloids in plant material, plant extracts, and pharmaceutical preparations is such that there are no predisposing analytical limitations, and any of the procedures described above can be used for the determination of cocaine.

The gravimetric method is recommended where relatively high concentrations are involved, but UV spectrophotometry is equally popular. The specificity of the method is insured by both a selective extraction of cocaine and the elimination of *cis*- and *trans*-cinnamoylcocaine by means of a potassium permanganate oxidation; this procedure does not affect cocaine[1] and probably the very small amount of tropacocaine present is also unaffected.

Quality control of commercial products is best performed by means of a complete chromatographic analysis which separates the cocaine from other contaminants such as cinnamoylcocaine and tropacocaine, and at the same time, provides for quantitation. High pressure liquid chromatography equipped with a UV detector provides the most suitable conditions for the quantitative determinations of cocaine. Columns of Mercksorb® S:60 (5 µm) and an elution solvent of chloroform-methanol or diethylether-methanol[64] are used.

Gas-liquid chromatography using columns of OV-1 at 225°C is a more sensitive procedure and has been used for the quantitation of cocaine in eye drops[76,106] or the quantitation of crude plant extracts[1,84] for cocaine and soluble contaminants, e.g., tropacocaine, *cis*-cinnamoylcocaine, and *trans*-cinnamoylcocaine.

Other amphoteric contaminants are not extracted by those solvents used for direct liquid-liquid extraction or for the elution of material previously adsorbed on Celite®.[8] When the need arises for the determination of these compounds in pharmaceutical preparations, they may be further concentrated in alcoholic solution from the aqueous residue remaining after the standard extraction of cocaine by application of the solvent-salt saturation technique.[32,62] Separation is achieved by any general chromatographic method suitable for separation of benzoylecgonine, cinnamoylecgonine, and ecgonine. Direct analysis of cocaine and its hydrolysis products, ecgonine and benzoylecgonine, is also possible by gas chromatography.[84]

DETERMINATION IN STREET SAMPLES

Street samples from the East Coast of the United States have been found to contain 2 to 5% cocaine and those from the West Coast between 14 to 92% (average 55%).[107] Hence, there is ample drug available for any method of determination. The main difficulty arises from the presence of large amounts of diluents which are almost always either sugars (e.g., dextrose, lactose) and/or local anesthetics introduced to simulate higher concentrations of cocaine. Of the latter group, benzocaine, lidocaine, procaine, and tetracaine are the more common.[107] However, caffeine[108] together with piperocaine and other drug mixtures such as pentobarbital, diphenhydramine, and acetaminophen have been used.[109,110]

The criteria for the choice of an analytical method will depend upon its selectivity for cocaine in presence of predominating quantities of those basic drugs used as diluents. These drugs should of course be simultaneously separated and identified in the analytical procedure.

Simple physical methods like the burn test or dissolution in methanol afford presumptive determination of sugar diluents as evidenced by the carbon left after burning or by the insoluble residue remaining in a methanolic solution. The detection of basic drugs used as diluents, however, requires such tests as the selective transfer of cocaine from a sodium bicarbonate solution to petroleum ether, or the determination of the specific density of cocaine powder which increases with the presence of diluents.*

Spectrophotometric methods and most chemical reactions cannot be applied directly to the sample. Emphasis should be given to those analytical techniques which provide separation of the components of the mixture; but these methods must also be capable of detecting other drugs of abuse which may be sold as cocaine in street

---

*1 oz. of "pure" cocaine should measure about 50 level, ¼-measuring teaspoons. If cut, the volume of the spoons will decrease.

samples. Based upon analysis of confiscated illicit material, the Drug Enforcement Administration reported that 8% of the street samples sold as cocaine only contained heroin, quinine, phencyclidine, procaine, amphetamine, and mescaline.[107,111-112]

Cobalt Thiocyanate Field Test

Cobalt thiocyanate, $Co(CNS)_2$, has been widely used as the principle reagent in field test kits for the detection of cocaine.[107,113] The older versions of this test were not specific, and even after the presence of opiates, antihistamines, and indole drugs were ruled out by negative findings with the Marquis and p-dimethylaminobenzoldehyde tests, a positive $Co(CNS)_2$ reaction could indicate the presence not only of cocaine, but of numerous other drugs such as tetracaine, dibucaine, phencyclidine HCl, pheniramine malate, and carbinoxamine malate.[114]

The cobalt thiocyanate reagent has been modified by the introduction of alcohols and acids so as to become more selective for cocaine.[115] Scott[116] has developed a three-step reaction sequence which significantly increases the selectivity for this drug and has been incorporated into commercial kits* for the field screening of drugs of abuse. This procedure involves the successive and carefully controlled application of the following to the test sample: (a) 2% aqueous cobaltous thiocyanate, diluted 1:1 with glycerine (formation of blue color); (b) concentrated hydrocloric acid (blue to pink color change); and (c) chloroform (chloroform layer turns blue). Scott states that of all the compounds tested, only pure cocaine yielded the indicated color reactions for all three steps.

Winek,[28] in a recent evaluation of Scott's method, pointed out the fact that certain drugs, each giving only one or two positive reactions in the sequence listed, could in combination produce a false positive reaction for cocaine. Thus, lidocaine in combination with phencyclidine or dibucaine or methapyrilene gave such false positive indications. The need for subsequent confirmation

of all positive findings using the $Co(CNS)_2$ test as well as all other field kits is emphasized.[28]

Recently Grant et al.[20] described a simple yet sensitive and specific field test for cocaine based upon the characteristic odor of methyl benzoate produced from the room temperature reaction of cocaine with methanolic sodium or potassium hydroxide reagent (1 g potassium or sodium hydroxide dissolved in 20 ml methanol). The dried test specimen is thoroughly moistened with the reagent, and after allowing excess alcohol to evaporate, the odor of the sample is noted. Of over 100 drugs tested for possible interference, only piperocaine (also a benzoate ester) gave a positive result. Certain amines such as amphetamine gave "weak, fishy odors." The sensitivity is claimed to be greater than that of existing field test kits. The sample and reagent must both be kept free of water, as this interferes with the test.

Microcrystal Tests

The noteworthy advantage of the use of microcrystal tests for the analysis of street samples is the availability of reagents that can detect cocaine with less interference from diluents. Sugars do not interfere at all, but other basic compounds can.

Gold chloride reagents in a phosphoric acid medium** are particularly recommended because they are poor precipitants for the anesthetic-type drugs which are the most common diluents used. Gold bromide in a mixture of acetic and sulphuric acids*** is highly recommended by Fulton[38] when procaine and other anesthetics are present. This reagent forms plates and also crystals that may be in the shape of a cross or of an X with ragged blade arms. Such observations can be made with a polarizing light microscope which is recommended for such tests. The crystals are dicroic, are salmon-colored or orange to colorless, and show birefringence and a positive elongation (if this property can be determined).

Aqueous 5% solutions of platinic chloride and lead iodide reagents are also included among the reagents of choice in the Analytical Manual of the Bureau of Narcotics and Dangerous Drugs.[8]

*K & K Laboratories, Plainview, New York.
**Dissolve 1 g of gold chloride ($HAuCl_4 \cdot 3H_2O$) in 20 ml of (1 + 2) phosphoric acid.[38]
***Dissolve 1 g of $HAuCl_4 \cdot 3H_2O$ and 1.5 ml of concentrated bromidric acid solution in 30 ml of diluted sulphuric acid (2 + 3). Add 30 ml of glacial acetic acid.[38]

Analysis After Separation

The best analytical methods for the determination of cocaine in street samples require prior extraction of the cocaine from fillers and adulterants.

Sugar fillers are insoluble in ethanol and other organic solvents. However when basic drugs are present, a special extraction may be required for the subsequent detection and quantitation of cocaine by any of the previously described analytical procedures.

Methylene chloride will extract cocaine in a very highly selective manner from mixtures containing procaine and other anesthetics. The best procedure though is the ion-pair elution of cocaine from a Celite® column.[11]

The column is packed with 4 g of Celite® 545 mixed with 2 ml of 1 M KNO$_3$ in O.1 N HCl.[117] A 50-mg sample dissolved in 1 ml of 1 M KNO$_3$ in O.1 N HCl is transferred onto the surface of the column which is now eluted with 45 ml of chloroform saturated with water. The eluant is collected in a 50-ml volumetric flask containing 5 ml of methanol and five drops of concentrated HCl. The volume is brought to 50 ml with chloroform, and this solution is then used for UV or IR determinations.[11]

The procaine and quinine retained on the column may be eluted with a triethylamine:chloroform solvent as described by Levine.[11,117]

When chromatographic methods are used for the qualitative or quantitative determination of cocaine, prior separation of the cocaine from other basic drugs is no longer necessary. Addition of alcohol to the sample, followed by filtration or centrifugation, is the only preparation required.

Thin-Layer Chromatography

Thin-layer chromatography is widely used for the detection of cocaine in seized illicit material. In general, the first screening will involve direct analysis using the standard O.25 mm silica gel plates, but micro-sheets[47] and micro-plates[118] may also be used.

The solvent systems shown in Table 2 are the most common, except for that of S-11. The degree of resolution shown is generally adequate for street samples, but it should be noted that solvent S-9 does not afford separation of morphine and quinine (not shown in table).

These solvent systems are useful mainly because most of the anesthetic drugs used as fillers for illicit cocaine do not interfere as may be seen in Table 4 (data obtained under the same conditions of chromatographic development as in Table 2).

One drawback of these systems is that cocaine and phencyclidine (PCP) are not resolved,[119] and hence, several other systems have been used to confirm the presence of cocaine. Methylene chloride:methyl ethyl ketone:ammonium hydroxide (90:10:0.8) was used for the separation of methadone, propoxyphene, methaqualone, cocaine, and phencyclidine.[48] The Analytical Manual of the Bureau of Narcotics and Dangerous Drugs[8] recommends the use of chloroform:dioxane:ethyl acetate:ammonium hydroxide (25:60:10:5), (also recommended by Choulis et al.[120]); ethyl acetate:benzene:ammonium hydroxide (60:35:5); and System S-9 described in Tables 2 and 4. Isopropanol:ethanol (80:20)[32] and ethanol:isopropanol:xylene:chloroform (12.5:12.5:25:50)[121] have also been suggested by other workers.

The sequence for detection of chromatographed drugs must be sufficiently sophisticated to account for the large variety of drugs of abuse and fillers that may be present in a seized material.

The first step is observation under ultraviolet light (294 nm and 350 nm), which will give an indication of the presence of LSD and other fluorescent drugs. Several spray sequences have been described for use after UV examination. Phillips and Gardiner[122] used the following: 1% iodine-methanol solution followed by light spraying with acidic iodoplatinate, and then appli-

TABLE 4

$R_f \times$ 100 Values of Cocaine and Other Components (Fillers and Adulterants) of Street Samples

	S-8[58,59]	S-9[11]	S-10[60]	S-11*[32]
Benzocaine	89	67		94
Butacaine	89			70
Caffeine			82	89
Cocaine	79	84	94	80
Holocaine	93			
Lidocaine	87			95
Procaine	70	45	70	70
Quinine		5		33
Strychnine	32		48	44
Tetracaine	55	11		77

*S-11 — chloroform:methanol (90:10) — a drop of ammonium hydroxide is spotted at the origin.
Other solvent systems are as described for Table 2.

cation of a solution containing 0.5 g of *p*-dimethylaminobenzaldehyde dissolved in 100 ml of 5% hydrochloric acid in ethanol (99% purity), followed by heating for 5 to 10 min at 105°.[14] However, more information may be obtained with the sequence: Ninhydrin spray, followed by heating of the plate for the detection of secondary amines; 5% sulphuric acid (which enhances both the fluorescence of quinine and the sensitivity of the subsequent iodoplatinate spray); UV examination; iodoplatinate reagent; and *p*-dimethylaminobenzaldehyde reagent followed by heating.[32]

Cocaine is readily detected by iodine and iodoplatinate sprays, and hence, some authors prefer to develop two separate chromatograms with one intended specifically for the application of the *p*-dimethylaminobenzaldehyde reagent for detection of LSD and other hallucinogenic drugs.[59]

Gas-Liquid Chromatography

The significant advantage of GLC for the analysis of seized material is its capability for quantitation of the components of street mixtures.

The New York City Police Department is currently developing an integrated system of GLC-mass spectrometry for the determination of the composition and dosage of its confiscated material.

Phencyclidine, whose resolution poses a problem in TLC, is easily separated from cocaine by GLC, but this requires maintaining the injection port temperature at 180°C to avoid thermal degradation of the PCP.[123]

The anesthetic drugs are also well resolved, except for the combinations piperocaine-procaine and cocaine-tetracaine chromatographed on SE-30 columns; but even here with efficient temperature programing and automated digital computation techniques applied to the areas of overlapping peaks, it is nevertheless possible to obtain quantitation within reasonable ranges of accuracy.[74]

The sensitivity and resolving power of GLC has made possible within the scope of the analysis the detection of such impurities or artifacts as *cis*- and *trans*-cinnamoylcocaine in cocaine samples[1] or ecgonine and benzoylecogonine in uncut cocaine samples. With regard to the latter two compounds, levels less than 0.1 and 0.3% respectively may be detected after derivatization.[84] These minor components may be used as parameters for tracing the origin of a sample.

The problem of distinguishing the cocaine peak from that of methaqualone on OV-17 columns may be solved through use of the derivatization techniques described above, in particular, the on-column reaction with trimethylanilinium hydroxide.[87]

In this manner, the choice of the column becomes less critical with respect to the determination of cocaine in the presence of the other drugs indicated in Table 3.

The use of different columns may be an alternative for the confirmation of the presence of cocaine, but Moffat et al.[124] have stated that the use of more than one stationary phase for the gas-liquid chromatography of basic drugs is of very limited value.

DETERMINATION IN BIOLOGICAL FLUIDS

The importance of the determination of cocaine and its metabolites in biological fluids comprises detecting and monitoring its use and abuse among addict populations,[125] tracing its course following application as a local surgical anesthetic, increasing the understanding of its pharmacologic, pharmacokinetic, and metabolic properties, and building a pharmacodynamic and toxicological basis to explain its role in drug-related deaths.

These factors, coupled with the increasing importance of cocaine as a drug of abuse, have prompted numerous investigations for newer, sensitive methods of analysis for cocaine and its metabolites. The focus on the special analytic requirements for the extraction of the water-soluble metabolites, ecgonine and benzoylecgonine, the application of immunoassay techniques (in particular, EMIT®) to these compounds, and the refinement of gas and thin-layer chromatographic methodology for both the parent drug and its metabolites have been the result of this attention.[73] Consequently, there has been a dramatic change from the infrequency with which cocaine analyses were included in previous standardized methodologies to the current emphasis on the inclusion of these compounds in current protocols for drug screening. An example of the consequence of this shift can be seen in the dramatic increase in the number of reported positive findings for cocaine and its metabolites in the Toxicological Laboratories of the Office of Chief Medical Examiner of New York City, i.e., 2 or 3 cases from 1968 to 1972, 23 cases in 1973, and 18 cases in 1974.

In addition to the problems cited above, the determination of cocaine and its metabolites encounters serious problems arising from the instability of cocaine present in tissue material stored over a period of time, its instability of high pH values, and from the presence of tissue components that may pose difficulties before and after derivatization of the compounds.

Price[126] observed that after 2 months storage at $4°C$, the cocaine levels in spleen and liver had fallen from 3 mg% to 0.2 mg%, and from 0.8 mg% to 0.08 mg%, respectively. Jatlow[77] reported that after 15- and 30-min periods at room temperature, the plasma cocaine levels decrease by 6.5% and 12.5% respectively. Furthermore, the rate of loss was approximately doubled at $37°C$. Even after 24 hr storage at $-15°C$ or on dry ice, the concentration was observed to decrease by a maximum of 30%.[77]

These observations make clear the necessity both for procuring as soon as possible all material for cocaine analysis, and for extending the analysis to the determination of the metabolites, particularly benzoylecgonine.

The therapeutic and toxic levels are not yet clearly delineated, but certain broad findings have been made.

Peak plasma values of 0.012 mg% to 0.47 mg% were found in individuals given therapeutic doses of 1.5 mg/kg of cocaine (intravenously) prior to surgery.[77]

The half-life of cocaine in plasma and brain of rats is 0.3 hr and 0.4 hr, respectively, following i.v. administration of 8 mg/kg doses.[127] The distribution in tissues in both dogs[130] and man[126] indicates that cocaine levels decrease in the order: spleen>kidney>liver>blood.

In cases of cocaine intoxication, blood concentrations of 0.8 mg%[126] and 0.2 mg%[128] were reported. However in two cases from New York City involving massive ingestion of cocaine, concentrations of 1.7 mg% (1.8 mg% lidocaine also present) and 8.5 mg% were observed.[21]

The metabolism of cocaine is extensive, with the formation of norcocaine,[127,129] which may be found in liver in cases of acute poisoning, and benzoylecgonine,[75,78,130,131] the principal

metabolite. Benzoylecgonine is further metabolized to benzoylnorecgonine, a partially conjugated phenolic derivative, and ecgonine.[131]

Excretion of cocaine and its metabolites is primarily through bile and urine. Free cocaine has been found in bile[21,126] in concentrations of 2.5 mg% following ingestion of 2 to 3g of cocaine.[126] Other metabolites of cocaine with R_f 0.7 and 0.49 in the System S 14 (Table 6) were found in bile.[21] The urine concentration after ingestion of 2 to 3 g of cocaine was 0.5 mg%,[126] this value agreeing with the concentration of 0.9 mg% found in a case of fatal intoxication.[132]

The concentration of cocaine after ingestion of therapeutic levels or after illicit use is lower and will depend upon the time elapsed after intake— 0.04 mg% in urine after inhalation 9 to 14 hr prior to collection of sample.[133] Wallace et al. reported 0.03 mg% during the 8-hr period following topical application of 250 mg of cocaine hydrochloride to nasal mucosa.[78] Under the same therapeutic conditions, the urinary concentration of benzoylecgonine ranged from 1.0 mg% to 12.4 mg%.[78] During the period 16 to 24 hr after ingestion, concentrations of benzoylecgonine and cocaine of 0 to 4.4 mg% and 0 to 0.01 mg%, respectively, were observed.[78]

This data are in agreement with that of Fish and Wilson,[75] who found that only 1 to 9% of a daily dose of cocaine (120 mg/day, i.v.) was excreted as the free base (urine concentrations in the range 0.2 to 0.8 mg%), with most of the drug excreted as benzoylecgonine.

Direct Analysis

The incorporation of immunological techniques into analytic methodology for the mass screening of drugs of abuse has resulted in the availability of a very simple method for the presumptive detection of benzoylecgonine in urine, i.e., the enzyme multiplied immunoassay technique (EMIT).

In the EMIT system, benzoylecgonine is bound to the enzyme, lysozyme, which lyses the peptidoglycan of bacterial cell walls and thereby decreases the turbidity of such a bacterial suspension. Upon injection into the bloodstream of experimental animals, this (benzoylecgonine-lysozyme) antigen will produce antibodies which may be isolated as an immune serum. Formation of the antigen-antibody complex results in an inhibition of the enzymatic activity. Free benzoylecgonine in the test solution will displace in a linear fashion, depending upon its concentration, some of the bound drug-enzyme complex. This in turn results in a reactivation of the enzyme and a corresponding decrease of the turbidity of a bacterial suspension.

This assay is sensitive (1.0 μg/ml) and highly specific for benzoylecgonine, with only ecgonine exhibiting significant cross reactivity (see Table 5),[89] a fact which enhances the sensitivity of the test for the presumptive prior use of cocaine.

Analysis After Extraction

The choice of an extraction procedure will be governed by whether cocaine or its metabolites are to be determined and will also depend upon which analytical method is to be followed after the extraction, with extracts intended for gas chromatography requiring much higher degrees of purity than those for thin-layer chromatography.

As with other alkaloids, cocaine may be extracted into organic solvents, including cyclohexane,[127] from aqueous alkaline media.[66] Ether is a good solvent for this purpose[75] despite conflicting reports as to its efficiency.[134,135] It should be emphasized that both rapid extraction and minimal contact with the basic solution are essential to prevent hydrolysis[75] which readily occurs in alkaline as well as in acidic media. The recovery of cocaine with chloroform as the solvent is 76.1% at pH 10.5 as contrasted with that of 93.3% at pH 9.5.[136] However, a double extraction procedure is always recommended for a general purpose analysis where other basic drugs are to be determined.

Successful separations may be achieved with the procedure of Wolen and Gruber,[137] which was made the basis for the analysis of methadone[138] and can be adapted for cocaine as well by lowering the pH of extraction. Four milliliters of plasma (or blood) adjusted to pH 9.8 are extracted twice with 5 ml of n-butyl chloride. The two butyl chloride phases are combined and extracted with 5 ml of 0.2 N H_2SO_4.* After centrifugation, the n-butyl chloride phase is aspirated and discarded. The acid phase is washed by shaking for 4 min with 5 ml of n-hexane, made alkaline (pH should be below 10), and extracted by shaking with 8 ml of chloroform for 5 min. After centrifugation for 3 min, the aqueous (upper) layer is aspirated and discarded. The chloroform is transferred to a 12-ml centrifuge tube and evaporated to dryness.

*Minor modification of the procedure of Inturrisi and Kaika.[138]

TABLE 5

Cross-Reactivity of Various Compounds in Urine with EMIT Assays* — EMIT Assays Equivalent to 1 μg/ml of Benzoylecgonine

Compound	μg/ml	RR[a]
Benzoylecgonine	1.0	1.000
Ecgonine	9.5	0.105
Ecgonine methyl ester	380	0.003
Cocaine	460	0.002
Homatropine	NR[b]	—
Morphine	NR[b]	—
Methadone	NR[b]	—

[a]RR, relative reactivity.
[b]NR, no reaction at concentrations of 500 to 1000 g/ml.
*excerpted from M. L. Bastos et al.[89]

Although a similar procedure could be used for the extraction of tissue homogenates, the impossibility of using high pH levels during extraction increases the chances of occurrence of troublesome emulsions. A better approach is the use of the nonionic Amberlite® XAD-2 resin for the extraction of aqueous homogenates obtained from 2 to 20 g of tissue,[127,139,140] the quantity required depending upon the subsequent choice of either gas-liquid or thin-layer chromatography.[141] Urine may also be conveniently extracted with XAD-2 columns. Chloroform:isopropanol (3:1) is used for elution, but to insure the complete removal of benzoylecgonine and benzoylnorecgonine from the resin, a further elution with methanol is required. Ecgonine and norecgonine are not adsorbed by the resin.[127]

Urine may also be conveniently analyzed by a single extraction with chloroform:isopropanol:1,2 dichloroethane (8:1:3)[39] or with chloroform:ethanol (8:2).[30] Using the latter procedure, recoveries of cocaine and benzoylecgonine of 93% and 65%, respectively, were reported.[30,78] Fifteen milliliters of chloroform-isopropanol (2:1 v/v) may be used to extract 2 ml of diluted urine, plasma (1:5 diluted) or tissue homogenate (20% in 0.9 saline) with reported recoveries of benzoylecgonine of 95.4 ± 0.3%, 91.0 ± 1.7%, 90.0 ± 0.6%, and 81.3 ± 0.9% from urine, plasma, brain, and liver respectively.[142] It may be noted that ecgonine has been isolated by liquid extraction using 12 times the aqueous volume of chloroform:methanol (68:32),[127] but this procedure is somewhat cumbersome.

The recovery of benzoylecgonine from relatively large volumes of urine may be optimized by the incorporation of a salt saturation step (e.g., addition of 5 g potassium carbonate to 25 ml urine) prior to extraction with a solvent such as chloroform:isopropanol (3:1).[48] Benzoylecgonine and the more polar ecgonine may be extracted together from urine or aqueous tissue extracts into solvents of relatively high polarity, provided sufficient electrolyte is present in the aqueous phase to effect salting-out of both these metabolites. Thus, saturation of a 10-ml aqueous phase with potassium carbonate will insure extraction of these compounds into 1 ml ethanol.[32] The extraction with chloroform:isopropanol (2:1) of K_2CO_3-saturated solutions provides recoveries of benzoylecgonine as high as 81.3% (liver), 90% (brain), and 91% (plasma),[142] as well as effecting recovery of ecgonine. The salting-out of 10 ml of urine may also be achieved by the addition of 9.0 ml of 95% ethanol, 10 g of a 1:1 mixture of KH_2PO_4: K_2HPO_4, followed by reextraction with 5 ml of ethanol.[62] This technique has the advantage of being carried out at lower pH, thereby avoiding saponification of the benzoylecgonine. A 3:2 mixture of sodium bicarbonate:potassium carbonate has also been used to effect salting-out.[143] Ethyl alcohol is the solvent usually used for salting-out extractions,[32,62] but 2-chloroethanol is a good alternative if the derivatization techniques (involving subsequent electron-capture G.C. detection) described below are carried out.

Liquid-solid extraction of previously lyophilized material may be used for the recovery of drugs that are not easily extractable with organic solvents.[144,145] This technique using methanol as the solvent was employed for the extraction of cocaine and metabolites from urine and tissue.[62,129]

A complete separation of cocaine and its metabolites, including ecgonine, may be achieved after derivatization. Moore[93] has proposed a direct derivatization technique for ecgonine and benzoylecgonine which involves the addition of 10 ml of a 10% solution of boron trichloride in 2-chloroethanol to 1 ml of urine in a test tube. The test tube is loosely plugged with cotton and immersed in a boiling water bath for 1 hr. After cooling, 10 ml of ice-cold water is added and the solution is extracted several times with 40-ml portions of diethyl ether. The ether extracts are

discarded and the aqueous solution alkalinized with ammonia and extracted with 4 to 5 portions of diethyl ether. The ether extracts are filtered through cotton and gently evaporated on a steam bath under a stream of air.

As applied to biological material, particularly tissue, the techniques of salting-out or of methanolic extraction of lyophilized material have been found to produce extracts that also contain large amounts of impurities. This necessitates subjecting the final extracts to chromatographic purification or to transformation of the desired compounds to other derivatives which more readily level themselves to purification and analysis. Preparative TLC has been suggested,[129] but the yield obtained is only 30%.[62] Derivatization of impure extracts to halogenated compounds capable of detection by electron-capture G.C., followed by solvent extraction, has been found to offer better recoveries and more accurate and sensitive quantitative analysis.

Thus the amphoteric water-soluble benzoylecgonine and ecgonine may be transformed into basic compounds by esterification of their respective carboxylic acid groups. The resulting derivatives may then be extracted from alkaline medium. This will afford pure extracts, provided the esterification is both preceded by solvent extraction removal of other basic compounds and followed by a similar step for the removal of neutral drugs.

Thin-Layer Chromatography

The choice of thin-layer chromatographic systems is considerably limited by the presence of tobacco alkaloids and their metabolites, caffeine, possible putrefaction products, and naturally occurring tissue and urine impurities. The Davidow System (S-13) — ethyl acetate:methanol: ammonium hydroxide (85:10:5)[146] — and its modifications[59] are widely used. The most commonly used solvent systems are those listed in Table 6 and the System S-11 (Table 2). System S-15 (Table 6), a modification of S-11, was developed for the detection of benzoylecgonine in urine, but it has very poor resolution for drugs with high R_f values.

The main problem with those solvent systems is that cocaine exhibits a high R_f in the same region of the chromatogram which contains other drugs of abuse, including methaqualone and propoxyphene. The required confirmation may be achieved using one or more of the following systems: Benzene:dioxane:ethyl ether:ammonium hydrox-

TABLE 6

$R_f \times 100$ Values of Drugs of Abuse

	S-12[57]	S-13[146]	S-14[149]	S-15[30]
Amphetamine	42	78	52	
Amitriptyline	79	98		90
Benzoylecgonine	~15			20
Chlorpheniramine	33	88	70	
Chlorpromazine	72	96	88	89
Cocaine	90	96	95	87
Codeine	30	54	42	
Cyclazocine	57		72	
Imipramine		95	85	
Meperidine	62	90	72	87
Mescaline			22	
Methadone	80	99	94	77
Methamphetamine	28		48	
Methapyrilene		94	86	
Methaqualone			95	
Methylphenidate	76	92	85	
Morphine	18	32	24	43
Nicotine	56	90		
Phenmetrazine	46		55	
Propoxyphene	94	90	98	93
Quinine	42	65	50	

S-12 — ethyl acetate:methanol:water:ammonium hydroxide (85:10:3:1) Merck plates

S-13 — ethyl acetate:methanol:ammonium hydroxide (85:10:3). Develop two blank plates just prior to development of the sample plate

S-14 — ethyl acetate:cyclohexane:ammonium hydroxide:methanol:water (70:15:2:8:0.5)

S-15 — chloroform:methanol:ammonium hydroxide (100:20:1) Uniplate—Analtech®

ide(50:40:5.5) for the differentiation of methadone, methadone metabolites, and cocaine;[83] and methylene chloride:methyl ethyl ketone:ammonium hydroxide (90:10:0.8);[48] Ethyl acetate:cyclohexane:ammonium hydroxide (50:40:0.1);[147] and chloroform:cyclohexane:dioxane:acetone:1N H_2SO_4 (20:20:20:20:0.3)[148] for the separation of cocaine, propoxyphene, and methadone.

The interference from other drugs is minimized when TLC is used for properly esterified cocaine metabolites,[89] i.e., derivatization of ecgonine and benzoylecgonine only after the biological material has been extracted with organic solvents. However, there is still interference from the presence of esterified biological artifacts which are separated with difficulty from esterified ecgonine derivatives. The chromatographic system, ethyl acetate:methanol:water (7:2:1), was used successfully to separate the butyl esters of benzoylecgonine, ecgonine, norbenzoylecgonine, and norecgonine,[89] but butylecgonine has the same R_f of morphine, which may be present after hydrolysis of morphine glucuronide. Clarification requires bidimensional chromatography using as the second solvent system the mixture: chloroform:acetone:ammonium hydroxide (5:94:1)[52,89] (Figure 6).

Following chromatographic development, cocaine and its metabolites or derivatives are best detected with a sequential application of Dragendorff 20% H_2SO_4-I_2 reagents[30] or Ludy Tenger reagent.[31] When detection of certain N-demethylated metabolites is required, the following procedure may be carried out without interfering with the subsequent use of the Dragendorff reagent. The plate is exposed for 15 min inside a closed chromatography tank to vapors generated by mixing 10 ml carbon disulfide and 10 ml concentrated ammonium hydroxide in a 150-ml beaker. The thiocarbamates that form with secondary amines are detected by lightly spraying with a 5% copper chloride solution.[32]

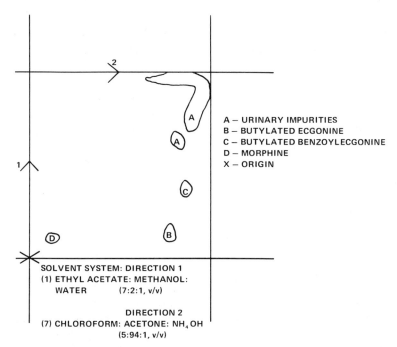

A — URINARY IMPURITIES
B — BUTYLATED ECGONINE
C — BUTYLATED BENZOYLECGONINE
D — MORPHINE
X — ORIGIN

SOLVENT SYSTEM: DIRECTION 1
(1) ETHYL ACETATE: METHANOL:
    WATER   (7:2:1, v/v)

                    DIRECTION 2
(7) CHLOROFORM: ACETONE: NH$_4$OH
        (5:94:1, v/v)

FIGURE 6.   Bidimensional thin-layer chromatography. Urine samples containing ecgonine and benzoylecgonine (10 μg/ml each) were saturated with potassium carbonate and extracted with ethanol. The ethanol extracts were butylated and then chromatographed. Control urines (no drug) were treated in a similar manner. The butylated extracts, as well as free morphine (10 μg), were applied at the origin, and the chromatogram was developed in two different solvent systems (two-dimensional chromatography). The solvent system used for the first dimension was ethyl acetate-methanol-water (7:2:1) (Solvent System No. 1) and that used for the second dimension was chloroform-acetone-ammonia (5:94:1) (Solvent System No. 7). A = urinary impurities; B = butylated ecgonine; C = butylated benzoylecgonine; D = morphine; X = origin. (From Bastos, M. L., Jukofsky, D., and Mulé, S. J., *J. Chromatogr.*, 89, 335, 1974. With permission.)

The detection of compounds containing NH groups by means of copper dithiocarbamate does not preclude the previous detection of primary amines by ninhydrin nor the subsequent detection of tertiary amines with the Dragendorff or iodo-platinate reagents.[32]

Gas-Liquid Chromatography

There are two main limitations to the use of GLC for the analysis of extracts obtained from biological material: the presence of interfering substances and the requirement of very high sensitivity for the GLC detection system.

The identification of the anticipated interfering compounds has been linked to the original biological material,[149,150] rubber stoppers,[103] and even the solvents or resins used for extraction. Minimizing this problem requires improvement in the degree of purity of the extracts and reduction in the size of the sample obtained from biological material.

The use of a Ni[63] electron-capture detector[85,86,93] for halogenated ecgonine derivatives or of a nitrogen specific detector[77] meets the demands for the high sensitivity required for the detection of small amounts of drugs and metabolites and is also less sensitive to most of the impurities that interfere with the gas chromatographic analysis.

The flame ionization detector has been used for detection of cocaine in urine and in blood for levels of this drug above 10 μg%.[130] This is above the therapeutical level, but complete studies involving cocaine may require sensitivities as low as 0.5 μg% obtainable with the nitrogen detector.[77]

The requirements for careful purification limit the application of the direct extraction technique using organic solvents to those cases where fresh biological material is available.[71,72,75]

However, cocaine has been successfully detected in urine[83] by extracting 2 ml of alkaline urine with 50 μl of chloroform. This procedure takes advantage of the extremely high chloroform/water partition coefficient of cocaine to effect transfer of most of the drug, but with most interfering materials left in the aqueous phase.[150]

The best results are those obtained after double extraction wherein cocaine is first extracted out at pH 9.7 by *n*-butyl chloride[138] or heptane:isoamyl alcohol (98:2)[77] and then back extracted into an aqueous 0.2 *N* acidic phase. The latter solution is now washed (hexane or heptane), alkalinized (pH below 10), and reextracted into organic solvents[77,138] using either a conventional technique or the microextraction with 50 μl of chloroform for a further enhancement of the purification.[151]

This double extraction procedure does not extract chlordiazepoxide, methaqualone, and other very weak bases. The problems relating to the choice of chromatographic conditions are now minimized by the absence of methaqualone which has the same retention time as cocaine on the OV-17 columns, commonly used for the detection of cocaine and its derivatives[77,78] (Table 3).

In the Toxicological Laboratories of the Office of Chief Medical Examiner in New York City, a 3% SE-30 column on 80-100 mesh Chromosorb W-HP is used for the screening of basic drugs in blood. This choice is based upon the fact that methadone, not cocaine, is the focal point of the investigations, the differentiation of cocaine from propoxyphene and amitriptyline being done by UV and TLC techniques.

OV-1 columns, which are similar to SE-30, have been used for the separation of fluoropropionylderivatives of ecgonine and benzoylecgonine,[85,86] but not for the silyl derivative of benzoylecgonine which has the same retention time as cocaine.[84]

Ultimately, a new column will have to be reserved for cocaine analysis, or alternately, the existing dual-column screening procedures utilizing OV-1 and Poly-A-103[70] will have to be extended to include the determination of cocaine. Gas-liquid chromatographic analysis will continue to be the best analytical method for blood, particularly when speed of analysis is essential, as in emergency toxicology, but also because of its usefulness in combination with immunoassay techniques and computerized mass spectrometer systems.

REFERENCES

1. **Moore, J. M.,** Identification of cis-trans-cinnamoylcocaine in illicit cocaine seizures, *J. Assoc. Off. Agric. Chem.,* 56, 1199, 1973.
2. **Toffoli, F. and Avico, U.,** Coca Paste, Residues from the industrial extraction of cocaine, ecgonine and anhydroecgonine, *Bull. Narcotics,* 17(4), 27, 1965.
3. **Clarke, E. G. C.,** *Isolation and Identification of Drugs,* Pharmaceutical Press, London, 1969.
4. **Findlay, S. P.,** The three-dimensional structure of the cocaines, Part I. Cocaine and pseudococaine, *J. Am. Chem. Soc.,* 76, 2855, 1954.
5. **Weast, R. C.,** Ed., *Handbook of Chemistry and Physics,* CRC Press, Cleveland, 1969.
6. **Jain, N. C.,** Mass Screening Methods, presented at the Meeting of American Academy of Forensic Sciences, Chicago, 1975.
7. **Oestreicher, P. M., Farmilo, C. G., and Levi, L.,** Part III, Section B., Ultraviolet spectra data for ninety narcotics and related compounds, *Bull. Narcotics,* 6(3–4), 42, 1954.
8. **Gunn, J. W., Sobol, S. P., and Moore, R. A.,** Analytical Manual, Bureau of Narcotics and Dangerous Drugs, Washington, D.C., 1975.
9. **Lous, P.,** Quantitative determination of barbiturates, *Acta Pharmacol. Toxicol.,* 6, 227, 1950.
10. **Toffoli, F. and Avico, U.,** Chemical evaluation of crude cocaine and of the residue after industrial extraction of cocaine therefrom, *R. C. Inst. Sup. Sanit.,* 26, 1011, 1963.
11. **Nakamura, G. R. and Parker, B. P.,** Assay of cocaine in the presence of procaine and quinine by column chromatography, *J. Chromatogr.,* 52, 107, 1970.
12. **Siek, T. J. and Osiewicz, R. J.,** Identification of drugs and other toxic compounds from their ultraviolet spectra. Part II. Ultraviolet absorption properties of thirteen structural groups, *J. Forensic Sci.,* 20, 1, 1975.
13. **Sunshine, I.,** Ed., *Handbook of Analytical Toxicology,* CRC Press, Cleveland, 1969.

14. **Mattson, L. N. and Holt, W. L.,** The colorimetric determination of barbiturates in pharmaceutical preparations, *J. Am. Pharm. Assoc. Sci. Ed.*, 38, 55, 1949.
15. **Frame, E. G., Russel, J. A., and Wilhelmi, A. E.,** The colorimetric estimation of amino nitrogen in blood, *J. Biol. Chem.*, 149, 255, 1943.
16. **Wood, I. A., Cochin, J., Fornefeld, E. J., McMahon, F. G., and Seevers, M. H.,** The estimation of amines in biological materials with critical data for cocaine and mescaline, *J. Pharmacol. and Exp. Ther.*, 101, 188, 1951.
17. **Delaville, I.,** Simple, rapid and sensitive technique for the detection of alkaloids and psychotropic amines in such physiological fluids as saliva and urine, *Ann. Biol. Clin.* (Paris), 20, 479, 1962.
18. **Philibert, H. and Martine, J.,** Determination of some ester alkaloids by formation of a ferric hydroxamate, *Bull. Soc. Pharm. Marseille*, 20, 61, 1971.
19. *Pharmacopeia of the United States,* 18th Revision, Mack Publishing, Easton, Pennsylvania, 1960.
20. **Grant, F. W., Martin, W. C., and Quackenbush, P. W.,** A single sensitive specific field test for cocaine based upon the recognition of the odour of methyl benzoate as a test product, *Bull. Narcotics*, 27(2), 33, 1975.
21. **Bastos, M. L., Valanju, N. N., and Hoffman, D. B.,** unpublished observations.
22. **Bastos, M. L.,** Microquimica de alguns alcaloides, *Bol. Inst. Quim. Agric. Rio de Janeiro*, 51, 35, 1957.
23. **Pezez, M.,** Revue des methodes d'identification de la cocaine, Nouvelle reaction coloree, *J. Pharm. Chim.*, 30, 200, 1939.
24. **Rathenasikam, E.,** A colour test for cocaine, *Analyst* (London), 75, 169, 1950.
25. **Rathenasikam, E.,** A colour test for amphetamine, *Analyst* (London), 76, 115, 1951.
26. **Tanker, M.,** Three new methods for colorimetric determination of cocaine, *Bull. Fac. Med. Istanbul*, 24, 542, 1961.
27. **Stanier, C.,** Use of cobalt thiocyanate in the analysis of organic bases, *Il Farmaco Ed. Prat.*, 29, 118, 1974.
28. **Winek, C. L. and Eastly, T.,** Cocaine identification, *Clin. Toxicol.*, 8, 205, 1975.
29. **Hider, C. L.,** The rapid identification of frequently abused drugs, *J. Forensic Sci.*, 11, 257, 1971.
30. **Wallace, J. E., Hamilton, H. E., Schwertner, H., and King, D. E.,** Thin layer chromatographic analysis of cocaine and benzoylecgonine in urine, *J. Chromatogr.*, 114, 433, 1975.
31. **Misra, A. L., Pontani, R. B., and Mulé, S. J.,** Separation of cocaine, some of its metabolites and congeners on glass fibre sheets, *J. Chromatogr.*, 81, 167, 1973.
32. **Bastos, M. L., Kananen, G. E., Young, R. M., Monforte, J. R., and Sunshine, I.,** Detection of basic organic drugs and their metabolites in urine, *Clin. Chem.*, 16, 931, 1970.
33. **Bamford, F.,** *Poisons, Their Isolation and Identification,* 3rd ed., J & A Churchill, London, 1951.
34. **Keenan, G. L.,** Notes on microscopy of some important alkaloids, *The Chem. Analyst*, 40, 4, 1951.
35. **Clarke, E. G. C. and Williams, M.,** Microchemical tests for the identification of alkaloids, *J. Pharm. Pharmacol.*, 7, 255, 1955.
36. **Whitmore, W. F. and Wood, C. A.,** Chemical microscopy of some toxicologically important alkaloids, *Mikrochemie*, 27, 249, 1939.
37. **Wagenaar, G. H.,** Microchemical alkaloid reactions with a new reagent containing lead iodide, *Pharm. Weekbl.*, 76, 276, 1939.
38. **Fulton, C. C.,** *Modern Microcrystal Tests for Drugs,* Interscience, New York, 1969.
39. **Valanju, N. N., Baden, M. M., Valanju, S. N., Mulligan, D., and Verma, S. K.,** Detection of biotransformed cocaine in urine from drug abusers, *J. Chromatogr.*, 81, 170, 1973.
40. **Butler, W. B.,** Methods of Analysis, Publ. #341, Internal Revenue Service, 1967.
41. **Stephenson, C. H.,** *Some Microchemical Tests for Alkaloids,* Lippincott, Philadelphia and London, 1921.
42. **Klementschitz, W. and Mathes, P.,** Paper chromatography of alkaloids, *Sci. Pharm.*, 20, 65, 1952.
43. **von Buchi, J. and Schumacher, H.,** Die Reinheitsprüfung der Alkaloide mit Hilfe der Papierchromatographie, *Pharm. Acta Helv.*, 32, 194, 1955.
44. **Sanchez, C. A.,** Analysis cromatografico de ecgonina en la orina de sujetos habituados a la mastigacion de la coca, *An. Fac. Farm. Bioquim. Lima*, 8, 82, 1957.
45. **Majlat, P. and Bayer, I.,** Separation of cocaine, benzoylecgonine and ecgonine by paper chromatography, *J. Chromatogr.*, 20, 187, 1965.
46. **Ortiz, R. V.,** Estudio de la distribuicion y metabolismo de la cocaine en la rata, *An. Fac. Quim. Farm. Santiago*, 18, 15, 1966.
47. **Sunshine, I., Filke, W. W., and Landesman, H.,** Identification of therapeutically significant organic bases by thin layer chromatography, *J. Forensic Sci.*, 11, 428, 1961.
48. **Jain, N. C., Leung, W. J., Budd, R. D., and Sneath, T. C.,** Thin layer chromatographic screening and confirmation of basic drugs of abuse in urine, *J. Chromatogr.*, 115, 519, 1975.
49. **Guven, K. C. and Altinkurt, T.,** Stability of cocaine solutions and identification of cocaine, ecgonine and benzoylecgonine by thin-layer chromatography, *Eczacilik Bul.*, 7, 119, 1965.
50. **Comer, J. P. and Comer, I.,** Application of thin-layer chromatography in pharmaceutical analyses, *J. Pharm. Sci.*, 56, 413, 1967.
51. **Noirfalise, A. and Mees, G.,** Chromatographie sur couche mince de quelques alkaloides et basis amines, *J. Chromatogr.*, 31, 594, 1967.
52. **Harrison, A. J. and Cook, A.,** A case history of drug addiction and a TLC system for the separation and identification of some drugs of addiction in sub-microgram amounts, *J. Forensic Sci. Soc.*, 9, 165, 1969.

53. **Noirfalise, A.,** Diagnosti chimique des intoxications par medicaments non stupefiants, *Acta Pharm. Jugosl.*, 3, 77, 1970.
54. **Baden, M. M., Valanju, N., Verma, S., and Valanju, S.,** Confirmed identification of biotransformed drugs of abuse in urine, *Am. J. Clin. Pathol.*, 57, 43, 1972.
55. **Jansen, G. A. and Bickers, I.,** Rapid method for simultaneous qualitative assay of narcotics, cocaine, quinine and propoxyphene in the urine, *South. Med. J.*, 64, 1072, 1971.
56. **Baselt, R. C. and Casarett, L. J.,** Detection of drugs in urine for methadone treatment programs, *J. Chromatogr.*, 57, 139, 1971.
57. **Mulé, S. J.,** Routine identification of drugs of abuse in human urine. I. Application of fluorometry, thin-layer and gas-liquid chromatography, *J. Chromatogr.*, 55, 255, 1971.
58. **Brown, J. K., Shapazian, L., and Griffin, G. D.,** Rapid screening for street drugs, *J. Chromatogr.*, 64, 129, 1972.
59. **Brown, J. K., Schingler, R. H., Chaubal, M. G., and Malone, M. H.,** A rapid screening procedure for some street drugs by thin layer chromatography. II. Cocaine, heroin, local anesthetics and mixtures, *J. Chromatogr.*, 87, 211, 1973.
60. **van Welsum, R. A.,** A simplified procedure for the identification of drugs from illicit street market by thin-layer chromatography, *J. Chromatogr.*, 78, 237, 1973.
61. **Moffat, A. C., Stead, A. H., and Salldon, K. W.,** Optimum use of paper, thin-layer and gas chromatography for the identification of basic drugs, *J. Chromatogr.*, 90, 19, 1974.
62. **Koontz, S., Besemer, D., Mackey, N., and Phillips, R.,** Detection of benzoylecgonine (cocaine metabolite) in urine by gas chromatography, *J. Chromatogr.*, 85, 75, 1973.
63. **Bohme, H., Stamm, H., and Tauber, E.,** Behaviour of alkaloid salt solutions on aluminum oxide columns. XI. Chromatographic determination of the purity of the hydrochlorides of lobeline, cocaine, pilocarpine and papaverine, *Arch. Pharm. Berlin*, 294, 794, 1961.
64. **Verporte, R., Svendsen, A. B., and Baerhein, A.,** High speed liquid chromatography of alkaloids, *J. Chromatogr.*, 100, 227, 1974.
65. **Chan, M. L., Whetsell, C., and McChesney, J. D.,** Use of high pressure liquid chromatography for the separation of drugs of abuse, *J. Chromatogr. Sci.*, 12, 512, 1974.
66. **Curry, A. S.,** *Advances in Forensic and Clinical Toxicology*, CRC Press, Cleveland, 1972.
67. **Moffat, A. C.,** Use of SE-30 as a stationary phase for the gas liquid chromatography of drugs, *J. Chromatogr.*, 113, 69, 1975.
68. **Skimner, R. F., Gallaher, E. J., Knight, J. B., and Bonelli, E. J.,** The gas chromatography-mass spectrometer as a new and important tool in forensic toxicology, *J. Forensic Sci.*, 17, 189, 1972.
69. **Goldbaum, L. R., Santinga, P., and Dominguez, A. M.,** A procedure for the rapid analysis of large number of urine samples for drugs, *Clin. Toxicol.*, 5, 369, 1972.
70. **Wells, J., Cimbura, G., and Koves, E.,** The screening of blood by gas chromatography for basic and neutral drugs, *J. Forensic Sci.*, 20, 382, 1975.
71. **Dahlstrom, B. and Paalzow, L.,** Quantitative determination of morphine in biological samples by gas-liquid chromatography and electron capture detection, *J. Pharm. Pharmacol.*, 27, 172, 1975.
72. **Sine, H. E., Kubasik, N. P. and Woytash, J.,** Simple gas-liquid chromatographic method for confirming the presence of alkaloids in urine, *Clin. Chem.*, 19, 340, 1973.
73. **Bastos, M. L. and Hoffman, D. B.,** Comparison of methods for detection of amphetamines, cocaine and metabolites, *J. Chromatogr. Sci.*, 12, 269, 1974.
74. **Elahi, N. and Cerrato, R.,** Rapid gas chromatographic method for the identification and quantitation of cocaine and cocaine substitutes, to be published.
75. **Fish, F. and Wilson, W. D. C.,** Gas chromatographic determination of morphine and cocaine in urine, *J. Chromatogr.*, 40, 164, 1969.
76. **Greenwood, N. D. and Guppy, I. W.,** A direct gas chromatographic method for determination of basic nitrogenous drugs in pharmaceutical preparations, *The Analyst* (London), 99, 313, 1974.
77. **Jatlow, P. I. and Balley, D. N.,** Gas chromatographic analysis for cocaine in human plasma with use of a nitrogen detector, *Clin. Chem.*, 21, 1918, 1975.
78. **Wallace, J. E., Hamilton, H. E., King, D. E., Bason, D. J., Schwertner, H. A., and Harris, S. C.,** Gas liquid chromatographic determination of cocaine and benzoylecgonine in urine, *Anal. Chem.*, 48, 34, 1976.
79. **Mathews, R. G., Schwartz, J. E., and Pettit, B. C.,** New polyamide liquid phases for gas chromatography, *J. Chromatogr. Sci.*, 8, 508, 1970.
80. **Mathews, R. G., Schwartz, R. D., Novotny, M., and Zlakis, A.,** Preparation and evaluation of isocyanate-based polyimides as liquid phases for gas chromatography, *Anal. Chem.*, 43, 1161, 1971.
81. **Jenden, D. J., Roch, M., and Booth, R.,** A new liquid phase for the gas chromatographic separation of amines and alkaloids, *J. Chromatogr. Sci.*, 10, 151, 1972.
82. **Wells, J., Cimbura, G., and Koves, E.,** The use of the liquid phase Poly A-103 in toxicology, *J. Chromatogr.*, 86, 225, 1973.
83. **Berry, D. J. and Grove, J.,** Improved chromatographic techniques and their interpretation for the screening of urine from drug dependent subjects, *J. Chromatogr.*, 61, 111, 1971.

84. **Moore, J. M.,** Gas chromatographic detection of ecgonine and benzoylecgonine in cocaine, *J. Chromatogr.*, 101, 215, 1974.

85. **Blake, J. W., Ray, R. S., Noonan, J. S., and Murdick, P. W.,** Rapid sensitive gas-liquid chromatographic screening procedure for cocaine, *Anal. Chem.*, 46, 288, 1974.

86. **Javaid, J. I., Dekirmenjian, H., Brunngraber, E. G., and Davis, J. M.,** Quantitative determination of cocaine and its metabolites benzoylecgonine and ecgonine by gas-liquid chromatography, *J. Chromatogr.*, 110, 141, 1975.

87. **Hammer, R. H., Templenton, J. L., and Panzik, H. L.,** Definitive GLC method of identifying cocaine, *J. Pharma. Sci.*, 63, 1963, 1974.

88. **Street, H. V.,** Characterization of drugs containing tertiary amine groups by application of the Hoffman degradation reaction and gas-liquid chromatography, *J. Chromatogr.*, 73, 73, 1972.

89. **Bastos, M. L., Jukofsky, D., and Mulé, S. J.,** Routine identification of cocaine metabolites in human urine, *J. Chromatogr.*, 89, 335, 1974.

90. **Felder, E., Tiepolo, U., and Mengassini, A.,** Method for the esterification of carboxylic acids in gas chromatographic analysis, *J. Chromatogr.*, 82, 291, 1973.

91. **Greeley, R. H.,** Rapid esterification for gas chromatography, *J. Chromatogr.*, 88, 229, 1974.

92. **Biondi, P. A. and Cagnasso, M.,** A procedure for boron-trifluoride catalysed esterification suitable for use in gas chromatographic analysis, *J. Chromatogr.*, 109, 389, 1975.

93. **Moore, J. M.,** Detection of ecgonine in urine, *Clin. Chem.*, 21, 1538, 1975.

94. **Brooks, J. B., Alley, C. C., and Liddle, J. A.,** Simultaneous esterification of carboxyl and hydroxyl groups with alcohols and heptafluorobutyric anhydride for analysis by gas chromatography, *Anal. Chem.*, 46, 1930, 1974.

95. **Blomquist, M., Bonnichsen, R., Fri, C. G., Marde, Y., and Ryhage, R.,** Gas chromatography-mass spectrometry as a routine procedure in forensic chemistry, *Zacchia*, 7, 399, 1971.

96. **Blomquist, M., Bonnichsen, R., Fri, C. G., Marde, Y., and Rhyage, R.,** Gas chromatography-mass spectrometry in forensic chemistry for identification of substances isolated from tissue, *Z. Rechtsmed.*, 69, 52, 1971.

97. **Law, N. C., Aandahl, V., Fales, H. M., and Milne, W. A.,** Identification of dangerous drugs by mass spectrometry, *Clin. Chim. Acta*, 32, 221, 1971.

98. **Finkle, B. S. and Taylor, D. M. A.,** GC/MS reference data system for the identification of drugs of abuse, *J. Chromatogr. Sci.*, 10, 312, 1972.

99. **Jenden, D. J. and Cho, A. K.,** Applications of integrated gas-chromatography/mass spectrometry in pharmacology and toxicology, *Annu. Rev. Pharmacol.*, 13, 371, 1973.

100. **Weil, L., Frimmel, F., and Quentin, K. E.,** Kombinierte gas-chromatographie/Massenspektrometrie:eine hochempfindliche Spezifizierungs methode, *Z. Anal. Chem.*, 268, 97, 1974.

101. **Seeley, C. C., Young, N. D., Holland, J. F., and Gates, S. C.,** Rapid computerized identification of compounds in complex biological mixtures by gas chromatography-mass spectrometry, *J. Chromatogr.*, 99, 507, 1974.

102. **Kimble, B. J., Cox, R. E., McPherron, R. V., Olsen, R. W., Roitman, E., Walls, F. C., and Burlingame, A. L.,** Real time gas chromatography – high resolution mass spectrography and its application to the analysis of physiological fluids, *J. Chromatogr. Sci.*, 12, 647, 1974.

103. **Costello, C. E., Hertz, H. E., Kakai, T., and Biemann, K.,** Routine use of a flexible gas chromatography-mass spectrometer computer system to identify drugs and their metabolism in body fluids of overdose victims, *Clin. Chem.*, 20, 255, 1974.

104. **Saferstein, R. and Chao, J. M.,** Identification of drugs by chemical ionization mass spectroscopy, *J. Assoc. Off. Anal. Chem.*, 56, 1234, 1973.

105. **Finkle, B. S., Foltz, R. L., and Taylor, D. M.,** A comprehensive GC-MS reference data system for toxicological and biomedical purposes, *J. Chromatogr. Sci.*, 12, 304, 1974.

106. **Greenwood, N. D.,** Examination of amine salts in eyedrops by gas-liquid chromatography, *J. Hosp. Pharm.*, 29, 240, 1971.

107. **Gupta, R. C., Montgomery, S. H., and Lundberg, G. D.,** Quantitative determination of street drugs in the Los Angeles area, *Clin. Toxicol.*, 7, 241, 1974.

108. **Moore, J.,** Cocaine and caffeine mixtures, *Microgram*, 3, 29, 1971.

109. **Lorch, S. K.,** Cocaine mixtures, *Microgram*, 7, 8, 1974.

110. **Lorch, S. K.,** Cocaine mixtures, *Microgram*, 7, 11, 1974.

111. **Johnson, D. W., Gunn, A., and Gunn, J., Jr.,** Dangerous drugs: adulterants, diluents and deception in street samples, *J. Forensic Sci.*, 17, 629, 1972.

112. **Drude, W.,** Adulteration of cocaine, *Sueddtsch. Apoth. Ztg.*, 89, 277, 1946.

113. **Young, J. L.,** The detection of cocaine in the presence of novocaine by means of cobalt thiocyanate, *Am. J. Pharm.*, 103, 709, 1931.

114. **Prall, J. D.,** Field test for cocaine, Drug Enforcement Administration, Laboratory Notes, June 1975.

115. **Alliston, G. V., Bartlett, A. F. F., Maunder, M. J. F., and Phillips, G. F.,** An improved test for cocaine, methaqualone and methadone with a modified cobalt (II) thiocyanate reagent, *Analyst* (London), 97, 263, 1972.

116. **Scott, L. J.,** Specific field test for cocaine, *Microgram*, 6, 11, 1973.

117. **Levine, J.,** Column extraction of alkaloids, *J. Assoc. Agric. Chem.*, 54, 488, 1965.

118. **Paul, J.,** Rapid separation of cocaine from codeine, heroin, 6-monoacetyl-morphine, morphine and quinine on microscopic slides, *Microchem. J.*, 18, 142, 1973.

119. **Jain, N. C.,** personal communication.
120. **Choulis, N. H.,** Separation and quantitations of mixtures of the most commonly abused drugs, *J. Pharm. Sci.*, 62, 112, 1973.
121. **Conine, F. and Paul, J.,** A thin-layer chromatographic procedure for the separation of aspirin, cocaine, caffeine, heroin, 6-monoacetylmorphine and morphine, *Microchem. Acta*, 443, 448, 1974.
122. **Phillips, G. F. and Gardiner, J.,** The chromatographic identification of psychoptropic drugs, *J. Pharm. Pharmacol.*, 21, 793, 1969.
123. **Sunshine, I., Forney, R. D., and Foltz, R. L.,** Quantitative Analysis of Phencyclidine in Biological Material, presented at the 7th International Meeting of Forensic Sciences, Zurich, 1975.
124. **Moffat, A. C., Stead, A. H., and Smalldon, K. W.,** A comparison of stationary phases for GLC of basic drugs, *J. Pharm. Pharmacol.*, 25, Suppl., 155, 1973.
125. **Chamber, C. D., Taylor, W. J., and Moffett, A. D.,** The incidence of cocaine abuse among methadone maintenance patients, *Int. J. Addict.*, 7, 427, 1972.
126. **Price, K. R.,** Fatal cocaine poisoning, *J. Forensic Sci.*, 14, 329, 1974.
127. **Misra, A. L., Nayak, P. K., Patel, M. N., Vadlamani, N. L., and Mulé, S. J.,** Identification of norcocaine as a metabolite of (^{3}H)-cocaine in rat brain, *Experientia*, 30, 1212, 1974.
128. **Griffin, B. R.,** Report on cocaine death, *Bull. Int. Assoc. Forensic Toxicol.*, 11, Case 4, 1975.
129. **Leighty, E. G. and Fentiman, A. F.,** Metabolism of cocaine to norcocaine and benzoylecgonine by an in vitro microsomal enzyme system, *Res. Commun. Chem. Pathol. Pharmacol.*, 8, 65, 1974.
130. **Wood, I. A., McMahon, F. C., and Seevers, M. H.,** Distribution and metabolism of cocaine in the dog and rabbit, *J. Pharmacol. Exp. Ther.*, 101, 200, 1951.
131. **Misra, A. L., Nayak, P. K., Bloch, R., and Mulé, S. J.,** Estimation and disposition of (^{3}H) benzoylecgonine and pharmacological activity of some cocaine metabolites, *J. Pharm. Pharmacol.*, 27, 784, 1975.
132. **Finkle, B. S.,** Cocaine fatalities, *Bull. Int. Assoc. Forensic Toxicol.*, 8, Case 3–4, 1972.
133. **White, J. M.,** Urine cocaine level in a case of cocaine use without gross intoxication, *Bull. Int. Assoc. Forensic Toxicol.*, 8, Case 6, 1972.
134. **Makisumi, S., Kotoku, S., Ota, H., Ishihara, F., Hino, M., and Nishi, K.,** Extraction of morphine with ether in the isolation procedure of Stas-Otto, *Yonago Acta Med.*, 3, 126, 1958.
135. **Debackere, M. and Laruelle, L.,** Isolation, detection and identification of some alkaloids or alkaloid-like substances in biological specimens from horses with special reference to doping, *J. Chromatogr.*, 35, 234, 1968.
136. **Mulé, S. J., Bastos, M. L., Jukofsky, D., and Saffer, E.,** Routine identification of drugs of abuse in human urine. II. Development and application of the XAD-2 resin column method, *J. Chromatogr.*, 63, 289, 1971.
137. **Wolen, R. L. and Gruber, C. M.,** Determination of propoxyphene in human plasma by gas chromatography, *Anal. Chem.*, 40, 1243, 1968.
138. **Inturrisi, C. E. and Kaika, R. F.,** A gas-liquid chromatographic method for the quantitative determination of methadone in human plasma and urine, *J. Chromatogr.*, 65, 361, 1972.
139. **Pranitis, P. A. F., Milzoff, J. R., and Stolman, A.,** Extraction of drugs from biofluids and tissue with XAD-2 resin, *J. Forensic Sci.*, 19, 917, 1974.
140. **Ibrahim, G., Andryauskas, S., and Bastos, M. L.,** Application of Amberlite XAD-2 resin for general toxicological analysis, *J. Chromatogr.*, 108, 107, 1975.
141. **Bastos, M. L., Jukofsky, D., Saffer, E., Chedekel, M., and Mulé, S. J.,** Modification of the XAD-2 resin column method for the extraction of drugs of abuse from human urine, *J. Chromatogr.*, 71, 549, 1972.
142. **Mulé, S. J.,** *Detection of cocaine metabolites*, CDC report, Toxicology, Drug abuse Survey III, Department of Health, Education, and Welfare, 1975.
143. **Aggarwal, V., Bath, R., and Sunshine, I.,** Technique for rapidly separating drugs from biological samples, *Clin. Chem.*, 20, 307, 1974.
144. **Broich, J. B., Hoffman, D. B., Goldner, S. J., Andryauskas, S., and Umberger, C. J.,** Liquid-solid extraction of lyophilized biological material for forensic analysis. I. Application to urine samples for detection of drugs of abuse, *J. Chromatogr.*, 63, 309, 1971.
145. **Hoffman, D. B., Umberger, C. J., Goldner, S., Andryauskas, S., Mulligan, D., and Broich, J. R.,** Liquid solid extraction of lyophilized biological materials for forensic analysis. II. Application to bile samples for the detection of drugs, *J. Chromatogr.*, 66, 63, 1972.
146. **Davidow, B., Li Petri, N., and Quame, B.,** A thin-layer chromatographic screening procedure for detecting drug abuse, *Am. J. Clin. Pathol.*, 50, 714, 1968.
147. **Kaistha, K. K. and Jaffe, J. H.,** TLC techniques for identification of narcotics, barbiturates and CNS stimulants in drug abuse urine screening program, *J. Pharm. Sci.*, 61, 679, 1972.
148. **Sunshine, I.,** personal communication.
149. **Niyogi, S. K. and Riedere, F.,** Interfering peaks in gas chromatographic seclusion screening of direct chloroform extracts of blood, *Acta Pharmacol. Toxicol.*, 19, 113, 1971.
150. **Ramsey, I. and Campbell, D. B.,** An ultra rapid method for the extraction of drugs from biological material, *J. Chromatogr.*, 63, 303, 1971.
151. **Goldbaum, L. R. and Dominguez, A. M.,** A system for the toxicological analysis of drugs in biological specimens, *Progress in Chemical Toxicology*, Vol. 5, Stolman, A., Ed., Academic Press, New York, 1974.

Detection and Identification

Analysis of Cocaine and Its Metabolites in Biological Fluids

ANALYSIS OF COCAINE AND ITS METABOLITES IN BIOLOGICAL FLUIDS

Peter Jatlow

TABLE OF CONTENTS

INTRODUCTION

The relative distribution and absolute concentrations of cocaine and its metabolites in plasma, urine, and tissues are sufficiently different to present distinctive analytical problems. With few exceptions, published procedures have been applied to either blood or urine but rarely to both. For this reason, the analysis of cocaine and its metabolites in each of these various biologic materials are discussed separately. Where procedures have been applied to multiple materials (i.e., plasma and tissue), it has been so indicated.

PLASMA

The parent drug (cocaine) can be measured in human plasma after its use, and in some animals its N-demethylated metabolite (norcocaine) has also been detected.[1,2] Plasma concentrations of the major water-soluble metabolites, benzoylecgonine and ecgonine, are too low for measurement, except possibly with tracer methodology.[3]

The successful analysis of cocaine, regardless of the procedure selected, must take into account certain fundamental information. Cocaine is rapidly hydrolyzed in vitro in human plasma. We have found that the in vitro half-life of cocaine in human plasma at 37°C can be as short as 35 min.[4] From 10 to 30% may be lost in 24 hr from plasma frozen conventionally or with Dry Ice®.[5] Unless specimens are extracted immediately, placed on ice in the event of short delays, or otherwise preserved, spuriously low cocaine concentrations will be found. We have found that the immediate addition of sodium fluoride (NaF) to plasma, to a final concentration of 0.14% NaF, will completely prevent the hydrolysis of cocaine for at least 2 hr at 37°C, and for at least 6 weeks at -15°C.[4] Loss of cocaine was also prevented by the addition of physostigmine or neostigmine. Our observation that cocaine is stable when added to plasma of patients with succinylcholine sensitivity further suggests that plasma cholinesterase is responsible for at least the in vitro hydrolysis of cocaine.

Cocaine has a pK_a of 8.6 and so is best extracted into organic solvents at alkaline pH.

Several reports[6,7] have emphasized that recovery of cocaine drops off at pH values above 10, presumably due to chemical hydrolysis.

Selection of a procedure for the analysis of cocaine in human plasma must also take into account the low concentrations found after its use. The quantities applied clinically for topical anesthesia result in peak plasma concentrations of 120 to 470 ng/ml.[8] The quantities abused in the "street" (intranasally) probably result in plasma concentrations of less than 100 ng/ml.[9] No data have been reported regarding the plasma concentrations in humans after intravenous use. Animal experiments on the other hand have used dosages as high as 100 mg/kg. Under such conditions there is greater latitude in selecting an analytical method.

Cocaine concentrations in plasma have been determined using gas chromatography, mass fragmentography, radioisotope tracers with thin-layer chromatography, and a dye binding-colorimetric procedure.

Colorimetry

Cocaine (and various other alkaloids) will bind halogenated sulfonph-thalein indicator dyes; the resultant colored complexes can be quantified spectrophotometrically.[10] This reaction is not specific and has been applied to other basic drugs. While at first such procedures may seem antiquated, their sensitivity, 0.5 to 1.0 μg/ml of plasma, is probably more than adequate for some animal studies where as much as 5 to 100 mg of cocaine per kilogram body weight may be administered. In the procedure published by Woods et al.,[10] alkalinized plasma (urine or tissue homogenates) was extracted with chloroform, dried by passage through a sucrose column, treated with bromocresol purple, and quantified at 410 nm. The authors reported a sensitivity of 1.0 μg cocaine/ml plasma which could be improved to 0.5 μg/ml if the drug was back extracted from the chloroform into dilute HCl and reextracted into a smaller volume of chloroform. Benzoylecgonine, ecgonine methyl ester and ecgonine were reported not to interfere.

Using this procedure Woods et al. studied cocaine concentrations following intravenous and subcutaneous administration to dogs.[11] Peak plasma concentrations of 2.6 and 4.6 μg/ml following 10 mg/kg i.v. and 15 mg/kg s.c., respectively, were well within the sensitivity of the procedure. Following 20 mg/kg i.v., brain concentrations reached 30 μg/kg. The convulsion-producing plasma concentrations of cocaine (in dogs) were reported to be 4.6 μg/ml. Woods et al.[10] also reported that erythrocyte to plasma ratios were 1.2 to 1.4:1, indicating that analysis of whole blood and plasma yields different results. Their data suggest that laboratories administering macro-quantities of cocaine to animals, which do not possess the equipment or technical experience required for other methodology, might do well to give this procedure a second glance. It is, however, not sufficiently sensitive to measure the concentrations achieved in humans after topical application of the usual anesthetic or abuse doses of cocaine.

Gas Chromatography

Although Fish's and Wilson's[12] original important observations on the metabolism and excretion of cocaine were obtained using gas chromatography with flame ionization detection, their measurements were made on urine. The concentrations of cocaine in plasma after human use are, for the most part, too low to measure accurately using a flame ionization detector. Jatlow and Bailey[5] have used a nitrogen-phosphorous ("alkali flame") detector for the gas chromatographic measurement of cocaine in plasma. This detector, which responds selectively to nitrogen-containing compounds, is about 100 times more sensitive than conventional flame ionization. The concept of this type of detector was originally described by Karmen and Guiffrida,[13] and its application to nitrogen-containing compounds refined by Kolb and Bischoff.[14] In the detector used for cocaine analysis a heated rubidium silicate glass bead is suspended above a conventional flame ionization detector. When nitrogen-containing compounds are burned in the low temperature flame, cyano ions are produced which elicit a response from the alkali flame detector. Plasma, buffered to pH 9.3 to 9.6 with carbonate-bicarbonate buffer was extracted with heptane-isoamyl alcohol (98:2) containing an internal standard. The drugs were back extracted into 0.1 N H_2SO_4, and the latter washed once with solvent. The acid was alkalinized with a carbonate-bicarbonate mixture and reextracted with heptane-isoamyl alcohol. After evaporation of the solvent, an aliquot of the residue was chromatographed isothermally at 255°C on 3% OV-17. A Perkin Elmer® Model 3920 gas chromatograph equipped with a nitrogen-phosphorous detector was used. The internal standard, the n-propyl ester of benzoylecgonine, was synthesized in the authors' laboratory by refluxing benzoylecgonine in acidified *n*-propanol. After concentration of the *n*-propanol, the derivative was purified and freed from unreacted benzoylecgonine by preparative thin-layer chromatography. Because of the detector's sensitivity to trace contaminants, considerable precautions in handling glassware and solvents were necessary.

The nitrogen detector was sufficiently sensitive to respond to picogram quantities of cocaine; however the total sensitivity of the procedure was limited by biological background which corresponded to about 0 to 2 ng/ml of cocaine in drug-free specimens. The precision (coefficients of variation) at plasma concentrations of 50 and 100 ng/ml was 3.0 and 5.1% respectively.

The described procedure was used to measure cocaine concentrations in human plasma after its intranasal application (Figure 1).[5,9] Following administration of 1.5 mg/kg of cocaine to surgical patients for local anesthesia, peak concentrations of 120 to 470 ng/ml were achieved in 30 to 60 min. In some patients cocaine was detected for as long as 6 hours, probably reflecting prolonged absorption due to persistence of cocaine on the mucosa. Lower concentrations were found in volunteers who received a smaller dose of cocaine.

Blake et al.[15] reported a procedure which is theoretically suitable for the determination of cocaine at the concentrations anticipated in human plasma. Cocaine was extracted with cyclohexane, and after evaporation of the solvent, reduced to 1,2-dihydroxymethyltropine by treatment with a saturated etheral solution of lithium aluminum hydride (LiAlH₄). After treatment with heptafluorobutyric anhydride, the heptafluorobutyrate derivative was extracted with cyclohexane and chromatographed on 3% OV-1 using an instrument with an electron-capture detector. Without concentration of the cyclohexane, a sensitivity of 20 to 30 ng/ml was obtained. Javid et al.[16] have adapted this procedure to the analysis of cocaine in plasma. After extraction of 0.1 ml of plasma, and reduction with LiAlH₄, the pentafluoropropionate derivative was prepared and analyzed on a gas chromatograph equipped with a [³H] electron-capture detector. Fifteen minutes following the injection of a rat with cocaine (20 mg/kg body weight), a sizeable cocaine peak was found (but not quantified) using this procedure. A

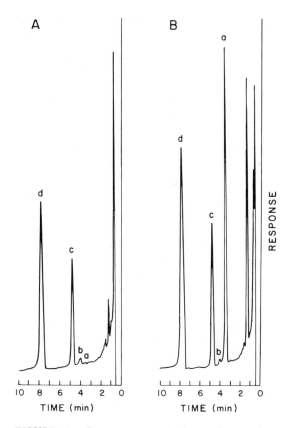

FIGURE 1. Chromatogram of plasma from patient before (A) and 20 min after (B) topical application of cocaine, 1.5 mg/kg body wt. The patient had also received diazepam. The peaks are (a) cocaine, or (in A) retention time corresponding to cocaine; (b) contaminant peak; (c) internal standard (propyl ester of benzoylecgonine); and (d) diazepam. (From Jatlow P. and Bailey, D., *Clin. Chem.*, 21, 1918, 1975. With permission.)

linear response following chromatography of 40 to 750 pg was reported. The authors indicated that benzoylecgonine was reduced by LiAlH₄ to the same dihydroxytropine derivative as cocaine. A derivative of ecgonine (and benzoylecgonine) suitable for gas chromatography was prepared by treatment with a 1:2 mixture of hexafluoroisopropanol and heptafluorobutyric anhydride. The authors did not, however, demonstrate the analysis of these latter compounds in biological material. Adequate but clean extraction of these polar cocaine metabolites from biological material is as much a problem as their subsequent chromatography.

Moore[17] has described preparation of the trimethylsilyl (TMS) derivatives of ecgonine and benzoylecgonine. The derivatives prepared with *N,O*-bis-(trimethylsilyl)-acetamide were chromatographed on OV-101 and OV-25. It should be noted that on OV-17, the stationary phase most commonly used for drug analysis, cocaine and benzoylecgonine-TMS failed to separate. Although no attempt was made by Moore to apply this technique to biological specimens, it potentially could be used once adequate and clean extraction of benzoylecgonine was achieved (no small problem). We have confirmed in our laboratory that the TMS derivative of benzoylecgonine has good chromatographic properties. Unfortunately, the derivatizing agent interacted with the rubidium silicate glass bead of our nitrogen detector, reducing sensitivity.

Hammer et al.[18] have reported that cocaine will react with trimethylanilinium hydroxide in the flash injector of the gas chromatograph to form a number of derivatives, including ecgonidine methyl ester. They recommend it for the confirmation of cocaine identification in street samples. It is difficult to see any potential application of this observation to the analysis of biologic samples.

Mass Spectrometry and Mass Fragmentography

As might be expected, mass fragmentography provides the most sensitive and specific assay for cocaine and some of its metabolites. Using mass fragmentography, Hawks[19] found a peak plasma concentration of 10 ng/ml after i.v. administration of 4 mg of cocaine to a human subject. He has also used mass fragmentography to detect both cocaine and N-demethylated cocaine (norcocaine) in the plasma of rhesus monkeys after administration of cocaine.[1] Using this technique Hawks determined that norcocaine (and cocaine) could be found in the brains of rhesus monkeys receiving 10 mg/kg of cocaine.[1]

Cocaine and norcocaine were extracted by Hawks (from a tissue homogenate in the case of brain) onto a column containing Amberlite® XAD-2 nonionic resin and eluted with chloroform-isopropanol (3:1). The eluate was evaporated and the residue, dissolved in dilute HCl, was washed with ethyl acetate, alkalinized, extracted with ethyl acetate, and submitted to mass fragmentography using chemical ionization. Cocaine-d-6, prepared in Hawks'[1] laboratory, was added immediately to the biological specimen or tissue homogenate and carried through the entire procedure. The analysis was carried out on 1% OV-17 and the quasi-molecular ions at m/e 310,

304, and 290 were monitored for cocaine-d-6, cocaine, and norcocaine respectively. The identity of these compounds was confirmed by rationing the intensity of the quasi-molecular ions to that of fragment ions at m/e 188, 182, and 168 and comparing their relative abundances to that of pure materials. The isotopic internal standard which was used for quantitation also served as a control for any deterioration of cocaine that may have occurred prior to analysis.

If rapid throughput of large numbers of specimens is not required, elaborate means may be used to recover the polar cocaine metabolites prior to chromatography. In establishing that cocaine was metabolized to norcocaine and benzoylecgonine by an in vitro rat liver microsomal preparation, Leighty and Fentimen[20] lyophilized their materials and extracted them with methanol, followed by fractionation with thin-layer chromatography. Spots corresponding to the compounds of interest were eluted and submitted to gas chromatography on 3% OV-17 and to gas chromatography-mass spectrometry using the chemical ionization mode. Norcocaine was analyzed as the free compound, and benzoylecgonine as its trimethylsilyl derivative prepared with N,O-bis-(trimethylsilyl)-trifluoroacetamide.

Thin-Layer Chromatography and Liquid Scintillation Spectroscopy

Mulé and co-workers[2,3,21-23] have developed procedures for the specific labeling of cocaine with tritium, and for its determination in biological materials at concentrations as low as 1 ng/ml. Following its administration to rats they studied the distribution of cocaine and its metabolites in plasma, urine, and tissues. Labeled cocaine and its metabolites were fractionated by a combination of differential solvent fractionation, column and thin-layer chromatography.

In several studies Mulé and co-workers[2,3,21,22] reported several facts relevant to the analysis of cocaine and its metabolites. Cocaine and norcocaine, but not their more polar metabolites, could be extracted by cyclohexane. Cocaine and benzoylecgonine but not ecgonine were extracted at pH 8 to 9 by chloroform. Cocaine and all of its metabolites, with the exception of ecgonine, were adsorbed to some extent onto Amberlite XAD-2 resin. Ecgonine could be extracted into chloroform-methanol (68:32, v/v). Using these principles they have identified cocaine, norcocaine, benzoylecgonine and benzoylnorectonine, in the brain of rats given specifically labeled [3H] cocaine. Tissue homogenates or other biological fluids at pH 7.5 were applied to Amberlite XAD-2 resin, eluted with methanol and fractionated on TLC, and radioscanned. Applying similar tracer techniques, the plasma half-lives of cocaine in acute and chronically treated rats were determined by Nayak et al.[22] (see chapter by A. L. Misra for details).

URINE

The analysis of cocaine and its metabolites in urine has received considerably more attention than has their determination in blood. This is probably explained by the considerable interest in the screening of urine for drugs of abuse. The concentration of cocaine in urine (although considerably less than its major metabolite, benzoylecgonine) is generally higher than in plasma and more amenable to detection by conventional methodology, such as gas chromatography with flame ionization detection, and thin-layer chromatography. Nonetheless, it should be realized that after human use, relatively little (less than 5%) is excreted as the parent drug. For example we have found that less than 2% of "street" cocaine users (abusers) identified by an immunological assay for benzoylecgonine have had a sufficiently high (1.0 μg/ml or greater) urinary cocaine concentration for detection by thin-layer chromatography.

Gas Chromatography

Fish and Wilson[12,24] described gas chromatography procedures for the analysis of cocaine and benzoylecgonine in urine which were used in one of the first studies of the human metabolism of cocaine. Alkalinized urine containing benzhexol (added as an internal standard) was extracted with diethyl ether. The ether was evaporated and an aliquot of the residue was chromatographed on 2.9% OV-17 isothermally at 185°C. Using flame ionization detection, a linear response was obtained over a range of 0.5 to 15 μg of cocaine per milliliter of urine. In their assay for benzoylecgonine, preformed cocaine was first extracted from an aliquot of urine as described above. The urine was subsequently submitted to continuous extraction with chloroform containing 5α-cholestane as an internal standard. After concentration of the chloroform extract by evaporation,

the benzoylecgonine was methylated to cocaine by treatment with an etheral solution of diazomethane. The residue was alkalinized, and the synthesized cocaine was extracted into ether and chromatographed as described. The authors indicated linearity over a range of 1 to 14 μg/ml of benzoylecgonine but did not report recovery data. Applying these procedures to the study of cocaine excretion in man after its parenteral use, they determined that 0.4 to 8.7% was excreted as the parent drug (with as expected, greater amounts in acid urine) and 35 to 54% as benzoylecgonine. Although traces of ecgonine were found in the urine using thin-layer chromatography, extraction efficiency was too poor to permit quantitation.

Adequate extraction of the polar metabolites of cocaine has been one of the major problems in developing procedures for their assay. Salt-solvent pairs have been applied by several investigators for this purpose. We have for example found that the system of Horning et al.,[25] which involves extraction with ethyl acetate following saturation of the aqueous phase with ammonium carbonate, permits fairly efficient extraction of benzoylecgonine. Such techniques will of course result in relatively "dirty" extracts which may require additional clean-up steps. Koontz et al.[26] extracted urine twice with chloroform, which was discarded, saturated the urine with a mixture of K_2HPO_4 and KH_2PO_4, and partitioned benzoylecgonine into 95% ethanol. After evaporation of the ethanol the residue was submitted to preparative thin-layer chromatography. Following development in methanol-ammonium hydroxide, benzoylecgonine (R_f 0.4) was eluted into water, which was evaporated, derivatized with DMF-dimethyl acetal, and chromatographed on 2.5% SE-30 at 200°C. Although the total analytical recovery was 30 to 40%, it is worth noting that the authors reported an extraction efficiency of 90 to 100% for the initial ethanol extraction. The authors validated their procedure on urines from known cocaine users and were able to detect concentrations of 1 μg/ml. While this procedure is much too cumbersome for routine screening, it may be applicable to pharmacologic studies, particularly if a tracer is added to monitor recovery. Koontz et al.[26] also investigated anion exchange chromatography for the extraction of benzoylecgonine. Although this approach is conceptually very attractive, they reported that it was less satisfactory than the more involved procedure using salt-solvent pair extraction and preparative thin-layer chromatography.

Wallace et al.[6] have reported a similar but simpler procedure for the gas chromatographic determination of cocaine and benzoylecgonine in urine. Benzoylecgonine and cocaine were extracted from urine with chloroform containing 20% ethanol (v/v). After evaporation of the solvent, the residue was treated with $4 M$ H_2SO_4 in methanol at $85°C$ for 10 min to effect methylation of benzoylecgonine. The acid-methanol was washed with ether to reduce endogenous contaminants, alkalinized with $NaHCO_3$, extracted with a small volume of chloroform containing butylanthraquinone as an internal standard, and chromatographed on 3% OV-17 at $200°C$. This procedure determined cocaine originally present together with that resulting from methylation of benzoylecgonine. If a separate estimate of unmetabolized cocaine was desired the methylation step was skipped. A total recovery of 65% was reported for benzoylecgonine, with a detection limit of approximately 0.4 $\mu g/ml$. The authors applied this procedure to urine from patients receiving cocaine for topical intranasal anesthesia and found levels of 10 to 12 $\mu g/ml$ of benzoylecgonine 8 hr after application of 250 mg. It should be noted that this was probably far in excess of the usual "street" dose. While this procedure is probably better suited to pharmacologic studies than large-scale screening, it does offer one of the few alternatives for confirmation of positive results obtained with immunologic procedures.

Preliminary studies in our laboratory, using the previously discussed nitrogen detector,[5] suggest that it could also be applied to the measurement of unmetabolized cocaine in urine at the relatively low concentrations anticipated. However, we have not yet thoroughly documented its application to urine. The extraction and derivatization procedure of Wallace et al.[6] for the assay of benzoylecgonine should also be amenable to use with a nitrogen detector.

Thin Layer Chromatography

Numerous procedures for the thin-layer chromatographic analysis of drugs of abuse using solvent-solvent extraction,[27,28] nonionic resins[29] and ion exchange papers[30] can be used to detect unmetabolized cocaine, *if it is present*. However, these are of limited value for this purpose since relatively few users of cocaine, even of comparatively massive doses, will excrete sufficient quantities of the parent drug to be detected by thin-layer chromatography. Numerous solvent systems for TLC development are available that will separate cocaine from other common basic drugs. These include modifications of the commonly used Davidow system.[27] For example, ethyl acetate-methanol-NH_4OH (85:10:0.5) will separate cocaine from methadone, important in drug abuse screening in support of treatment programs. In many development systems in common use, the major polar metabolites of cocaine (i.e., benzoylecgonine and ecgonine) do not migrate appreciably, remaining near the origin. However development systems have been described which are suitable for the analysis of benzoylecgonine. Misra et al.[31] have studied the separation of cocaine and its derivatives by thin-layer chromatography and they describe six solvent systems which, used in proper combination, can achieve separation of cocaine, benzoylecgonine, benzoylnorecgonine, ecgonine, ecgonine methyl ester, and norecgonine (Table 1).

Although potassium iodoplatinate is most commonly used to detect alkaloids on thin-layer chromatograms, several observers have noted that Dragendorff's reagent, or modifications thereof,

TABLE 1

Chromatographic Mobilities on Gelman® ITLC (Silica Gel) of Cocaine and Some of Its Metabolites and Congeners in Different Solvent Systems

S_1 = Chloroform-acetone-conc ammonia (5:94:1); S_2 = benzene-ethyl acetate-methanol-conc ammonia (80:20:1.2:0.1); S_3 = chloroform-acetone-diethylamine (5:4:1); S_4 = ethyl acetate-methanol-conc ammonia (17:2:1); S_5 = ethyl acetate-methanol-conc ammonia (15:4:1); S_6 = n-butanol-acetic acid-water (35:3:10).

	S_1	S_2	S_3	S_4	S_5	S_6
			$R_f \times 100$			
Cocaine	98	98	98	98	98	83
Benzoylecgonine	0	0	29	50	73	88
Ecgonine methyl ester	98	64	98	98	98	66
Ecgonine	0	0	33	11	28	48
Benzoylnorecgonine	0	0	12	30	46	95
Norecgonine	0	0	12	4	15	75

From Misra, A. L., Pontani, R. B., and Mulé, S. J., *J. Chromatogr.*, 81, 167, 1973. With permission.

provides superior sensitivity toward cocaine metabolites. Misra et al.[31] applied Ludy Tenger reagent which is a modification of Dragendorff's reagent. Wallace et al.[32] exposed the chromatograms to iodine vapor following treatment with Dragendorff's reagent. We have found that sensitivity for detection of benzoylecgonine and ecgonine can be greatly enhanced by spraying the plate with Dragendorff's reagent followed by 5% potassium nitrite.

Bastos et al.[33] have reported a thin-layer chromatography procedure in which cocaine metabolites are butylated to facilitate both their extraction and chromatographic separation. After an initial clean-up extraction with chloroform-ethanol, urine was saturated with potassium carbonate and the drugs salted out into ethanol. The ethanol extract was treated with butanolic HCl, and the butylated derivatives were extracted into cyclohexane and submitted to thin-layer chromatography. Under these conditions a sensitivity of 3 to 5 μg/ml was achieved for butylated benzoylecgonine and ecgonine. Correlation with an immunological assay (EMIT®) was excellent, most discrepancies being explained by the greater sensitivity of the latter procedure. This procedure was developed primarily for drug-abuse screening of cocaine.

More recently, Wallace et al.[32] have reported a simpler thin-layer chromatographic procedure for the detection of cocaine and underivatized benzoylecgonine. Cocaine and benzoylecgonine were extracted together from urine with chloroform-ethanol, and the solvent residue was chromatographed in chloroform:methanol:NH$_4$OH (100:20:1). Detection was achieved by treating the chromatogram in sequence with Dragendorff's reagent, dilute sulfuric acid, and iodine vapor. The authors indicate that extraction efficiency was independent of pH under the conditions of the assay. They reported recoveries of 95 and 65%, and sensitivities of 0.1 and 0.25 μg/ml for cocaine and benzoylecgonine respectively. They also emphasized the considerable enhancement of sensitivity obtained with their sequence of detection reagents as compared to traditional iodoplatinate spray.

Valanju et al.[34] reported that if extraction was performed with chloroform-isopropanol-1,2 dichloroethane (8:1:3) as part of a general thin-layer chromatographic procedure for drugs of

abuse, sufficient benzoylecgonine was extracted to yield a sensitivity of 3 to 5 μg benzoylecgonine per milliliter of urine. Confirmation was achieved by eluting the benzoylecgonine spot and submitting it to immunologic (EMIT) assay or microcrystal tests.

Immunoassay[35]

Enzyme multiplied immunoassay technique (EMIT)*[36] — This assay is probably the only presently available practical assay suited to large-scale screening of urines for evidence of cocaine use. It is a competitive protein-binding immunoassay, in which an enzyme rather than an isotope is used as a label. In this case, benzoylecgonine is bonded to lysozyme. The enzyme drug complex, an anti-benzoylecgonine antibody, a suspension of bacteria, and an aliquot of urine are mixed. If no benzoylecgonine is present in the specimen, the enzyme drug complex is antibody bound and inactivated. If sufficient benzoylecgonine is present it competes for antibody binding sites and displaces the enzyme drug complex which is now available to act on the substrate, resulting in clearing of the turbid bacterial suspension. The rate of this reaction, which is followed spectrophotometrically, is a function of the concentration of benzoylecgonine at concentrations of 1 to 4 μg/ml. Unlike traditional radioimmunoassay, no step is required to separate free from bound drug, and the entire analysis may be completed in less than a minute. The practical sensitivity in routine use is about 1 μg of benzoylecgonine per milliliter of urine. There is slight cross reactivity with ecgonine (about 10%) and almost none with cocaine (about 0.2%).[35] Other drugs, including other tropine alkaloids, have been reported not to interfere. It is fortunate that this assay is relatively free from interferences or false positives because no practical confirmatory procedure of equal sensitivity has been available. The thin-layer chromatographic procedure recently reported by Wallace et al.[32] and discussed earlier may turn out to be useful for this purpose. The EMIT procedure can be used for semi-quantitative estimation of benzoylecgonine. Applying it to the analysis of timed urines from individuals receiving various doses of topical (intranasal) cocaine, we have determined that urinary benzoylecgonine concentrations peak after 6 to 12 hr and are usually undetectable by 24 hr.[37]

*Syva Corp., Palo Alto, California.

Radioimmunoassay (RIA) — An RIA procedure for benzoylecgonine is presently under development by Roche Laboratories, but is not yet (at the time of this writing) available. The detection limit for purposes of routine drug screening is stated to be 100 ng/ml,[38] but it may be considerably less.

Hemagglutination Assay (HI) — Antibody and other reagents for the HI assay of benzoylecgonine are commercially available.* The principle is the same as that for other types of HI assays. Erythrocytes covalently bonded to benzoylecgonine are incubated with specific antibody and an aliquot of urine. If benzoylecgonine is present, it binds or masks some of the antibody, thus inhibiting the agglutination and leaving unaggluti-

nated erythrocytes which settle out and form a characteristic pellet. The antibody is stated to show greater cross reactivity with ecgonine and unmetabolized cocaine, theoretically increasing its sensitivity for detection of cocaine use.[39] However, if the urinary benzoylecgonine concentration is below the detection limit of the HI assay, it is unlikely that significant quantities of cocaine will be present.

ACKNOWLEDGMENT

Supported by National Institute on Drug Abuse Contract ADM NIDA 45-74-164 and in part by Grant NIDA 10294.

*Technam Assoc., Park Forrest South, Illinois.

REFERENCES

1. Hawks, R. L., Kopin, I. J., Colburn, R. W., and Thoa, N. B., Norcocaine; a pharmacologically active metabolite of cocaine found in brain, *Life Sci.,* 15, 2189, 1974.
2. Misra, A. L., Nyak, P. K., Patel, M. N., Vadlamani, N. L., and Mulé, S. J., Identification of norcocaine as a metabolite of (^{3}H)-cocaine in rat brain, *Experientia,* 30, 1312, 1974.
3. Misra, A. L., Vadlamani, N. L., Bloch, R., Nyak, P. K., and Mulé, S. J., Physiologic disposition and metabolism of (^{3}H) ecgonine (cocaine metabolite) in the rat, *Res. Commun. Chem. Pathol. Pharmacol.,* 8, 55, 1974.
4. Jatlow, P., Barash, P. L., Van Dyke, C., and Byck, R., Impaired hydrolysis of cocaine in plasma from succinylcholine sensitive individuals, *Clin. Res.,* (abstr.), 24, 255A, 1976.
5. Jatlow, P. and Bailey, D., Gas chromatographic analysis of cocaine in human plasma, with use of a nitrogen detector, *Clin. Chem.,* 21, 1918, 1975.
6. Wallace, J. E., Hamilton, H. E., King, D. F., Bason, D. J., Schwertner, H. A., and Harris, S. C., Gas-liquid chromatographic determination of cocaine and benzoylecgonine in urine, *Anal. Chem.,* 48, 34, 1976.
7. Bastos, M. L. and Hoffman, D. B., Comparison of methods for detection of amphetamines, cocaine and metabolites, *J. Chromatogr. Sci.,* 12, 269, 1974.
8. Van Dyke, C., Barash, P. G., Jatlow, P., and Byck, R., Cocaine: plasma concentrations after intranasal application in man, *Science,* 191, 859, 1976.
9. Van Dyke, C., Byck, R., Jatlow, P., and Barash, P. G., unpublished observations.
10. Woods, L. A., Cochin, J., Fornefeld, E. J., McMahon, F. G., and Seevers, M. H., The estimation of aminos in biological materials with critical data for cocaine and mescaline, *J. Pharmacol. Exp. Ther.,* 101, 188, 1951.
11. Woods, L. A., McMahon, F. G., and Seevers, M. H., Distribution and metabolism of cocaine in the dog and rabbit, *J. Pharmacol. Exp. Ther.,* 101, 200, 1951.
12. Fish, F. and Wilson, W. D. C., Excretion of cocaine and its metabolites in man, *J. Pharm. Pharmacol.,* 21, 1355, 1969.
13. Karmen, A. and Guiffrida, L., Enhancement of the response of hydrogen flame ionization detector to compounds containing halogen and phosphorous, *Nature,* 201, 1204, 1964.
14. Kolb, B. and Bischoff, J., A new design of a thermionic nitrogen and phosphorous detector, *J. Chromatogr. Sci.,* 12, 625, 1974.
15. Blake, J. W., Ray, R. S., Noonan, J. S., and Murdock, P. W., Rapid, sensitive, gas-liquid chromatographic screening procedure for cocaine, *Anal. Chem.,* 46, 288, 1974.
16. Javid, J. I., Dekirmenjian, H., Brunngraber, E. G., and Davis, J. M., Quantitative determination of cocaine and its metabolites benzoylecgonine and ecgonine by gas-liquid chromatography, *J. Chromatogr.,* 110, 141, 1975.

17. **Moore, J. M.,** Gas chromatographic determination of ecgonine and benzoylecgonine in cocaine, *J. Chromatogr.,* 101, 215, 1974.

18. **Hammer, R. H., Templeton, J. L., and Panzik, H. L.,** Definitive GLC method of identifying cocaine, *J. Pharm. Sci.,* 63, 1963, 1974.

19. **Hawks, R.,** personal communication.

20. **Leighty, E. G. and Fentimen, A. F., Jr.,** Metabolism of cocaine to norcocaine and benzoylecgonine by an in vitro microsomal system, *Res. Commun. Chem. Pathol. Pharm.,* 8, 65, 1974.

21. **Nayak, P. K., Misra, A. L., and Mulé, S. J.,** Physiological disposition of and biotransformation of (^{3}H)-cocaine in acute and chronically-treated rats, *Fed. Proc.,* 34, 781, 1975.

22. **Nayak, P. K., Misra, A. L., and Mulé, S. J.,** Physiologic disposition and metabolism of (^{3}H)-cocaine in the rat, *Fed. Proc.,* 33, 527, 1974.

23. **Nayak, P. K., Misra, A. L., Patel, M. N., and Mulé, S. J.,** Preparation of radiochemically pure, randomly labeled and ring-labeled [^{3}H] cocaine, *Radiochem. Radioanal. Lett.,* 16, 167, 1973.

24. **Fish, F. and Wilson, W. D. C.,** Gas chromatographic determination of morphine and cocaine in urine, *J. Chromatogr.,* 40, 164, 1969.

25. **Horning, M. G., Gregory, P., Nowlin, J., Stafford, M., Letratanangkoon, C., Butler, C., Stillwell, W. G., and Hill, R. M.,** Isolation of drugs and drug metabolites from biological fluids by use of salt-solvent pairs, *Clin. Chem.,* 20, 282, 1974.

26. **Koontz, S., Besemer, D., Mackey, N., and Phillips, R.,** Detection of benzoylecgonine (cocaine metabolite) in urine by gas-liquid chromatography, *J. Chromatogr.,* 85, 75, 1973.

27. **Davidow, B., Petri, N. L., and Quame, B.,** A thin-layer chromatographic screening procedure for detecting drugs of abuse, *Am. J. Clin. Pathol.,* 50, 714, 1968.

28. **Bastos, M. L., Kananen, G. E., Young, R. M., Monforte, J. R., and Sunshine, I.,** Detection of basic organic drugs and their metabolites in urine, *Clin. Chem.,* 16, 931, 1970.

29. **Mulé, S. J., Bastos, M. L., Jukofsky, D., and Saffer, E.,** Routine identification of drugs of abuse in human urine, *J. Chromatogr.,* 63, 289, 1971.

30. **Kaistha, K. K., Tadrus, R., and Janda, R.,** Simultaneous detection of a wide variety of commonly abused drugs in a urine screening program using thin-layer identification techniques, *J. Chromatogr.,* 107, 359, 1975.

31. **Misra, A. L., Pontani, R. B., and Mulé, S. J.,** Separation of cocaine, some of its metabolites and congeners on glass fiber sheets, *J. Chromatogr.,* 81, 167, 1973.

32. **Wallace, J. E., Hamilton, H. E., Schwertner, H., King, D. E., McNay, J. L., and Blum, K.,** Thin-layer chromatographic analysis of cocaine and benzoylecgonine in urine, *J. Chromatogr.,* 114, 433, 1975.

33. **Bastos, M. L., Jukovsky, D., and Mulé, S. J.,** Routine identification of cocaine metabolites in human urine, *J. Chromatogr.,* 89, 335, 1974.

34. **Valanju, N. N., Baden, M. M., Valanju, S. N., Mulligan, D., and Verma, S. K.,** Detection of biotransferred cocaine in urine from drug abusers, *J. Chromatogr.,* 81, 170, 1973.

35. **Mulé, S. J., Bastos, M. L., and Jukofsky, D.,** Evaluation of immunoassay methods for detection in urine of drugs subject to abuse, *Clin. Chem.,* 20, 243, 1974.

36. **Rubinstein, K. E., Schneider, R. S., and Vilman, E. F.,** "Homogeneous" enzyme immunoassay. A new immunochemical technique, *Biochem. Biophys. Res. Commun.,* 47, 846, 1972.

37. **Van Dyke, C., Jatlow, P., Barash, P. G., and Byck, R.,** unpublished observations.

38. **Nutley, N. J.,** Roche Laboratories, personal communication.

39. Technical Bulletin, Technam Assoc., Park Forrest South, Illinois.

Disposition and Biotransformation

Disposition and Biotransformation of Cocaine

DISPOSITION AND BIOTRANSFORMATION OF COCAINE

Anand L. Misra

TABLE OF CONTENTS

INTRODUCTION

Cocaine (methyl-3β-hydroxy-1-αH, 5αH-tropane-2β carboxylate-3-benzoate), pk_a 8.70, is a potent central nervous system stimulant of relatively short duration, low margin of safety, and high systemic toxicity ($LD50$ i.v. in rats and rabbits 17.5 and 17 mg/kg respectively; fatal dose i.p. in rats 100 mg/kg). It is much less toxic by oral ingestion than by other routes of administration. Its intense euphoriant action leads to a very high degree of psychic dependence.[1-8] Craving for cocaine is more apparent by intravenous and not by oral route of administration. Cocaine has little or no tolerance and physical dependence liability, and considerable evidence has been presented[1-9] for a reverse tolerance or increase in sensitivity to cocaine on repeated dosing. This sensitization persisted unabated for a couple of weeks after complete withdrawal of cocaine. In spite of several studies,[10-20] there is a paucity of detailed information on the biological disposition and metabolism of cocaine in acute and chronic states in experimental animals, particularly in species (e.g., dogs and monkeys) which exhibit psychological effects so characteristic of chronic cocainism in man.

This chapter deals with dispositional and metabolic aspects of cocaine in rat, dog, and monkey in acute and chronic states, with a view to assess the possible relationship and significance of these parameters to the acquired sensitivity and systemic toxicity to cocaine in these species on chronic treatment.

DISPOSITION AND METABOLISM OF [³H] COCAINE IN RATS

Materials and Methods

The method for the preparation of randomly labeled and ring-labeled [³H] cocaine has been described earlier.[21] In our studies, randomly labeled [³H] cocaine, which was isotopically stable in vivo and had high specific activity, was used for the tissue distribution studies, and ring-labeled [³H] cocaine with lower specific activity was used for the excretion studies in view of the metabolic lability of methyl ester and benzoyl groups of cocaine. Other details on method of estimation of cocaine in biofluids and tissues, recoveries, specificity of extraction procedure,[22] radioscanning of thin-layer radiochromatograms (Gelman®ITLC, silica gel sheets), and counting procedures, etc. have previously been described.[23,24]

Distribution of [³H] cocaine in Tissues and Biofluids of Rats After Intravenous Injection

The data on the distribution of [³H] cocaine after a single 8 mg/kg intravenous injection in male Wistar rats appear in Figure 1. The peak levels of cocaine in brain, plasma, and other tissues occurred within 15 min. Highest concentrations of cocaine were observed in spleen followed by kidney, lung, brain, and testes. Liver and fat had lower concentrations as compared to these tissues. Muscle, heart, and plasma had still lower levels of [³H] cocaine. These levels declined sharply and 4 hr after injection were very low in brain and absent from plasma. After 6 hr cocaine disappeared completely from brain, heart, muscle, testes, and fat. The values in spleen, kidney, lung, intestine, and liver 6 hr post-injection ranged between 0.03 to 0.09 μg/g. No persistence of cocaine in rat brain was observed with this dose. The half-life of cocaine in rat brain and plasma with this dose was 0.4 and 0.3 hr respectively. After a 10 mg/kg convulsive dose of [³H] cocaine by intravenous injection in the rat, the levels of cocaine in rat brain and plasma were 35 μg/g and 5 μg/ml respectively within 2 min of injection. N-Dealkylation of cocaine to norcocaine was observed in rat brain within 1 to 2 min after 10 mg/kg i.v. dose of cocaine. High lipid solubility of cocaine (apparent partition coefficient in the concentration range 0.1 to 1 μg/ml in 1-octanol-0.1 M phosphate buffer, pH 7.4, 7.6 ± 0.1 [S.E.M.]) played an important role in rapid entry of cocaine into rat brain. The high brain to plasma ratio (12 to 8) between 0.25 to 2 hr post-injection of 8 mg/kg i.v. dose indicated a marked affinity of cocaine for the tissues.

Biliary Excretion Studies in the Rat

These studies[22] after 5 mg/kg i.v. injection in the rat showed that cocaine was very rapidly metabolized, and unchanged cocaine was excreted in very small amounts in bile (Figure 2) up to 3.5 hr post-injection. The excretion of total radioactivity comprising metabolites of cocaine was high at 0.5 and 0.5 to 1 hr and gradually declined thereafter. Total radioactivity as mean percentage of dose excreted in rat bile was approximately 36 in 3.5 hr post-injection.

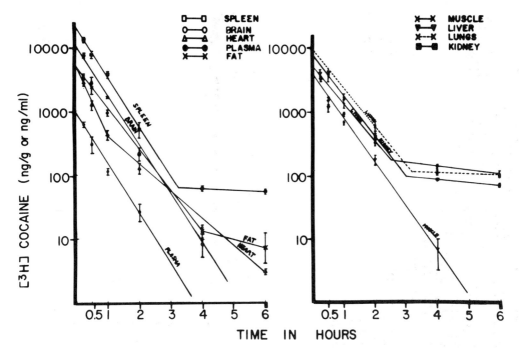

FIGURE 1. Distribution of [³H] cocaine in tissues and biofluids of male Wistar rats after a single 8 mg/kg intravenous injection (n = 3).

Distribution of [³H] Cocaine in Tissues and Biofluids of Acutely and Chronically Treated Rats After Subcutaneous Injection

The mobilization of cocaine from the injection site after a 20 mg/kg subcutaneous injection in acutely and chronically treated male Wistar rats (Figure 3) was rapid, in spite of the fact that local vasoconstriction effect of cocaine could limit its absorption. No significant differences were observed in relative rates of disappearance of cocaine from the subcutaneous site in the two groups.[22]

No significant differences were observed in plasma-protein binding of cocaine (mean value, 33.4 to 38.6%) in vitro at ambient temperature (25°C) in control, acutely, and chronically treated rats using an earlier procedure.[24] In view of the relatively small degree of plasma-protein binding of cocaine and its elimination primarily by biotransformation, binding of lipophilic cocaine to tissues may play a more important role in determining its overall pharmacokinetics than the plasma-protein binding.

Data on the comparative distribution of [³H] cocaine in acutely and chronically treated rats following a 20 mg/kg subcutaneous injection are given in Figure 4. In acute animals, a characteristic pattern of gradual increase in cocaine concentration to a peak at 4 hr was observed for plasma,

brain, and most tissues, with the exception of heart and fat, where peak levels occurred at 0.5 and 2 hr respectively. Metabolism of cocaine by liver resulted in much lower levels in this tissue. The sustained peak plasma levels between 1 to 4 hr, which were lower than those in other tissues, represented a state of relative equilibrium between absorption from the subcutaneous site and detoxication mechanisms. An abrupt fall in levels of cocaine occurred from plasma and most tissues at 4 and 6 hr, resulting in very low levels in brain, testes, and plasma at 12 hr and the absence of drug at 24 hr. The fairly rapid disappearance of cocaine from rat brain and plasma is similar to that observed earlier by us with thebaine,[24,25] a morphine congener and stimulant with little or no tolerance and physical dependence liability. In contrast, the opioid depressant drugs[23,26-28] (e.g., morphine and methadone) with high tolerance and physical dependence liability persisted in the CNS in small concentrations for prolonged periods, even after a single subcutaneous injection.

Peak levels of cocaine in brain and plasma of chronically treated rats occurred between 1 to 2 hr post-injection (Figure 4), and a shift in cocaine levels from 4 to 2 hr in brain and 4 to 1 hr in plasma occurred in chronically treated rats. However, no significant differences were observed in

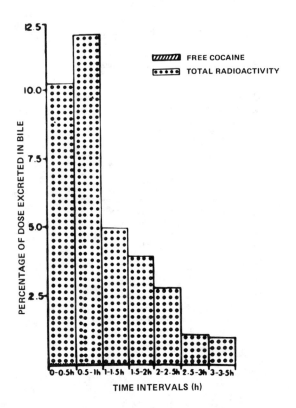

DATA REPRESENT MEAN VALUES FROM 2 ANIMALS.
EXPERIMENT TERMINATED AFTER 3-5 h.

FIGURE 2. Biliary excretion of [³H] cocaine and total radioactivity after a 5 mg/kg intravenous injection in male Wistar rats.

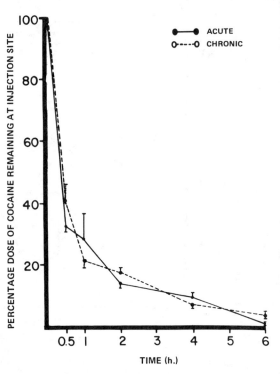

FIGURE 3. Comparative rates of disappearance of [³H] cocaine from subcutaneous site in acutely and chronically treated rats after 20 mg/kg subcutaneous injection (n = 5 in each group). For chronic experiments, the animals were given s.c. injection of 20 mg/kg dose of nonradioactive cocaine twice daily for 3 weeks, then with same dose of labeled cocaine twice daily for 2 days before the terminal injection of same dose of labeled cocaine.

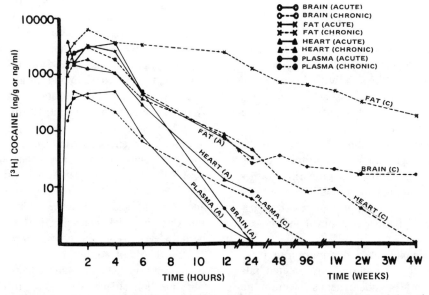

FIGURE 4. Comparative distribution of [³H] cocaine in tissues and biofluids of acutely and chronically treated rats after 20 mg/kg subcutaneous injection (n = 5 in each group). Other details on chronic treatment as given in footnote of Figure 3.

peak levels of cocaine in brain and plasma in two groups. Cocaine was not detectable in plasma of chronically treated rats 24 hr post-injection and barely detectable in heart and testes at 48 and 96 hr. Comparatively high levels of cocaine were sequestered in fat of chronically treated rats, and these declined gradually over a period of 4 weeks to 0.18 μg/g. Although the relatively poor blood supply to fat depots slows the transfer of cocaine from blood to fat, enough cocaine is finally transferred in 2 hr to bring the fat depots in both groups to their equilibrium concentrations. The half-life of cocaine in fat in acutely and chronically treated rats was 1.8 to 2.0 hr. The sequestration of cocaine in substantial amounts in fat depots of chronically treated rats, in contrast to the acute, provided a slow and prolonged release and may account for its persistence in brain in small amounts in this group. The equilibrium of cocaine in other tissues of the acute animals occurred only after the attainment of equilibrium in heart and fat. The pharmacokinetics of cocaine after subcutaneous injection in the rat is complicated by the prolonged course of its absorption from the subcutaneous site and the redistribution phenomena occurring during this phase. The approximate half-life of cocaine in brain and plasma of acute animals was 0.8 and 1 hr respectively, and that in brain, plasma, and tissues of chronically treated rats was 1.8, to 2.0 hr respectively.

The brain to plasma ratios of cocaine in chronically treated rats after 20 mg/kg subcutaneous injection were in general higher than those in the acute animals, with the exception at 1 hr when peak levels of cocaine occurred in plasma in the chronic group. The data indicated an altered distribution of cocaine in the chronic group.

The rise and fall of cocaine levels in rat brain coincided roughly with the change of levels in plasma and suggested that (a) cocaine was probably present in the CNS in the interstitial compartment, (b) its penetration into and exit out of the cell in the CNS must be fairly rapid, and (c) any significant intracellular or extracellular binding in the CNS must be freely reverisble.

Metabolites of Cocaine in Rat Brain

Norcocaine, benzoylecgonine, benzoylnorecgonine, and ecgonine were shown[29] to be the metabolites of cocaine in brains of both acutely and chronically treated rats. Norcocaine represented approximately 15% of the values expressed as

cocaine in brain in Figure 1 and approximately 10% of those expressed as cocaine in brain in Figure 4. In chronic experiments, the content of norcocaine[22] in brain of rats injected with a 20 mg/kg s.c. dose of [^{3}H] cocaine was approximately 20% of that expressed as cocaine (Figure 3). Rat liver microsomal enzymes in vitro have been reported[30,31] to convert cocaine to norcocaine and benzoylecgonine. The half-life of benzoylecgonine and ecgonine in rat brain following a 10 mg/kg intravenous injection of these compounds was 1.3 and 7.8 hr respectively; that in plasma was 0.8 and 3.8 hr respectively.[32,33] This may imply a slower clearance of these polar metabolites from rat brain. Our studies[32] on the pharmacological activity of these metabolites after intravenous and intracisternal injection in the rat showed that norcocaine, like cocaine, possessed potent stimulant activity by both routes of administration, while benzoylecgonine and benzoylnorecgonine were active only by the intracisternal route, and ecgonine and ecgonine methyl ester were inactive by both routes of administration. Benzoylnorecgonine was approximately ten times more potent intracisternally as compared to benzoylecgonine in the rat.[32]

Urinary and Fecal Excretion of Cocaine and its Metabolites in Acutely and Chronically Treated Rats

Comparative data on the urinary and fecal excretion of cocaine and total radioactivity in the two groups are given in Figure 5. Cocaine was metabolized very rapidly in the rat and only 1 to 1.5% of the dose was excreted unchanged in the rat urine and feces, with maximum excretion occurring within 24 hr in the two groups. The excretion of metabolites continued for several days as reflected by the values of total radioactivity which were similar in the acute (49.3% of the dose) and the chronic group (51.6%). Significant differences, however, were observed in the two groups relative to the excretion of total radioactivity in feces, the values in the chronic group being consistently higher (35.6% of the dose) than those in the acute group (22.1%). Cumulative total radioactivity in urine and feces in the chronic group was significantly higher (87.5% of the dose) as compared to the acute (71.4%).

Urinary Metabolites of Cocaine in Acutely and Chronically Treated Rats

Column and thin-layer chromatographic

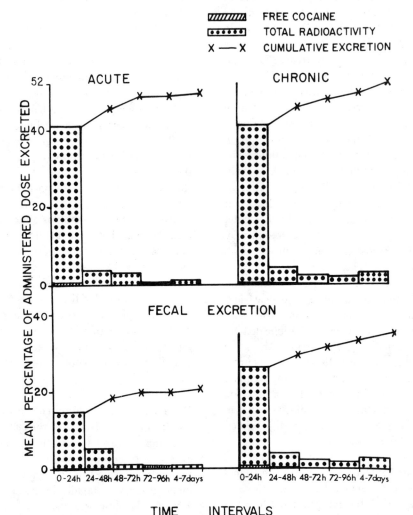

FIGURE 5. Comparative urinary and fecal excretion of free cocaine and total radioactivity in acutely and chronically treated rats after 20 mg/kg s.c. injection of [³H] cocaine (n = 5 in each group). (From Nayak, P. K., Misra, A. L., and Mulé, S. J., *J. Pharmacol. Exp. Ther.*, 196, 556, 1976. With permission.)

studies[34] on pooled urine of rats injected sub-cutaneously with a 20 mg/kg dose of [³H] cocaine provided evidence for the presence of benzoylecgonine, benzoylnorecgonine, ecgonine, and ecgonine methyl ester as urinary metabolites in addition to unmetabolized cocaine. Norcocaine and norecgonine were not detected as urinary metabolites. Tentative evidence was also obtained for a phenolic metabolite (*p*-aromatic hydroxylation) and ring-hydroxylated metabolites (hydroxy groups presumably in the 6,7 position of the pyrrolidine ring). Such hydroxylation probably occurs before the hydrolysis of cocaine or norcocaine to polar benzoylecgonine or benzoylnorecgonine. In our study,[22] evidence for glucuronide conjugation of these metabolites was not obtained. The pattern of urinary metabolites in acutely and chronically treated rats was qualitatively similar, with somewhat higher excretion of benzoylecgonine and ecgonine methyl ester in the chronic group as compared to the acute. The known and hypothetical metabolic pathways of cocaine in the rat are outlined in Figure 6.

DISPOSITION AND METABOLISM OF COCAINE IN THE DOG

Distribution of Cocaine in Acutely and Chronically Treated Dogs[35]

Beagle dogs of either sex (6 to 10 kg) were given intravenous injection of 5 mg/kg (free base) dose of [3H] cocaine. This dose produced mild excitation, restlessness, anxious behavior, rapid respiration, some rise of body temperature, muscle tremors for a few minutes, salivation and pupillary dilatation, but no convulsions. An intravenous dose of 10 mg/kg produced very severe convulsions and hyperexcitation. For the chronic study, beagle dogs were administered a 5 mg/kg dose of nonradioactive cocaine subcutaneously twice daily for 6 weeks, followed by the radioactive dose (5 mg/kg) by intravenous injection. Comparative data on the distribution of cocaine in tissues and body fluids of acutely and chronically treated dogs after 5 mg/kg i.v. injection of [3H] cocaine appear in Figure 7. The values of cocaine in plasma, muscle, heart, fat, duodenum, spleen, lung, and kidney were higher in the chronic as compared to the acute group. The values of cocaine in liver were lower in the chronic group up to 2 hr post-injection and somewhat higher than those in the acute at later times. In the chronic group, the values of cocaine in bile were lower initially (0.5 and 1 hr), higher at 2 and 4 hr, and again dropped lower than those in the acute group at later times. Comparatively faster disappearance of cocaine occurred from bile 4 hr post-injection in the chronic as compared to the acute group. Cocaine disappeared from plasma in the two groups by 12 hr, and with the exception of bile and liver, other tissues had very low levels of cocaine 24 hr post-injection. The levels of cocaine in bile and liver 1 week post-injection were in the range of 50 to 80 ng/ml or g respectively. The half-lives of cocaine in plasma, liver, kidney, spleen, and heart in the acute dogs were 1.2, 2.2, 1.8, 1.8, and 2.0 hr respectively, and in the chronic group, 1.1, 1.8, 1.2, 1.3, and 1.2 hr respectively.

The values of total radioactivity in plasma and fat were higher in the chronic group, but those in liver, kidney, lung, and spleen were lower in the

chronic as compared to the acute study. No changes in the levels of total radioactivity occurred in muscle in the two groups at earlier times.[35]

Data on the distribution of cocaine in selected anatomic areas of the CNS of the acutely and chronically treated dogs [35] appear in Figure 8. With the exception of cerebrospinal fluid, the levels of free cocaine in general were higher in the chronic group in all areas of the CNS as compared to the acute. Cocaine did not persist in the CNS of dog in the two groups, and by 12 to 24 hr post-injection, complete disappearance of cocaine occurred from all areas of the CNS in both groups. The half-lives of cocaine in selected areas of the CNS of the acute dogs were in the range 1.5 to 1.6 hr, and in the chronic group, 1.2 to 1.5 hr. There was no change in the half-life of cocaine in the cerebrospinal fluid and the spinal cord. The lack of persistence of cocaine in the CNS and plasma of the dog in two groups is similar to that observed for the rat.[22] The rise and fall of cocaine levels in the CNS of the dog coincided roughly with changes in plasma levels of cocaine. This suggested that penetration of cocaine into and exit out of the cell in the CNS must be fairly rapid and any extra- or intracellular binding in the CNS must be freely reversible.

The brain to plasma ratios of cocaine (Figure 9) showed no significant differences at 0.5 and 1 hr, were lower in the chronic group at 2 and 4 hr post-injection as compared to the acute, and indicated an altered distribution of cocaine in the chronic group.[35] The CSF to plasma ratios of cocaine (Figure 10) were significantly higher in the acute as compared to the chronic group up to 2 hr, but showed no significant differences thereafter.[35]

The total radioactivity values were significantly higher in the areas of the CNS of chronically treated dogs as compared to the acute up to 24 hr, and they tended to reach similar levels thereafter due to rapid metabolism and elimination of cocaine and its metabolites in chronically treated dogs. Significant amounts of radioactivity persisted in selected areas of the CNS of the chronically treated dogs 1 week post-injection, long after the disappearance of cocaine and norcocaine from these areas.

Metabolism of Cocaine in Brain of Acutely and Chronically Treated Dogs[35]

As previously observed in the rat,[22] norcocaine, benzoylecgonine, benzoylnorecgonine,

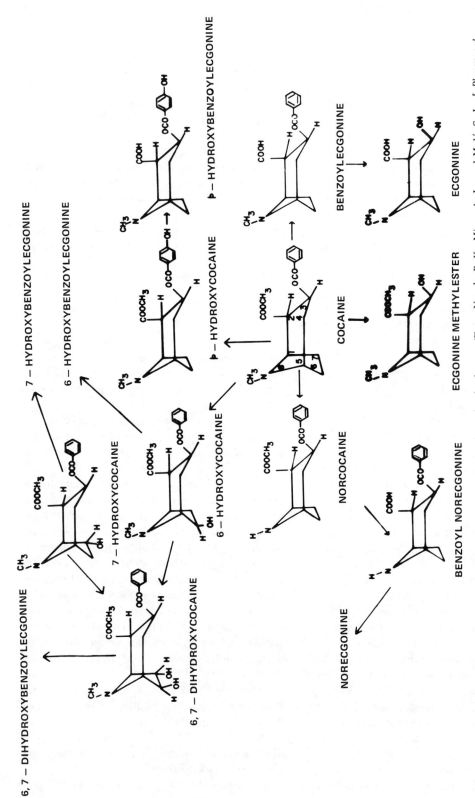

FIGURE 6. The known and hypothetical metabolic pathways of cocaine in the rat. (From Nayak, P. K., Misra, A. L., and Mulé, S. J., *J. Pharmacol. Exp. Ther.*, 196, 556, 1976. With permission.)

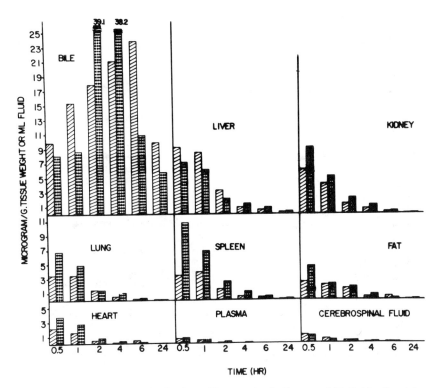

FIGURE 7. Comparative distribution of free cocaine in tissues and biofluids of acutely (slanted-line bar) and chronically treated (dotted bar) dogs after 5 mg/kg intravenous injection of [³H] cocaine. Each figure represents the mean value from two dogs sacrificed at various times, and duplicate determinations were performed on the individual tissues of each animal and the results averaged. For chronic experiments, beagle dogs were injected s.c. with a 5 mg/kg dose of nonradioactive cocaine twice daily for 6 weeks, then with a 5 mg/kg s.c. dose of randomly labeled [³H] cocaine twice daily for 2 days, followed by a terminal injection of the same dose by i.v. route.

and ecgonine were identified as metabolites of cocaine in the dog brain in the two groups. At later times, however, only benzoylecgonine and benzoylnorecgonine were present in the dog brain. The amounts of norcocaine as percentage of cocaine values in brain (Figure 11) were higher in the chronic as compared to the acute group. The half-life of norcocaine in the brain of dogs injected with 5 mg/kg i.v. dose of [³H] cocaine was 1 hr for the fast phase and 3.3 hr for the slower phase. Norcocaine did not persist in the CNS of the dog, and its rate of disappearance in brain was similar to that of cocaine. In brains of chronically treated dogs, benzoylnorecgonine was approximately four times that in the acute at 0.5 hr and twice that at the 4- and 24-hr periods, while benzoylecgonine was approximately one-third the amount in the acute group at 0.5 hr and approximately twice that at the 4- and 24-hr periods. Ecgonine concentration was several times higher in brains of chronically treated dogs as compared to the acute

0.5 hr post-injection. Although the lower lipid solubility of polar benzoylecgonine[32] and benzoylnorecgonine (apparent partition coefficients at 25°C in 1-octanol-M/15 phosphate buffer, pH 7.4, 0.15, and 0.21 respectively) prevented their penetration through the blood-brain barrier in adequate concentration, direct metabolism of cocaine and norcocaine in brain could lead to significant amounts of these metabolites in the selected anatomic areas of the CNS of the dog.

Urinary and Fecal Excretion of [³H] Cocaine and Total Radioactivity in Acutely and Chronically Treated Dogs[35]

The excretion profile of cocaine and total radioactivity in acutely and chronically treated dogs is given in Figure 12. As previously observed,[15] cocaine was rapidly metabolized in the dog and a comparatively small fraction of the dose was

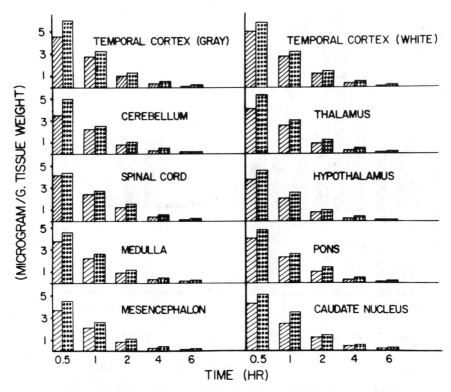

FIGURE 8. Comparative distribution of free cocaine in selected areas of the CNS of the acutely (slanted-line bar) and chronically treated (dotted bar) dogs after 5 mg/kg intravenous injection of [³H] cocaine. Other details as in footnote of Figure 7.

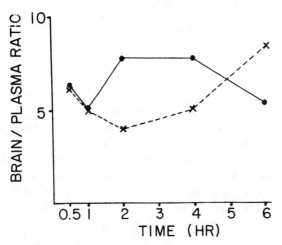

FIGURE 9. The brain to plasma ratio of mean concentration of cocaine in acutely (solid line) and chronically treated (dotted line) dogs after 5 mg/kg intravenous injection of [³H] cocaine. Data represent mean values obtained from the ratio of concentration of cocaine in ten selected anatomic areas of brain to plasma at different times post-injection. Other details as in footnote of Figure 7. (From Misra, A. L., Patel, M. N., Alluri, V. R., Mulé, S. J., and Nayak, P. K., *Xenobiotica,* in press, 1976. With permission.)

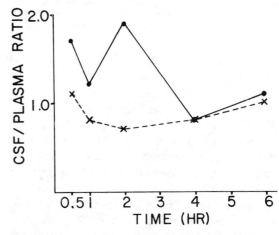

FIGURE 10. The CSF to plasma ratio of mean concentrations of cocaine in acutely (solid line) and chronically treated (dotted line) dogs after 5 mg/kg intravenous injection of [³H] cocaine. Other details as in footnote of Figure 7. (From Misra, A. L., Patel, M. N., Alluri, V. R., Mulé, S. J., and Nayak, P. K., *Xenobiotica,* in press, 1976. With permission.)

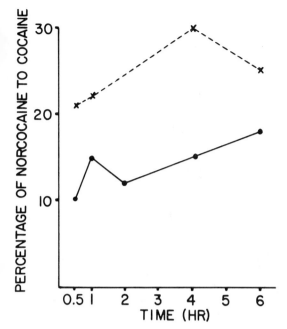

FIGURE 11. The ratio of amounts of norcocaine to cocaine in brain of acutely (solid line) and chronically treated (dotted line) dogs after 5 mg/kg intravenous injection of [^{3}H] cocaine. Ratios were determined from radioscans of the brain extracts processed by the method of extracting cocaine from tissues and biofluids. Other details as in footnote of Figure 7. (From Misra, A. L., Patel, M. N., Alluri, V. R., Mulé, S. J., and Nayak, P. K., *Xenobiotica*, in press, 1976. With permission.)

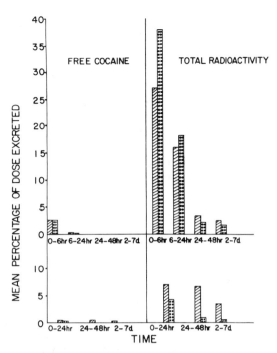

FIGURE 12. Comparative urinary (top) and fecal (bottom) excretion of cocaine and total radioactivity in two acutely (slanted-line bar) and two chronically treated (dotted bar) dogs after 5 mg/kg intravenous injection of ring-labeled [^{3}H] cocaine. The values represent mean percentage of dose excreted at different times in two dogs. The same dogs used in acute experiments were subcutaneously injected with a 5 mg/kg dose of nonradioactive cocaine twice daily for 6 weeks, then with a 5 mg/kg i.v. dose of ring-labeled [^{3}H] cocaine for the chronic experiments.

excreted unchanged in urine and feces. The excretion of cocaine as mean percentage of dose in urine and feces of two acute dogs was 3.0 and 1.4, and in the chronically treated dogs, 2.8 and 0.3 respectively. Major excretion of total radioactivity occurred in urine within 24 hr in both groups, but excretion of total radioactivity continued for several days. There was comparatively higher excretion of total radioactivity in urine as percentage of dose in the chronic (60%) as compared to the acute group (49%). Cumulative percentages of total radioactivity in urine and feces in the two groups, however, were very similar.

Comparative Profile of Urinary Metabolites of Cocaine in Acutely and Chronically Treated Dogs[3][5]

Data on the comparative metabolic profile of cocaine are given in Figure 13. Norcocaine, benzoylnorecgonine, benzoylecgonine, norecgonine, ecgonine methyl ester, and ecgonine were identified as urinary metabolites of cocaine in both groups. Approximately 6 to 7% of the dose was present as unidentified metabolites in 48-hr

urine in both groups. There were no significant differences in mean percentages of norcocaine, ecgonine methyl ester, and unidentified metabolites. Benzoylnorecgonine and ecgonine were present in higher amounts, and benzoylecgonine and norecgonine in lower amounts, in the acute as compared to the values in the chronically treated dogs.

DISPOSITION AND METABOLISM OF [^{3}H] COCAINE IN THE MONKEY

Pharmacokinetic Studies on [^{3}H] Cocaine in Monkeys after Intravenous Injections

Although several studies have been reported on the self-administration of cocaine in the monkey,[7][8] detailed information on the pharmacokinetics and metabolism of cocaine in this species in the acute and chronic states is lacking. In our laboratory, studies were carried out

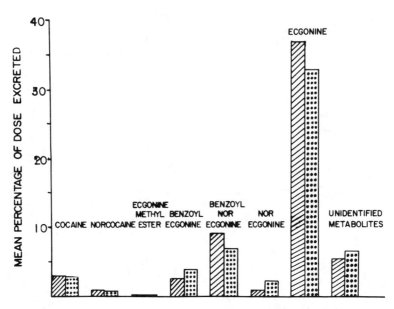

FIGURE 13. Comparative profile of urinary metabolites of cocaine in two acutely (slanted-line bar) and two chronically treated (dotted bar) dogs after 5 mg/kg intravenous injection of ring-labeled [³H] cocaine (the details on chronic treatment of dogs as given in the footnote of Figure 12). Data represent mean values from two dogs in each group. The mean percentages of dose excreted in 48 hr after injection of labeled cocaine in acute and chronic dogs were 58 and 56.2, respectively.

using different intravenous doses (5, 3, and 1 mg/kg) of [³H] cocaine in the monkey. Female monkeys were catheterized with Bardex-Foley® indwelling catheters (size 8, 12 Fr.) and transferred to a restraining chair. With a 5 mg/kg intravenous injection of [³H] cocaine to the monkey, severe convulsions were observed within 5 min of administration of drug, along with the spasmodic lateral movements of the head. These effects and hyperthermia lasted for 1 hr, and this was followed by a depression phase in which the monkey went into shock and died of respiratory arrest approximately 2.5 hr after the injection of cocaine. Analysis of tissues and biofluids removed immediately after the death gave the following values (μg/g or ml) of free cocaine: liver 0.42, spleen 0.67, kidney 0.25, pancreas 2.78, heart 0.30, lung 1.13, bile 10.88, cerebrospinal fluid 0.27, and plasma 0.03. The values (μg/g) of free cocaine in selected areas of the CNS of the monkey were as follows: temporal cortex (gray) 0.60, temporal cortex (white) 0.58, cerebellum 0.50, spinal cord 0.53, hypothalamus 0.52, thalamus 0.51, medulla 0.59, pons 0.61, mesencephalon 0.53, and caudate nucleus 0.49. The approximate half-life of cocaine in plasma ob-

tained up to the time of death was approximately 1 hr.

With a 3 mg/kg intravenous injection of [³H] cocaine to the monkey, convulsions were observed within 15 min of administration and the effects lasted for about 30 min. After 50 min, the hyperthermic monkey (43°C) went into severe depression and died of respiratory arrest 1.5 hr after administration of cocaine. Attempts to revive the animal by lowering the body temperature were unsuccessful. The levels of free cocaine (μg/g or ml) in tissues and biofluids of this monkey removed immediately after death were as follows: liver 0.41, spleen 0.80, kidney 0.48, pancreas 1.71, heart 0.33, lung 0.87, bile 13.67, cerebrospinal fluid 0.20, and plasma 0.01. The values of free cocaine (μg/g) in selected anatomic areas of the CNS of the monkey were as follows: Temporal cortex (gray) 0.56, temporal cortex (white) 0.57, cerebellum 0.57, spinal cord 0.56, hypothalamus 0.51, thalamus 0.51, medulla 0.51, pons 0.66, mesencephalon 0.54, and caudate nucleus 0.55.

Metabolites of Cocaine in the Brain of Monkeys

Analysis of brains of monkeys administered a 3 or 5 mg/kg intravenous injection of [³H] cocaine removed immediately after death showed the presence of norcocaine, benzoylecgonine, and benzoylnorecgonine as metabolites. The formation of norcocaine as a metabolite of cocaine in the brain of monkeys has been reported recently.[36] The ratio of the amounts of benzoylnorecgonine to benzoylecgonine in brain with 5 mg/kg i.v. injection was 3:2 and that with 3 mg/kg i.v. injection 1:3 respectively.

Pharmacokinetic Studies in Acutely and Chronically Treated Monkeys Injected Intravenously with 1 mg/kg Dose of [³H] Cocaine

In chronic experiments, two female monkeys were administered 1 mg/kg s.c. dose of cocaine twice daily for one week, 2 mg/kg s.c. dose twice daily for the following week, and 3 mg/kg s.c. dose twice daily for the third week followed by an intravenous injection of 1 mg/kg dose of [³H] cocaine. Comparative data on the distribution of [³H] cocaine in acute and chronically treated monkeys are given in Table 1. In both groups, the plasma values showed a biphasic pattern between 5 min to 1 hr. The approximate half-life of cocaine in two acute experiments was 1.3 and 1.2 hr respectively; that in the chronically treated monkeys was 1.0 and 0.8 hr respectively. The peak plasma levels of cocaine and total radioactivity values were also much lower in the chronically

treated monkeys as compared to the acute, and significant amounts (38 to 85 ng/ml) of total radioactivity persisted in the plasma of chronically treated monkeys 48 hr after injection. Cocaine was either absent or present in barely detectable concentrations in plasma 6 hr after injection in both groups.

Administration of 1 mg/kg dose of [³H] cocaine by intravenous injection in another monkey produced restlessness and excitement immediately after injection, and these effects lasted for approximately 45 min as previously observed in other monkeys with a similar dose. However, this monkey went into a severe post-stimulatory depression 1 hr after injection and died of respiratory arrest 1 hr and 45 min after injection. Intravenous injection of 5% glucose or lowering of body temperature, etc. during the depression phase did not revive the animal. The exact cause of death in these monkeys is not known. A sensitivity to cocaine or lack of adaptation to the primate chair and consequent stress during the onset of convulsions could possibly be involved. The levels of free cocaine (μg/g or ml) in tissues and biofluids of monkey removed immediately after death were as follows: liver 0.17, spleen 0.08, kidney 0.13, pancreas 0.68, heart 0.14, lung 0.27, bile 5.54, cerebrospinal fluid 0.07, and plasma 0.008. The values (μg/g) in selected

TABLE 1

Distribution[a] of [³H] Cocaine and Half-lives in Plasma of Acutely and Chronically Treated[b] Monkeys After 1 mg/kg (Free Base) Dose by i.v. Injection[c]

	5 min	10 min	20 min	0.5 hr	1 hr	2 hr	4 hr	6 hr	Half-lives[d] (hr)
Acute									
(A)	45	16	20	37	32	15	5	2	1.3
(B)	97	84	67	90	49	9	5	3	1.2
Chronic									
(A)	26	15	23	11	17	6	2	0	1.0
(B)	19	17	20	15	21	16	2	0	0.8

[a]Each figure represents the average of duplicate determinations in ng per ml plasma from two female monkeys (A) and (B).

[b]For chronic experiments, the same monkeys were administered 1 mg/kg dose of nonradioactive cocaine subcutaneously twice daily for one week, 2 mg/kg dose twice daily for the following week, 3 mg/kg dose twice daily for the third week, followed by 1 mg/kg dose of [³H] cocaine by i.v. injection.

[c]This dose produced restlessness and excitement but no convulsions in the monkeys immediately after injection.

[d]Correlation coefficient r = −0.997, −0.919 for data in the acute experiments, P < 0.05. Correlation coefficient r = −0.985, −0.974 for data in the chronic experiments, P < 0.05.

areas of the CNS of the monkey were as follows: temporal cortex (gray) 0.25, temporal cortex (white) 0.27; cerebellum 0.26, spinal cord 0.33, hypothalamus and thalamus 0.23, medulla 0.25, pons 0.32, mesencephalon 0.26, and caudate nucleus 0.26.

Urinary and Fecal Excretion of Free Cocaine and Total Radioactivity After 1 mg/kg Intravenous Injection in Acutely and Chronically Treated Monkeys

In acute experiments, the percentage of dose excreted in two female monkeys as free cocaine in urine and feces collected over a period of 96 hr post-injection was (a) 0.2 and 0.2, and (b) 5.1 and 0.1, respectively. The total radioactivity values in urine and feces for these monkeys were (a) 43.2 and 6.1, and (b) 67.6 and 3.8%, respectively. The same monkeys on chronic treatment with cocaine excreted (a) 0.5 and 0.1, and (b) 7.0 and 0.1%, respectively as free cocaine in urine and feces. The total radioactivity values as percentage of dose in urine and feces in the chronic group were (a) 42.7 and 9.5, and (b) 69.6 and 4.6, respectively. Major excretion of free cocaine and total radioactivity occurred within 24 hr.

Urinary Metabolites of Cocaine in the Monkey

In addition to small amounts of unchanged cocaine, minor amounts (< 0.1%) of norcocaine, ecgonine methyl ester, benzoylnorecgonine (33%), and benzoylecgonine (5%) were identified as urinary metabolites in pooled urine of monkeys collected over a period of 96 hr post-injection of a 1 mg/kg i.v. dose of [^{3}H] cocaine.

THE IMPLICATIONS OF DISPOSITION AND BIOTRANSFORMATION ON THE ACQUIRED SENSITIVITY TO COCAINE AND ITS SYSTEMIC TOXICITY IN EXPERIMENTAL ANIMALS ON CHRONIC TREATMENT

Chronic treatment of dogs and monkeys with cocaine has been reported to produce increased sensitization (instead of tolerance) which persisted unabated for 2 weeks or more after the discontinuance of cocaine.[1,3,4] Tolerance to and physical dependence on cocaine have not been reported to develop on repeated dosing.[1-9] In our study, dogs chronically treated with 5 mg/kg s.c. doses of cocaine twice daily for 20 weeks and suddenly withdrawn for 2 days did not show any withdrawal symptoms or after-depression. Resumption of 5 mg/kg s.c. dose produced severe convulsions, prostration, incoordination, extensor rigidity, and death within 1 hr of injection. Recent studies have shown that toxic and behavioral effects of cocaine did not depend exclusively on catecholamine release.[37,38]

In all three species (rats, dogs, and monkeys) studied by us, cocaine was shown to be very rapidly metabolized, and the metabolites in brain were identified as norcocaine, benzoylecgonine, benzoylnorecgonine, and ecgonine. Cocaine and norcocaine did not persist in the CNS of these animals in acute or chronic states 12 to 24 hr post-injection, and the decay of norcocaine in the CNS was similar to that of cocaine. Benzoylecgonine and benzoylnorecgonine persisted in the CNS long after the disappearance of cocaine or norcocaine. These polar metabolites also formed distinct molecular complexes with calcium ions[39] and possessed potent stimulant activity after intracisternal injection in the rat. Benzoylnorecgonine was approximately ten times more potent as a stimulant compared to benzoylecgonine.[32] Alteration or displacement of neuronal membrane-bound Ca^{2+} (which normally keeps the membrane in a condensed state) by benzoylnorecgonine and benzoylecgonine could conceivably cause a conformational change in membrane proteins, leading to changes in permeability to Na^+ and K^+, depolarization of membrane, and excitatory effects. Concurrently, a reduction in the Ca^{2+}-binding sites on membrane proteins could also interfere with release or uptake of neurotransmitters.

Previous work[40-43] has shown that the interaction of lipophilic cocaine with neural membrane phospholipids through electrostatic and nonpolar forces produces alteration in ordering and fluidity of nonpolar regions, marked inhibition in the functioning of membrane as a cation exchange site, and displacement of Ca^{2+} from membrane sites at which it participates in the generation of action potential. Changes in brain tissue respiration, oxidative phosphorylation,[44] and cerebral metabolism[45] have also been reported with cocaine. Increased partitioning, therefore, of lipophilic cocaine and its metabolite norcocaine into the hydrocarbon domains of neural membrane and high affinity binding coupled with hyperthermia (which enhances its toxicity[46]) may modify the membrane function and its structural integrity, and consequently alter the energy metabolism of the nerve tissue. Furthermore, higher doses or repeated administration of cocaine could conceivably lead to the oxidation in vivo of cocaine to the fairly stable and highly reactive nitroxide free radical. Such an oxidation reportedly[47] occurs at ambient temperature with hydrogen peroxide, and nitroxide free radicals are known[48] to be reduced to the corresponding norcompounds with membrane-SH groups. The mechanistic scheme for the formation of such a free radical, its binding with neural membrane proteins and phospholipids, and its dissociation as a result of reduction with membrane-SH groups are outlined in Figure 14.

A most interesting property of cocaine is the potentiation of adrenergic responses and lack of potentiation in denervated organs. The "unitary" hypothesis[49-58] of cocaine action postulates that cocaine blocks a specialized nerve membrane transport system for sympathomimetic amines, prevents their inactivation by uptake and storage, and thus diverts larger amounts of amines to appropriate tissue receptor, therefore potentiating the response. Although the inhibition of uptake of norepinephrine by cocaine has been confirmed for the peripheral tissues, brain norepinephrine uptake is unaffected.[59] Other workers[60-62] have suggested that the block of norepinephrine uptake may not be an important factor in the supersensitivity produced by cocaine, and a direct action on the effector cells leads to hyperresponsiveness. The changes in effector cells following denervation may be of the same type as those produced by cocaine, and they are maximal by the time sensitization is fully developed.[62] Most of these experiments on supersensitivity to norepinephrine have been performed on isolated tissue preparations in vitro, and it is not certain to what extent these tissues metabolize cocaine to benzoylecgonine and benzoylnorecgonine. These metabolites form distinct molecular complexes with Ca^{2+}, which is known to participate in a

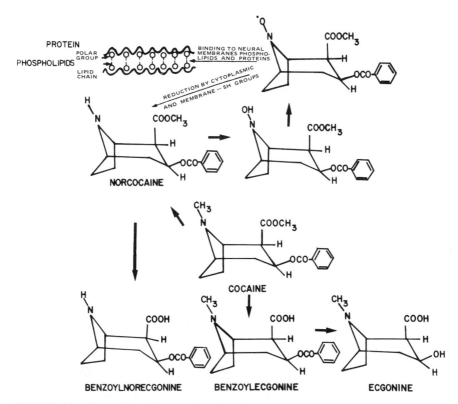

FIGURE 14. Metabolic pathways of cocaine in brain of rats, dogs, and monkeys and the mechanistic scheme for the formation of nitroxide free radical, its binding with neural membrane proteins and phospholipids, and its dissociation as a result of reduction with membrane-SH groups.

number of nerve functions at the membrane level, e.g., in excitation of neuronal membranes,[63] potassium transport,[64] release of neurotransmitter substances,[65,66] and intracellular mediation of catecholamine response through the cyclic AMP system.[67] Studies[68] on binding of [³H] cocaine to guinea pig vas deferens in vitro showed complete uptake within 8 min, with 90% radioactivity being washed out after 4 min and little additional washout occurring after 16 min, indicating a specifically bound radioactive cocaine or its metabolite.

ACKNOWLEDGMENT

The work reported in this chapter was supported by U. S. Army Medical Research and Development Command contract No. DA DA-17-73-C-3080. The author wishes to thank Dr. S. J. Mulé, P. K. Nayak, V. V. Giri, M.-N. Patel, V. R. Alluri, R. Bloch, and N. L. Vadlamani for their contribution to this work.

REFERENCES

1. Tatum, A. L. and Seevers, M. H., Experimental cocaine addiction, *J. Pharmacol. Exp. Ther.*, 36, 401, 1929.
2. Downs, A. W. and Eddy, N. B., The effect of repeated doses of cocaine in the rat, *J. Pharmacol. Exp. Ther.*, 46, 199, 1932.
3. Downs, A. W. and Eddy, N. B., The effect of repeated doses of cocaine in the dog, *J. Pharmacol. Exp. Ther.*, 46, 195, 1932.
4. Gutierrez-Noriega, C. and Zapata-Ortiz, V., Cocainismo experimental. I. Toxicologia general Acostumbramiento y sensibilization, *Rev. Med. Exp.* (Lima), 3, 279, 1944.
5. Eddy, N. B., Halbach, H., Isbell, H., and Seevers, M. H., Drug dependence, its significance and characteristics, *Bull. W.H.O.*, 32, 721, 1965.
6. Kosman, M. E. and Unna, K. R., Effect of chronic administration of amphetamine and other stimulant drugs on behaviour, *Clin. Pharmacol. Ther.*, 9, 240, 1968.
7. Deneau, G. A., Yanagita, T., and Seevers, M. H., Self-administration of psychoactive substances by the monkey – a measure of psychological dependence, *Psychopharmacologia* (Berlin), 16, 30, 1969.
8. Seevers, M. H., Psychologic dependence defined in terms of individual and social risks in *Psychic Dependence*, Goldberg, L. and Hoffmeister, F., Eds., Springer-Verlag, Berlin, 1973, 25.
9. Grode, J., Über die Wirkung längerer Cocain Darreichung bei Tieren, *Arch. Exp. Pathol. Pharmakol.*, 67, 172, 1912.
10. Oeklers, H. A. and Raetz, W., Über das Schicksal des Cocains im Tierkörper, *Arch. Exp. Pathol. Pharmakol.*, 170, 246, 1933.
11. Oelkers, H. A., Wirkung des Cocains auf den Organismus, *Arch. Exp. Pathol. Pharmakol.*, 170, 265, 1933.
12. Oelkers, H. A. and Vincke, E., Untersuchungen über die Ausscheidung von Cocain, *Arch. Exp. Pathol. Pharmakol.*, 179, 341, 1935.
13. McIntyre, A. R., Renal excretion of cocaine in a case of acute cocaine poisoning, *J. Pharmacol. Exp Ther.*, 57, 133, 1936.
14. Langecker, H. and Lewitt, K., Über die Entgiftung von Cocain und Percain, sowie von Atropin im Organismus, *Arch. Exp. Pathol. Pharmakol.*, 190, 492, 1938.
15. Woods, L. A., McMahon, F. G., and Seevers, M. H., Distribution and metabolism of cocaine in the dog and rabbit, *J. Pharmacol. Exp. Ther.*, 101, 200, 1951.
16. Sanchez, C. A., Chromatographic analysis of ecgonine in urine of subjects habitually chewing coca leaves, *An. Fac. Farm. Bioquim. Univ. Nac. Major San Marcos*, 8, 82, 1957.
17. Werner, G., Metabolism of tropane alkaloids in some mammals, *Planta Med.*, 9, 293, 1961.
18. Montesinos, F., Metabolism of cocaine, *Bull. Narcotics (U.N.)*, 17, 11, 1965.
19. Ortiz, R. V., Distribution and metabolism of cocaine in the rat, *An. Fac. Quim. Farm. Univ. Chile*, 18, 15, 1966.
20. Fish, F. and Wilson, W. D. C., Excretion of cocaine and its metabolites in man, *J. Pharm. Pharmacol.*, 21, 135 S, 1969.
21. Nayak, P. K., Misra, A. L., Patel, M. N., and Mulé, S. J., Preparation of radio-chemically pure randomly-labeled and ring-labeled [³H] cocaine, *Radiochem. Radioanal. Lett.*, 16, 167, 1974.
22. Nayak, P. K., Misra, A. L., and Mulé, S. J., Physiological disposition and biotransformation of [³H] cocaine in acutely and chronically-treated rats, *J. Pharmacol. Exp. Ther.*, 196, 556, 1976.

23. **Misra, A. L., Mulé, S. J., Bloch, R., and Vadlamani, N. L.,** Physiological disposition and metabolism of levo methadone-1-^{3}H in nontolerant and tolerant rats, *J. Pharmacol. Exp. Ther.,* 185, 287, 1973.

24. **Misra, A. L., Pontani, R. B., and Mulé, S. J.,** Pharmacokinetics and metabolism of [^{3}H] thebaine in the rat, *Xenobiotica,* 4, 17, 1974.

25. **Misra, A. L., Pontani, R. B., and Mulé, S. J.,** Relationship of pharmacokinetic and metabolic parameters to the absence of physical dependence liability on thebaine, *Experientia,* 29, 1108, 1973.

26. **Misra, A. L., Mitchell, C. L., and Woods, L. A.,** Persistence of morphine in central nervous system of rats after a single injection and its bearing on tolerance, *Nature,* 232, 48, 1971.

27. **Misra, A. L. and Mulé, S. J.,** Persistence of methadone-^{3}H and metabolite in rat brain after a single injection and its implications on pharmacological tolerance, *Nature,* 238, 155, 1972.

28. **Misra, A. L., Bloch, R., Vadlamani, N. L., and Mulé, S. J.,** Physiological disposition and biotransformation of levo-methadone-1-^{3}H in the dog, *J. Pharmacol. Exp. Ther.,* 188, 34, 1974.

29. **Misra, A. L., Nayak, P. K., Patel, M. N., Vadlamani, N. L., and Mulé, S. J.,** Identification of norcocaine as a metabolite of [^{3}H] cocaine in rat brain, *Experientia,* 30, 1312, 1974.

30. **Ramos-Aliaga, R. and Chiriboga, J.,** Enzymatic N-demethylation of cocaine and nutritional status, *Arch. Latinoam. Nutr.,* 20, 415, 1970.

31. **Leighty, E. C. and Fentiman, A. F., Jr.,** Metabolism of cocaine to norcocaine and benzoylecgonine by an *in vitro* microsomal enzyme system, *Res. Commun. Chem. Pathol. Pharmacol.,* 8, 65, 1974.

32. **Misra, A. L., Nayak, P. K., Bloch, R., and Mulé, S. J.,** Estimation and disposition of [^{3}H] benzoylecgonine and pharmacological activity of some cocaine metabolites, *J. Pharm. Pharmacol.,* 27, 784, 1975.

33. **Misra, A. L., Vadlamani, N. L., Bloch, R., Nayak, P. K., and Mulé, S. J.,** Physiological disposition and metabolism of [^{3}H] ecgonine (cocaine metabolite) in the rat, *Res. Commun. Chem. Pathol. Pharmacol.,* 8, 55, 1974.

34. **Misra, A. L., Pontani, R. B., and Mulé, S. J.,** Separation of cocaine, some of its metabolites and congeners on glass-fibre sheets, *J. Chromatogr.,* 81, 167, 1973.

35. **Misra, A. L., Patel, M. N., Alluri, V. R., Mulé, S. J., and Nayak, P. K.,** Disposition and metabolism of [^{3}H] cocaine in acutely and chronically-treated dogs, *Xenobiotica,* in press, 1976.

36. **Hawks, R. L., Kopin, I. J., Colburn, R. W., and Thoa, N. B.,** Norcocaine: a pharmacologically active metabolite of cocaine found in brain, *Life Sci.,* 15, 2189, 1974.

37. **Hatch, R. C. and Fischer, R.,** Cocaine-elicited behaviour and toxicity in dogs after pretreatment with synaptic blocking agents morphine or diphenylhydantoin, *Pharmacol. Res. Commun.,* 4, 383, 1972.

38. **Simon, P., Sultan, Z., Chermat, R., and Broissier, J. R.,** La Cocaine: Une substance amphetaminique? Un problem de psychopharmacologie experimentale, *J. Pharmacol.* (Paris), 3, 129, 1972.

39. **Misra, A. L. and Mulé, S. J.,** Calcium-binding property of cocaine and some of its active metabolites: formation of molecular complexes, *Res. Commun. Chem. Pathol. Pharmacol.,* 11, 663, 1975.

40. **Hauser, H., Penkett, S. A., and Chapman, D.,** Nuclear magnetic resonance spectroscopic studies of cocaine hydrochloride and tetracaine hydrochloride at lipid-water interfaces, *Biochim. Biophys. Acta,* 183, 466, 1969.

41. **Seeman, P.,** The membrane actions of anesthetics and tranquilizers, *Pharmacol. Rev.,* 24, 583, 1972.

42. **Singer, M. A.,** Interaction of local anesthetics and salicylates with phospholipid membranes, *Can. J. Physiol. Pharmacol.,* 51, 785, 1973.

43. **Feinstein, M. B. and Paimre, M.,** Specific reaction of local anesthetics with phosphodiester groups, *Biochim. Biophys. Acta,* 115, 33, 1966.

44. **Kuzhman, M. I.,** Disturbance of energy metabolism of nerve tissue by local anesthetics and its role in the metabolism of local anesthetics, *Eksp. Khir. Anesteziol.* (U.S.S.R.), 14, 62, 1969; *Chem. Abstr.,* 71, 79492 J, 1969.

45. **Rogers, K. J. and Nahorski, S. R.,** Depression of cerebral metabolism by stimulant doses of cocaine, *Brain Res.,* 57, 255, 1973.

46. **Peterson, D. I. and Hardinge, M. G.,** The effects of various environmental factors on cocaine and ephedrine toxicity, *J. Pharm. Pharmacol.,* 19, 810, 1967.

47. **Rozantsev, E. G. and Sholle, V. D.,** Products from the oxidation of cocaine and other narcotics of tropane series, *Dokl. Akad. Nauk* (U.S.S.R.), 187, 1319, 1969; *Chem. Abstr.,* 71, 128619 S, 1973.

48. **Giotta, G. J. and Wang, H. H.,** Reduction of nitroxide free radicals by biological materials, *Biochem. Biophys. Res. Commun.,* 46, 1576, 1972.

49. **MacMillan, W. H.,** A hypothesis concerning the effect of cocaine on the action of sympathomimetic amines, *Br. J. Pharmacol. Chemother.,* 14, 385, 1959.

50. **Muscholl, E.,** Effect of cocaine and related drugs on the uptake of noradrenaline by heart and spleen, *Br. J. Pharmacol. Chemother.,* 16, 352, 1961.

51. **Furchgott, R. F., Kirepekar, S. M., Ricker, M., and Schwab, A.,** Actions and interactions of norepinephrine, tyramine and cocaine on aortic strips of rabbit and left atria of guinea pig and cat, *J. Pharmacol. Exp. Ther.,* 142, 39, 1963.

52. **Kopin, I. J.,** Storage and metabolism of catecholamines: the role of monoamine oxidase, *Pharmacol. Rev.,* 16, 179, 1964.

53. **Trendelenburg, U.,** Supersensitivity by cocaine to dextrorotatory isomers of norepinephrine and epinephrine, *J. Pharmacol., Exp. Ther.,* 148, 329, 1965.

54. Whitby, L. G., Hertting, G., and Axelrod, J., Effect of cocaine on the disposition of noradrenaline labeled with tritium, *Nature* 187, 604, 1960.

55. Dengler, H. J., Spiegel, H. E., and Titus, E. O., Effect of drugs on the uptake of isotopic norepinephrine by cat tissues, *Nature,* 191, 816, 1961.

56. Iversen, L. L., The uptake of noradrenaline by the isolated perfused rat heart, *Br. J. Pharmacol. Chemother.,* 21, 523, 1963.

57. Malmfors, T., Studies on adrenergic nerves. The use of rat and mouse iris for direct observations on their physiology and pharmacology at cellular and subcellular levles, *Acta Physiol. Scand.,* 64, Suppl. 248, 1, 1965.

58. Von Zwieten, P. A., Widhalm, S., and Hertting, G., Influence of cocaine and of pretreatment with reserpine on the pressor effect and the tissue uptake of injected dl-catecholamines-2-^{3}H, *J. Pharmacol. Exp. Ther.,* 149, 50, 1965.

59. Glowinski, J. and Axelrod, J., Effect of drugs on the uptake, release and metabolism of [^{3}H] norepinephrine in rat brain, *J. Pharmacol. Exp. Ther.,* 149, 43, 1965.

60. Maxwell, R. A., Wastila, W. B., and Eckhardt, S. B., Some factors determining the response of rabbit aortic strips to dl-norepinephrine-7-^{3}H hydrochloride and the influence of cocaine, guanethidine and methyl phenidate on these factors, *J. Pharmacol. Exp. Ther.,* 151. 253, 1966.

61. Kasuya, Y. and Goto, K., The mechanism of supersensitivity to norepinephrine induced by cocaine in rat isolated vas deferens, *Eur. J. Pharmacol.,* 4, 355, 1968.

62. Kalsner, S. and Nickerson, M., Mechanism of cocaine potentiation of responses to amines, *Br. J. Pharmacol.,* 35, 428, 1969.

63. Singer, I. and Tasaki, I., *Biological Membranes,* Chapman, D., Ed., Academic Press, New York, 1968, 347.

64. Blum, R. M. and Hoffman, J. F., Calcium-induced potassium transport in human red cells: Localization of Ca-sensitive site to the inside of the membrane, *Biochem. Biophys. Res. Commun.,* 46, 1146, 1972.

65. Katz, B., Ed., *Nerve, Muscle and Synapse,* McGraw Hill, New York, 1966.

66. Heuser, J. and Miledi, R., Effect of lanthanum ions on function and structure of frog neuromuscular junction, *Proc. R. Soc. London Ser. B,* 179, 247, 1971.

67. Greengard, P., McAfee, D. A., and Kebabian, J. W., *Advances in Cyclic Nucleotide Research,* Greengard, P., Robinson, A., and Paoletti, R., Eds., Raven Press, New York, 1, 337, 1972.

68. Marks, B. H., Dutta, S., and Hoffman, R. F., Cocaine-[^{3}H] binding by the isolated guinea pig vas deferens, *Arch. Int. Pharmacodyn.,* 168, 28, 1967.

Effect on Biogenic Amines

Cocaine and Its Effect on Biogenic Amines

COCAINE AND ITS EFFECT ON BIOGENIC AMINES*

Antonio Groppetti and Anna Maria Di Giulio

TABLE OF CONTENTS

*Supported in part by CNR Grant CT 75.00537.04.

INTRODUCTION

Cocaine is known as a powerful central nervous system (CNS) stimulant drug. In this respect it shares with d-amphetamine several behavioral effects. Like amphetamine, cocaine increases locomotor activity and body temperature,[1,2] elicits stereotyped behavior[3-5] and turning towards the lesioned side in animals with unilateral lesion of the dopaminergic nigro-striatal pathway,[6] reduces food intake,[7] induces desynchronized electroencephalogram (EEG), and increases the multiple unit activity at the reticular formation;[8] in addition, its toxicity is enhanced by aggregation.[9] In man, cocaine produces euphoria, anorexia, perceptual and affective changes at low doses, and paranoid psychoses at higher doses.[10-12] Both total and rapid eye movement (REM) sleep are significantly reduced by cocaine.[13] Chronic use of cocaine does not lead to physical dependence. However, unlike amphetamine, tolerance to the excitatory effects does not develop (see chapter by M. Matsuzaki) with prolonged use of this drug; on the contrary, there is evidence of an increased severity of the symptoms with repeated daily injections.[1,10,14-18]

Much evidence has linked brain catecholamines (CA) to the CNS stimulant effects of d-amphetamine;[19] less information in this regard is instead available for cocaine. In fact, although behavioral studies support the idea that this drug may interact with noradrenergic and dopaminergic neurons, evidence so far presented is often incomplete and sometimes contradictory. Moreover, only few attempts have been made to establish which of the monoamines, norepinephrine (NE) or dopamine (DM), is involved in mediating single behavioral effects elicited by cocaine. Recently it has been shown that also the serotoninergic system is affected by cocaine. This chapter will review the interactions between cocaine and these neurotransmitter monoamines.

EFFECTS OF COCAINE ON NORADRENERGIC NEURONS

Peripheral Effects

In 1960 Withby et al.[20] reported that cocaine, when given to anesthetized cats (5 mg/kg i.v.), prevented the accumulation of injected [³H] norepinephrine (³H-NE) into heart, spleen, and adrenal glands, suggesting that cocaine reduced the uptake of circulating NE into these tissues. Since then, a large number of in vitro and in vivo studies performed on a variety of peripheral tissues such as isolated cat colon,[21] cat nictitating membrane,[22] rat and rabbit aorta,[23-25] rabbit ear central artery strips,[26] guinea pig vas deferens,[27] rat iris,[28] and rat salivary glands,[29] in addition to cat,[24,30,31] rat,[23,32-34] guinea pig,[24] and rabbit heart,[35] cat[30,31] and rat[32] spleen, and cat adrenal glands,[30] have substantiated these findings.

According to Iversen, who has provided evidence for the existence of two different mechanisms of norepinephrine uptake,[36-38] cocaine is a potent inhibitor of the uptake of trace amounts of NE (uptake$_1$), but has little effect on the uptake of NE at higher concentrations (uptake$_2$).[37,38] Site of its action is the neuronal membrane, while it is less effective in inhibiting uptake by granular membrane.[39] Moreover, the uptake of NE by sympathetic cell bodies appears to be considerably less sensitive to inhibition by cocaine than the uptake of this transmitter by sympathetic nerve endings.[28,29] The inhibition of NE uptake is not reflected by alteration of neurotransmitter content in peripheral organs.

Callingham and Cass[40] have reported that doses of cocaine ranging from 10 to 50 mg/kg s.c. did not alter the NE content of the heart and spleen of rats, an observation which has been confirmed and extended to other peripheral tissues either in acute[21,41-43] or chronic experiments.[42,44] In this respect, cocaine differs from amphetamine which is known to decrease tissue concentration of NE.[45-49]

Normal tissue levels of NE present after cocaine administration despite inhibition of the uptake process suggest that compensatory mechanisms, such as reduction of monoaminooxidase (MAO) activity or increase synthesis or decreased release of NE, have been operating in the neurons in order to maintain the steady-state levels of the amine.

The finding that cocaine does not affect MAO activity rules out the first hypothesis.[50] On the other hand, an increase of NE synthesis in peripheral tissues is not supported by experimental evidence indicating that cocaine has no effect on the levels of ¹⁴C-norepinephrine synthetized from labeled tyrosine in the guinea pig vas deferens in vitro.[27] Moreover, neither the activity of tyrosine hydroxylase nor that of dopamine β-hydroxylase, measured in homogenates of this tissue, were affected by cocaine.[27] On the contrary, Prioux-Guyonneau et al. have shown that in rats injected with ³H-NE, the rate of disappearance of the labeled amine from the heart is decreased by cocaine treatment, and that the rate of decline of NE from the heart of mice pretreated with α-methyl-tyrosine is also decelerated by cocaine administration, suggesting that the rate of NE synthesis may be reduced by this drug.[43]

However, a decreased release of NE from heart nerve terminals should also be considered as an alternative interpretation of the latter data. In fact, inhibition of the rate of NE synthesis, associated with inhibition of NE uptake, would be expected to result in a marked fall in NE tissue concentrations. The findings that NE levels as well as the activity of catabolic enzymes, monoamino oxidase and catechol-O-methyltransferase,[20,50] are not affected by cocaine suggest that this drug, more likely, inhibits the release of NE from structures in which this neurotransmitter is stored. Consistent with this hypothesis is the evidence presented by Costa et al. indicating that cocaine, as well as desmethylimipramine, depresses the spontaneous release of ³H-NE from granules in rat heart.[21] In addition, cocaine decreases NE released from isolated tissues by sympathetic nerve stimulation.[21,51,52] Also, the overflow of dopamine β-hydroxylase induced by nerve stimulation in the perfused spleen of dog and cat is reduced by cocaine.[53,54] Recently, it has been postulated that the release of NE by nerve stimulation is regulated through a negative feed-back control mechanism mediated by presynaptic alpha receptors.[55-62] Since cocaine increases the concentration of NE at the neuroeffector junction by inhibiting its uptake, it has been suggested that this drug enhances the presynaptic inhibition of the transmitter released by nerve stimulation.[57,62]

In the light of these observations, the reported

increase in the output of urinary norepinephrine and epinephrine (E) in animals treated with cocaine[42] may be explained by an increase in the outflow of unmetabolized amines from synaptic junctions, as a result of inhibition of NE and E uptake by nerve terminals. Also in this context cocaine differs from amphetamine which, at least when given at high doses, increases CA urinary output by releasing the transmitter from tissue stores.[63] Even more striking are the differences between the two drugs when comparing the findings of long-term experiments. In fact, while during chronic amphetamine treatment, there was (after an initial increase in urinary CA levels) a gradual decrease in CA outflow,[49] during continued cocaine administration for 2 weeks, the urinary excretion did not indicate any tolerance to the catecholamine increased output of the drug.[42]

Central Effects

Similar to what is observed in peripheral tissues, cocaine fails to alter NE concentrations in the brain. In fact, besides earlier findings by Higuchi et al.[41] that show a slight reduction of NE levels in brain of rabbits given intravenous cocaine (2 mg/kg), most of the reports in the literature agree that cocaine, within a large range of doses, does not affect significantly NE concentrations in the whole brain of mice[43,64,65] and rats,[42,66,67] as well as in the rat telediencephalon[68] and hypothalamus.[67,69] Moreover, despite convincing evidence that cocaine inhibits NE uptake in peripheral nerve terminals, contradictory results have been reported for the brain between in vitro and in vivo studies. Cocaine was shown to decrease the radioactivity which can be accumulated into brain slices of cat incubated in Krebs bicarbonate medium containing ^{3}H-NE.[31] Similar results have been obtained from studies on isolated rat pineals,[70] brain slices of mice,[71] mouse synaptosomes,[72] where cocaine showed from 1 to 3% of the activity of desmethylimipramine, and on chopped rat brain, where cocaine was as active as desmethylimipramine and amphetamine in inhibiting neuronal uptake of ^{3}H-NE.[73]

Although results from in vitro studies indicate that, as in the peripheral nervous system, cocaine inhibits NE uptake in the brain, results of in vivo experiments do not support this conclusion. No evidence has been reported, in fact, showing that cocaine, when directly injected to animals, inhibits brain NE uptake. Glowinski and Axelrod[74]

showed that cocaine given to rats (15 mg/kg) failed to affect the brain concentrations of intraventricularly injected [^{3}H]norepinephrine, while reserpine, amphetamine, and guanetidine markedly reduced it. Moreover, brain slices of mice treated with doses of cocaine up to 40 mg/kg took up tritiated NE to the same extent as saline treated animals.[71] This suggested that cocaine may not have the same actions in the intact brain as it does in brain slices or in the peripheral nervous system.[74] The effect of cocaine on the regulation of brain norepinephrine synthesis is also controversial. It has been reported that cocaine (20 mg/kg i.p.) does not affect the accumulation rate of ^{14}C-NE synthetized in mice brain following administration of labeled tyrosine.[75]

In agreement with these findings, other investigators have indicated that cocaine, given intravenously to rats at a dose of 3 mg/kg 10 min after intraventricular or intravenous injection of [^{3}H]tyrosine and 15 min before killing, does not alter the incorporation rate of the labeled precursor into telediencephalic[68] or hypothalamic[71] NE, while increasing the striatal formation of [^{3}H]dopamine.[68,69] These results are consistent with in vivo studies by Carr and Moore, who failed to demonstrate changes in the efflux rate of ^{3}H-NE into cat cerebral perfusate after cocaine.[76] In contrast with these observations Bralet and Lallemant[67] have recently reported that cocaine (10 mg/kg i.m.) given 30 min before intravenous administration of [^{3}H]tyrosine and 60 or 90 min before killing, reduces the amount of ^{3}H-NE synthetized from the labeled amino acid in the whole brain and in the hypothalamus of the rat. In addition, these investigators showed that in rats pretreated with α-methyltyrosine, cocaine decreases the rate of disappearance of brain norepinephrine and similar results have been reported also in mice.[43,75] The discrepancy of these findings does not allow at present any positive conclusion that might not be accounted for in the differences in the experimental design, e.g., animal strain dosage or route of administration, duration of exposure to drug, etc.

Moreover, because of differences in the injection schedules (in some experiments [^{3}H]tyrosine being administrated before, and in others, after cocaine), an eventual interference of this drug with uptake and distribution of the labeled amino acid could be a major determinant of the observed inconsistencies. Discrepancies in turnover studies utilizing rate of transmitter disappearance after synthesis inhibition or incorporation rate from a labeled precursor have already been reported. Thus, Fekete and Borsy[75] showed that in mice given α-methyltyrosine, chlorpromazine, a drug which increases dopamine synthesis,[77-79] reduced the decline of brain dopamine concentrations, and they suggested that the rate of transmitter disappearance after synthesis inhibition might not always be the best indicator of changes in synthesis rate and utilization of the neurotransmitter.

EFFECTS OF COCAINE ON DOPAMINERGIC NEURONS

In contrast with the relatively large amount of information concerning cocaine-NE interaction, only a few studies have been reported so far on the effect of this drug on dopaminergic neurons. In 1967 Ross and Renyi[71] provided evidence that cocaine inhibited dopamine uptake in brain slices in similar concentrations as those active on NE, while imipramine-like drugs inhibit the dopamine uptake only in concentrations 100 times greater than those which block NE uptake. A few years later Farnebo and Hamberger[56] showed that cocaine increases the electrical field stimulation induced overflow of labeled dopamine from neostriatal brain slices previously incubated with [^{3}H] dopamine, and they have suggested that an inhibition of the transmitter uptake and/or an increase of release from DM terminals may cause this effect. These data are consistent with more recent findings showing that cocaine, in a manner similar to amphetamine, increases 3-methoxytyramine (3-MT) levels in rat striatum (Table 1). 3-MT, in fact, appears to be a reliable indicator of impulse-induced release of dopamine since it is exclusively formed from dopamine released into the synaptic cleft.[81]

The observation that 3-MT formation can be almost completely abolished by axotomy of dopaminergic neurons adds further support to this hypothesis.[82] The increased 3-MT concentrations found in rat striatum after cocaine administration should reflect, therefore, an increased accumulation of dopamine into neuronal junction due to either increased release or uptake inhibition into nerve terminals or both.

Since it has been reported that drugs known to inhibit reuptake processes in the central dopaminergic neurons, such as benzotropine,[83,84] do

TABLE 1

Effect of Cocaine and d-Amphetamine on 3-Methoxytyramine (3-MT) Concentrations in Rat Striatum

Treatment*	Dose mg/kg i.v.	3-MT mμmol/g ± S.E.
Saline	–	0.234 ± 0.006
Cocaine	3	0.389 ± 0.073**
d-Amphetamine	1	0.380 ± 0.015**

*Drugs or saline were given i.v. to rats 10 min before killing. The animals were sacrificed by exposure to microwave radiations. 3-MT was measured in striatum of single animals by mass-fragmentographic method (Galli et al.[80]). Five animals per group were used.
**$P < 0.01$ relative to controls. The significance of the differences between groups was calculated according to Student's t test.

not increase 3-MT accumulation in the brain of rats pretreated with monoaminoxidase inhibitors, it seems more likely that the higher concentrations of 3-MT found in striatum of cocaine treated rats may be due to increased release of the neurotransmitter instead of to a decreased reuptake. Consistent with this view is the observation that cocaine increases the turnover rate of striatal dopamine. In fact, it has been shown that in rats treated with cocaine (3 mg/kg i.v.), the incorporation rate of injected labeled tyrosine into striatal DM is higher than in saline treated animals.[68] In addition, in similar experimental conditions, the concentrations of labeled 3-MT are increased (Figure 1), suggesting that cocaine may increase the release of newly synthetized dopamine. On the other hand, since no alteration of brain DM and homovanillic acid concentrations have been reported after cocaine administration,[66,68,75,86-88] the existence of a balance between inhibition of uptake and increased release on one side, and enhanced synthesis on the other side, has to be postulated in cocaine treated animals, in order to maintain steady-state levels of the endogenous stores of the neurotransmitter.

The cocaine interference with DM neurons is also suggested by a series of behavioral findings. In fact, it has been shown that α-methyltyrosine inhibits both hypermotility and stereotyped behavior induced by cocaine,[5,12,89] while p-chlorophenylalanine has no effect.[12,90] Moreover, it has been reported that reserpine blocks the increased locomotor activity in cocaine treated

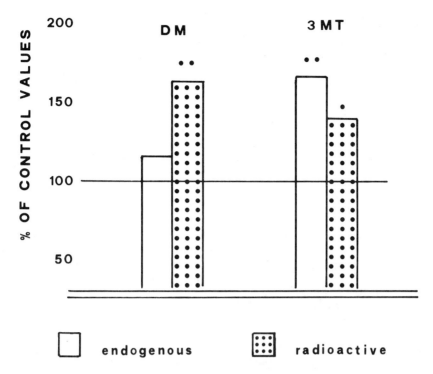

FIGURE 1. Effect of cocaine on endogenous and radioactive striatal dopamine (DM) and 3-methoxytyramine (3-MT) in rats injected with labeled tyrosine. Cocaine (3 mg/kg) or saline was given i.v. to rats 11 min before killing. 3-5, [^{3}H]tyrosine (50 Ci/mmol) was injected, 10 μCi in each ventricle, through chronically implanted polyethylene cannulas, 10 min before killing. The animals were sacrificed by exposure to microwave radiations. Endogenous and radioactive DM and 3-MT were determined according to the methods devised by Galli et al.[80] and Di Giulio et al.[85] Fourteen animals per group were used. The data are expressed as percent of control values. $^*P < 0.05$; $^{**}P < 0.01$ relative to controls. The significance of the differences between groups was calculated according to Student's t test.

mice.[2,5,91,92] L-Dopa, but not dihydroxyphenyl-serine or 5-hydroxytryptophan, can restore this activity.[2,91] In agreement with these findings, drugs known to block dopaminergic receptors antagonize cocaine induced hypermotility and stereotypy.[75,92] Also, cocaine-anorexia, in a manner similar to amphetamine,[69,93] is reduced by pimozide (Table 2).

It would appear, therefore, that brain DM plays an important role in regulating behavioral effects of cocaine. From this point of view, cocaine and d-amphetamine could share an identical mechanism of action. Evidence has been given, however, suggesting that the similarity between the two drugs may not be so close. In fact, it has been reported that haloperidol antagonized cocaine only when given at high, depressant doses. When this neuroleptic drug was given at nondepressant doses, it did not modify significantly the stimulant effect of cocaine, while d-amphetamine

was antagonized.[94] Similarly, Simon et al. failed to demonstrate that α-methyltyrosine affects cocaine induced hypermotility in mice at doses that inhibit amphetamine effects,[90,94] and they have suggested that the action of cocaine on catecholamines may not be sufficient to explain its behavioral effects.

EFFECTS OF COCAINE ON SEROTONINERGIC NEURONS

It has been recently reported that the rate of serotonin (5-HT) accumulation in brain of rats given pargyline is decreased by cocaine.[94] In addition, the rise of brain 5-hydroxyindolacetic acid (5-HIAA) that follows probenecid administration is slower in cocaine-treated than in control animals.[95] A decreased accumulation of [^{3}H] serotonin in brain of mice given [^{3}H]tryptophan intravenously has also been shown after cocaine

TABLE 2

Effect of Pimozide Pretreatment on Cocaine and d-Amphetamine Induced Anorexia in Rat

	Food Intake	
Treatment*	Saline	Pimozide
Saline	4.12 ± 0.35	4.44 ± 0.82
Cocaine	1.04 ± 0.21	2.00 ± 0.13**
d-Amphetamine	1.23 ± 0.27	2.88 ± 0.55**

*Cocaine (3 mg/kg i.v.) and d-amphetamine (1.5 mg/kg i.p.) were given 15 min before food presentation. Pimozide (0.25 mg/kg i.p.) was given 4 hr before food presentation. Rats were trained to eat 4 hr/day. Six animals per group were used. Food intake, expressed as g of food eaten/100 g of body weight ± S.E., was measured 1 hr after food presentation.

**P < 0.01 relative to non-Pimozide-treated animals. The significance of the differences between groups was calculated according to Student's t test.

administration (30 mg/kg i.p.).[96] These findings have been interpreted to mean that cocaine inhibits the turnover rate of brain 5-HT. In view of the reported cocaine inhibition of tryptophan uptake into rat septal synaptosomes,[97] it is likely that a reduced availability of the precursor amino acid, tryptophan, into the neuronal biosynthetic units may be responsible for the decreased brain 5-HT synthesis by cocaine. Inhibition of 5-HT uptake in the brain has also been reported by in vitro and in vivo studies with cocaine.[98,99] In this respect, cocaine is as potent as desmethylimipramine and amitryptiline, while amphetamine is not active. On the other hand, no significant effect on the whole brain concentrations as well as on total and free plasma levels of tryptophan has been found.[95]

Similarly, no alteration of brain 5-HT levels has been reported.[95,96] A time-related decrease in 5-HIAA concentrations was instead observed in the whole brain of rat following the acute administration of cocaine (20 mg/kg s.c.).[95] Although the role of brain 5-HT in mediating behavioral effects of cocaine has not yet been established, it seems likely that the inhibition of uptake and/or synthesis rate of brain 5-HT produced by cocaine may be responsible for some of the pharmacological differences between this drug and d-amphetamine.

Thus, the reported psychotomimetic-like behavioral and postural changes observed in chicks after high doses of cocaine[100] could be attributed to alteration of the serotoninergic system. Brain 5-HT, in fact, has often been linked to CNS effects of psychotomimetic drugs.[101,102]

CONCLUSIONS

Results from several biochemical studies have shown that cocaine affects important processes involved in the regulation of the functional activity of monoaminergic neurons in the periphery as well as in the CNS. Probably, the most convincing evidence of cocaine interaction with noradrenergic neurons has been provided by the discovery of an inhibitory effect of this drug on the uptake of norepinephrine in peripheral tissues.

It has been suggested that the potentiation of responses to nerve stimulation or to exogenous NE in presence of cocaine is related predominantly to the higher concentration of the transmitter in the proximity of the adrenergic receptor, as a result of uptake inhibition.[103] Both release of NE from nerve terminals and rate of NE synthesis may also be reduced by cocaine in peripheral tissues. Less convincing evidence is instead available to suggest an interaction of the drug with central noradrenergic neurons. Inhibition of NE uptake in the brain has been demonstrated only by in vitro studies, whereas no data have been presented showing that cocaine, when given directly to animals, inhibits brain NE uptake. Also, the effect of cocaine on brain NE turnover is controversial, an area which surely needs further research. In contrast to elusive results on the effects on brain NE neurons, more consistent data indicate that cocaine interferes with brain dopaminergic neurons. It increases the rate of synthesis and inhibits the uptake of brain dopamine. Striatal concentrations of 3-methoxytyramine are also ehnahced by cocaine, suggesting an increased release of the neurotransmitter into the synaptic cleft. Behavioral findings indicate that, in a manner similar to amphetamine, stereotyped behavior, increased locomotor activity, as well as anorexia induced by cocaine may depend at least in part on an activation of the dopaminergic system.

Although collectively these data indicate a strong similarity between cocaine and amphetamine, there is evidence that the biochemical profiles of these two drugs are not identical. Unlike amphetamine, cocaine does not affect NE tissue concentrations, while it inhibits both the uptake and the synthesis of the neurotransmitter — two processes on which *d*-amphetamine is completely ineffective. Differences between the two drugs have also been suggested by some inconsistencies reported from behavioral studies.

REFERENCES

1. **Goodman, L. S. and Gilman, A.,** *The Pharmacological Basis of Therapeutics,* 5th ed., Macmillan, New York, 1975.
2. **Van Rossum, J. M., Van der Schott, J. B., and Hurkmans, J. A.,** Mechanism of action of cocaine and amphetamine in the brain, *Experientia,* 18, 229, 1962.
3. **Fog, R.,** Stereotyped and non-stereotyped behavior in rats induced by various stimulant drugs, *Psychopharmacologia,* 14, 299, 1969.
4. **Willner, J. H., Samach, M., Angrist, B. M., Wallach, M. B., and Gershon, S.,** Drug induced stereotyped behavior and its antagonism in dogs, *Comm. Behav. Biol.,* 5, Part A, 135, 1970.
5. **Wallach, M. B. and Gershon, S.,** The induction and antagonism of central nervous system stimulant-induced stereotyped behavior in the cat, *Eur. J. Pharmacol.,* 18, 22, 1972.
6. **Christie, J. E. and Crow, T. J.,** Possible role of dopamine-containing neurons in the behavioral effects of cocaine, *Br. J. Pharmacol.,* 42, 643, 1971.
7. **Monnier, M.,** Topic action of psychotropic drugs on the electrical activity of cortex, rhinencephalon and mesodiencephalon, in *Psychotropic Drugs,* Garattini, S. and Ghetti, V., Eds., Elsevier, Amsterdam, 1957, 217.
8. **Wallach, M. B. and Gershon, S.,** A neuropsychopharmacological comparison of d-amphetamine, l-dopa and cocaine, *Neuropharmacology,* 10, 743, 1971.
9. **Lal, H. and Chessick, R. D.,** Lethal effects of aggregation and electric shock in mice treated with cocaine, *Nature,* 208, 295, 1965.
10. **Kosman, M. E. and Unna, K. R.,** Effects of chronic administration of the amphetamines and other stimulants on behavior, *Clin. Pharmacol. Ther.,* 9, 240, 1968.
11. **Bejerot, N.,** A comparison of the effects of cocaine and synthetic central stimulants, *Br. J. Addict.,* 65, 35, 1970.
12. **Post, R. M.,** Cocaine psychoses: a continuum model, *Am. J. Psychiatry,* 132(3), 225, 1975.
13. **Post, R. M., Gillin, J. C., Wyatt, R. J., and Goodwin, F. K.,** The effects of orally administered cocaine on sleep of depressed patients, *Psychopharmacologia,* 37, 59, 1974.
14. **Tatum, A. L. and Seevers, M. H.,** Experimental cocaine addiction, *J. Pharmacol. Exp. Ther.,* 36, 401, 1929.
15. **Gutierrez-Noriega, C. and Zapata-Ortiz, V.,** Cocainismo experimental. Toxicologia general acostumbramiento y sensibilization, *Rev. Med. Exp.,* 3, 280, 1944.
16. **Downs, A. W. and Eddy, N. B.,** The effect of repeated doses of cocaine on the rat, *J. Pharmacol. Exp. Ther.,* 46, 199, 1932.
17. **Downs, A. W. and Eddy, N. B.,** The effect of repeated doses of cocaine on the dog, *J. Pharmacol. Exp. Ther.,* 46, 195, 1932.
18. **Eddy, N. B., Halbach, H., Isbell, H., and Seevers, M. H.,** Drug dependence: Its significance and characteristics, *Bull. W.H.O.,* 32, 721, 1965.
19. **Costa, E. and Garattini, S., Eds.,** *Amphetamines and Related Compounds,* Raven Press, New York, 1970.
20. **Whitby, L. G., Hertting, G., and Axelrod, J.,** Effect of cocaine on the disposition of noradrenaline labelled with tritium, *Nature,* 187, 604, 1960.
21. **Costa, E., Boullin, D. J., Hammer, W., Vogel, W., and Brodie, B. B.,** Interactions of drugs with adrenergic neurons, *Pharmacol. Rev.,* 18, 577, 1966.
22. **Trendelenburg, U.,** Mechanisms of supersensitivity and subsensitivity to sympathomimetic amines, *Pharmacol. Rev.,* 18, 629, 1966.
23. **Bralet, J., Cohen, Y., and Valette, G.,** Action de l'ephédrine et de la cocaïne sur la réponse tensionelle et sur la fixation cardiovasculaire de la noradrénaline chez le rat, *Biochem. Pharmacol.,* 15, 793, 1966.
24. **Furchgott, K. F., Kirpekar, S. M., and Schwab, A.,** Actions and interactions of norepinephrine, tyramine and cocaine on aortic strips of rabbit and left atria of guinea pig and cat, *J. Pharmacol. Exp. Ther.,* 142, 39, 1963.
25. **Shibata, S., Kuchii, M., Hattori, K., and Fujiwara, M.,** The effect of cocaine on the ^{3}H-norepinephrine uptake by cold stored aorta from rabbit, *Jpn. J. Pharmacol.,* 24(1), 151, 1974.
26. **De la Lande, J. F. and Waterson, J. G.,** Site of action of cocaine in the perfused artery, *Nature,* 214, 313, 1967.

27. Johnson, D. G., Thoa, N. B., and Kopin, I. J., Inhibition of norepinephrine biosynthesis by chlorpromazine in the guinea-pig vas deferens, *J. Pharmacol. Exp. Ther.,* 177, 146, 1971.
28. Hanbauer, I., Johnson, D. G., Silberstein, S. D., and Kopin, I. J., Pharmacological and kinetic properties of uptake of (3H)-norepinephrine by superior cervical ganglia of rats in organ culture, *Neuropharmacology,* 11, 857, 1972.
29. Fisher, J. E. and Synder, S., Disposition of norepinephrine-H[3] in sympathetic ganglia, *J. Pharmacol. Exp. Ther.,* 150, 190, 1965.
30. Hertting, G., Axelrod, J., and Whitby, L. G., Effect of drugs on the uptake and metabolism of ^{3}H-norepinephrine, *J. Pharmacol. Exp. Ther.,* 134, 146, 1961.
31. Dengler, H. S., Spiegel, H. E., and Titus, E. O., Effects of drugs on uptake of isotopic norepinephrine by cat tissue, *Nature,* 191, 816, 1961.
32. Muscholl, E., Effect of cocaine and related drugs on the uptake of noradrenaline by heart and spleen, *Br. J. Pharmacol.,* 16, 352, 1961.
33. Bralet, J., Lallemant, A. M., and Beley, A., The effect of treatment by cocaine on the fixation and liberation of noradrenaline in different peripheral organs of the rat, *Arch. Int. Pharmacodyn. Ther.,* 209(1), 118, 1974.
34. Iversen, L. L., Ed., *The Uptake and Storage of Noradrenaline in Sympathetic Nerves,* Cambridge University Press, London, 1967, 147.
35. Starke, K., Montel, H., and Schumann, H. J., Influence of cocaine and phenoxybenzamine on noradrenaline uptake and release, *Naunyn-Schmiedebergs Arch. Pharmacol.,* 270, 210, 1971.
36. Iversen, L. L., The uptake of noradrenaline by the isolated perfused rat heart, *Br. J. Pharmacol.,* 21, 523, 1963.
37. Iversen, L. L., The uptake of catecholamines at high perfusion concentrations in the rat isolated heart: a novel catecholamine uptake process, *Br. J. Pharmacol.,* 25, 18, 1965.
38. Iversen, L. L., Inhibition of noradrenaline uptake by drugs, *J. Pharm. Pharmacol.,* 17, 62, 1965.
39. Von Euler, U. S. and Lishajko, F., Effects of some drugs on the release of noradrenaline from isolated nerve granules, *Biochem. Pharmacol.,* 9, 77, 1962.
40. Callingham, B. A. and Cass, R., The effects of bretylium and cocaine on noradrenaline depletion, *J. Pharm. Pharmacol.,* 14, 385, 1962.
41. Higuchi, H., Matsuo, T., and Shimamoto, K., Effects of metamphetamine and cocaine on the depletion of catecholamine of the brain, heart and adrenal gland in rabbit by reserpine, *Jpn. J. Pharmacol.,* 12, 48, 1962.
42. Gunne, L. M. and Jonsson, J., Effects of cocaine administration on brain, adrenal and urinary adrenaline and noradrenaline in rats, *Psychopharmacologia,* 6, 125, 1964.
43. Prioux-Guyonneau, M., Cohen, Y., Bralet, J., Jacquot, C., and Rapin, J., Effects of cocaine on the release and turnover of noradrenaline, *J. Pharmacol.* (Paris), 6, 5, 1975.
44. Farrant, J., Interactions between cocaine, tyramine and noradrenaline at the noradrenaline store, *Br. J. Pharmacol.,* 20, 540, 1963.
45. McLean, J. R. and McCartney, M., Effect of *d*-amphetamine on rat brain noradrenaline and serotonin, *Proc. Soc. Exp. Biol. and Med.,* 107, 77, 1961.
46. Sanan, S. and Vogt, M., Effect of drugs on the noradrenaline content of brain and peripheral tissues and its significance, *Br. J. Pharmacol.,* 18, 109, 1962.
47. Moore, K. E., Toxicity and catecholamine releasing action of d- and l-amphetamine in isolated and aggregated mice, *J. Pharmacol. Exp. Ther.,* 142, 6, 1963.
48. Gunne, L. M. and Lewander, T., Long-term effects of some dependence-producing drugs on the brain monoamines, *Molecular Basis of Some Aspects of Mental Activity,* Vol. 2, Academic Press, London-New York, 1967, 75.
49. Lewander, T., Urinary excretion and tissue levels of catecholamines during chronic amphetamine intoxication, *Psychopharmacologia,* 13, 394, 1968.
50. Eisenfeld, A. J., Axelrod, J., and Krakoff, L., Inhibition of the extraneuronal accumulation and metabolism of norepinephrine by adrenergic blocking agents, *J. Pharmacol. Exp. Ther.,* 156, 107, 1967.
51. Hukovic, S. and Muscholl, E., Die Noradrenalin-abgabe aus dem isolierten kaninchenherzen bei sympathischer nervenrizung und ihre pharmakologische beeinflussung, *Naunyn-Schmiedebergs Arch. Pharmakol.,* 244, 81, 1962.
52. Langer, S. Z., The metabolism of (^{3}H)-noradrenaline released by electrical stimulation from the isolated nictitating membrane of the cat and from the vas deferens of the rat, *J. Physiol.* (London), 208, 515, 1970.
53. De Potter, W. P., Chubb, I. W., Put, A., and De Schaepdryve, A. F., Facilitation of the release of noradrenaline and dopamine β-hydroxylase at low stimulation frequencies by α-blocking agents, *Arch. Int. Pharmacodyn. Ther.,* 193, 191, 1971.
54. Cubeddu, L. X., Barnes, E. M., Langer, S. Z., and Weiner, N., Release of norepinephrine and dopamine-β-hydroxylase by nerve stimulation. I. Role of neuronal and extraneuronal uptake and alpha presynaptic receptors, *J. Pharmacol. Exp. Ther.,* 190, 431, 1974.
55. Langer, S. Z., Adler, E., Emero, M. A., and Stefano, F. J. E., The role of alpha receptor in regulating noradrenaline overflow by nerve stimulation, XXVth International Congress on Physiological Sciences, 1971, 335.
56. Farnebo, L. O. and Hamberger, B., Drug-induced changes in the release of ^{3}H-monoamines from field stimulated rat brain slices, *Acta Physiol. Scand.* (suppl), 371, 35, 1971.
57. Enero, M. A., Langer, S. Z., Rothlin, R. P., and Stefano, F. J. E., Role of α-adrenoceptor in regulating nordrenaline overflow by nerve stimulation, *Br. J. Pharmacol.,* 44, 672, 1972.

58. **Starke, K.,** Influence of extracellular noradrenaline on the stimulation-evoked secretion of noradrenaline from sympathetic nerves: Evidence for an α-receptor mediated feed-back inhibition of noradrenaline release, *Naunyn-Schmiederbergs Arch. Pharmakol.,* 275, 11, 1972.

59. **Enero, M. A. and Langer, S. Z.,** Influence of reserpine-induced depletion of noradrenaline on the negative feed-back mechanism for transmitter release during nerve stimulation, *Br. J. Pharmacol.,* 49, 214, 1973.

60. **Langer, S. Z.,** The regulation of transmitter release elicited by nerve stimulation through a presynaptic feed-back mechanism, in *Frontiers in Catecholamine Research,* Usdin, E. and Snyder, S., Eds., Pergamon Press, New York, 1973, 543.

61. **Dubocovich, M. and Langer, S. Z.,** Negative feed-back regulation of noradrenaline release by nerve stimulation in the perfused cat's spleen: differences in potency of phenoxybenzamine in blocking the pre and post synaptic adrenergic receptors, *J. Physiol.* (London), 237, 505, 1974.

62. **Langer, S. Z.,** Presynaptic regulation of catecholamine release, *Biochem. Pharmacol.,* 23, 1973, 1974.

63. **Biscardi, A. M., Carpi, A., and Orsingher, O. A.,** Urinary excretion of catecholamines in the rat after their liberation by reserpine or dexamphetamine, *Br. J. Pharmacol.,* 23, 529, 1964.

64. **Smith, C. B.,** Effects of d-amphetamine upon brain amine content and locomotor activity of mice, *J. Pharmacol. Exp. Ther.,* 147, 96, 1965.

65. **Grabarits, F., Lal, H., and Chessick, R. D.,** Effects of cocaine on brain NE in relation to toxicity and convulsions in mice, *J. Pharm. Pharmacol.,* 18, 131, 1966.

66. **Baird, J. R. C. and Lewis, J. J.,** The effects of cocaine amphetamine and some amphetamine-like compounds on the *in vivo* levels of noradrenaline and dopamine in the rat brain, *Biochem. Pharmacol.,* 13, 1475, 1964.

67. **Bralet, J. and Lallemant, A. M.,** Influence of cocaine on synthesis and release of brain noradrenaline, *Arch. Int. Pharmacodyn. Ther.,* 217, 332, 1975.

68. **Costa, E., Groppetti, A., and Naimzada, M. K.,** Effects of amphetamine on the turnover rate of brain catecholamines and motor activity, *Br. J. Pharmacol.,* 44, 742, 1972.

69. **Groppetti, A., Zambotti, F., Biazzi, A., and Mantegazza, P.,** Amphetamine and cocaine on amine turnover, in *Frontiers in Catecholamine Research,* Usdin, E. and Snyder, S., Eds., Pergamon Press, New York, 1973, 917.

70. **Holz, R. W., Deguchi, T., and Axelrod, J.,** Stimulation of serotonin N-acetyltransferase in pineal organ culture by drugs, *J. Neurochem.,* 22, 205, 1974.

71. **Ross, S. B. and Renyi, A. L.,** Inhibition of the uptake of tritiated catecholamines by antidepressant and related agents, *Eur. J. Pharmacol.,* 2, 181, 1967.

72. **Carmichael, F. J. and Israel, Y.,** In vitro inhibitory effects of narcotic analgesics and other psychotropic drugs on the active uptake of norepinephrine in mouse brain tissue, *J. Pharmacol. Exp. Ther.,* 186, 253, 1973.

73. **Rutledge, C. O., Azzaro, A. J., and Ziance, R. J.,** Dissociation of amphetamine-induced release of norepinephrine from inhibition of neuronal uptake in isolated brain tissue, in *Frontiers in Catecholamine Research,* Usdin, E. and Snyder, S., Eds., Pergamon Press, New York, 1973, 973.

74. **Glowinski, J. and Axelrod, J.,** Effect of drugs on the uptake release and metabolism of ^{3}H-norepinephrine in the rat brain, *J. Pharmacol. Exp. Ther.,* 149, 43, 1965.

75. **Fekete, M. and Borsey, J.,** Chloropromazine-cocaine antagonism: its relation to changes of dopamine metabolism in the brain, *Eur. J. Pharmacol.,* 16, 171, 1971.

76. **Carr, L. A. and Moore, K. F.,** Release of norepinephrine and normetanephrine from cat brain by central nervous system stimulants, *Biochem. Pharmacol.,* 19, 2671, 1970.

77. **Pletscher, A. and Da Prada, M.,** Veräuderungen des cerebralen dopamin-Metabolisms durch Psychopharmaca, *Helv. Physiol. Acta,* 24, C45, 1966.

78. **Sharman, D. F.,** Changes in the metabolism of 3,4-dihydroxyphenylethylamine (dopamine) in the striatum of the mouse induced by drugs, *Br. J. Pharmacol.,* 28, 153, 1966.

79. **Nybök, N., Borzecki, Z., and Sedvall, G.,** Accumulation and disappearance of catecholamines formed from tyrosine-^{14}C in mouse brain: effect of some psychotropic drugs, *Eur. J. Pharmacol.,* 4, 395, 1968.

80. **Galli, C. G., Eves, T., Cattabeni, F., Spano, P. F., Algeri, S., Di Giulio, A. M., and Groppetti, A.,** A mass fragmentographic assay of 3-methoxytyramine in rat brain areas, *J. Neurochem.,* in press, 1976.

81. **Carlsson, A. and Lindqvist, M.,** Effect of chloropromazine or haloperidol on formation of 3-methoxytyramine and normethanephrine in mouse brain, *Acta Pharmacol. Toxicol.,* 20, 140, 1963.

82. **Kehr, W., Carlsson, A., and Lindqvist, M.,** Biochemical aspects of dopamine agonists, in *Advances in Neurology,* Vol. 9, Calne, D. B., Chase, T., and Barbeau, A., Eds., Raven Press, New York, 1975, 185.

83. **Coyle, J. T. and Snyder, S. H.,** Antiparkinsonian drugs: inhibition of dopamine uptake in the corpus striatum as a possible mechanism of action, *Science,* 166, 899, 1969.

84. **Farnebo, L. O., Fuxe, K., Hamberger, B., and Ljungdahl, H.,** Effect of some antiparkinsonian drugs on catecholamine neurons, *J. Pharm. Pharmacol.,* 22, 737, 1970.

85. **Di Giulio, A. M., Groppetti, A., Ponzio, F., Algeri, S., Cattabeni, F., Galli, C. C., and Spano, P. F.,** Measurement of dopamine metabolites specific activity in rat striatum: a new method to study dopaminergic neuronal activity, *J. Pharm. Pharmacol.,* in press, 1976.

86. **Scheel-Kruger, J.,** Behavioral and biochemical comparison of amphetamine derivatives, cocaine, benztropine and tricyclic antidepressant drugs, *Eur. J. Pharmacol.,* 18, 63, 1972.

87. Holzer, G. and Hornykiewicz, O., Uber den dopamin (Hydroxytyramine) stoffwechsel in gehirn der ratte, *Naunyn-Schmiedebergs Arch. Pharmakol.*, 237, 27, 1959.

88. Bernheimer, H. and Hornykiewicz, O., Wirkung von Phenotiazin derivaten auf den dopamin (3-Hydroxy-tyramine) stoffwechsel in Nucleus caudatus, *Naunyn-Schmiedebergs Arch. Pharmakol.*, 251, 135, 1965.

89. Menon, M. K., Dandiya, P. C., and Bapna, J. S., Modification of the effect of some central stimulants in mice pretreated with α-methyl-1-tyrosine, *Psychopharmacologia*, 10, 437, 1967.

90. Simon, P., Psychopharmacological profile of cocaine, in *Frontiers in Catecholamine Research*, Usdin, E. and Snyder, S., Eds., Pergamon Press, New York, 1973, 1043.

91. Van Rossum, J. M., Significance of dopamine in psychomotor stimulant action, *Proc. 2nd Pharmacol. Meeting*, Vol. 2, Trabucchi, E., Paoletti, R., and Canal, N., Eds., Macmillan, London, 1964, 115.

92. Galambos, E., Pfeifer, A. K., György, L., and Molnar, J., Study on the excitation induced by amphetamine, cocaine and alphamethyl-tryptamine, *Psychopharmacologia*, 11, 122, 1967.

93. Barzaghi, F., Groppetti, A., Mantegazza, P., and Muller, E. E., Reduction of food intake by apomorphine: a pimozide-sensitive effect, *J. Pharm. Pharmacol.*, 25, 911, 1973.

94. Simon, P., Sultan, Z., Chermat, R., and Boissier, J. R., La cocaine, une substance amphétaminique? Un problème de psychopharmacologie expérimentale, *J. Pharmacol.* (Paris), 3, 129, 1972.

95. Friedman, E., Gershon, S., Rotrose, J., Effects of acute cocaine treatment on the turnover of 5-hydroxytryptamine in the rat brain, *Br. J. Pharmacol.*, 54(1) 61, 1975.

96. Schubert, J., Fyrö, B., Nybäck, H.. and Sedvall, G., Effects of cocaine and amphetamine on the metabolism of tryptophan and 5-hydroxytryptamine in mouse brain in vivo, *J. Pharm. Pharmacol.*, 22, 860, 1970.

97. Knapp, S. and Mandell, A. J., Narcotic drugs: effects on the serotonin biosynthetic-system of the brain, *Science*, 177, 1209, 1972.

98. Ross, S. B. and Renyi, A. L., Accumulation of tritiated 5-hydroxytryptamine in brain slices, *Life Sci.*, 6, 1407, 1967.

99. Segawa, T., Kuruma, I., Takatsuka, K., and Takagi, H., The influence of drugs on the uptake of 5-hydroxytryptamine by synaptic vesicles of rabbit brain stem, *J. Pharm. Pharmacol.*, 20, 800, 1968.

100. Wallach, M. B., Friedman, E.. and Gershon, S., Behavioral and neurochemical effects of psychotomimetic drugs in neonate chicks, *Eur. J. Pharmacol.*, 17, 259 1972.

101. Andén, N. E., Corrodi, H., Fuxe, K., and Hokfelt, T., Evidence for a central 5-hydroxytyptamine receptor stimulation by lysergic acid diethylamide, *Br. J. Pharmacol.*, 34, 1, 1968.

102. Aghajanian, G. K., Foote, W. E., and Sheard, M. H., Action of psychotogenic drugs on single mid brain raphe neurons, *J. Pharmacol. Exp. Ther.*, 171, 178, 1970.

103. Langer, S. Z. and Enero, M. A., The potentiation of responses to adrenergic nerve stimulation in the presence of cocaine: its relationship to the metabolic fate of released norepinephrine, *J. Pharmacol. Exp. Ther.*, 191, 431, 1974.

Behavior, Psychic, Neuropharmacologic and Physiologic Aspects

Pharmacokinetics of Intravenous Cocaine Self-injection

PHARMACOKINETICS OF INTRAVENOUS COCAINE SELF-INJECTION

John Dougherty and Roy Pickens

TABLE OF CONTENTS

INTRODUCTION

In 1968, Pickens and Thompson published the first comprehensive study of intravenous cocaine self-injection in rats.[21] In that study, rats were fitted with chronic intravenous cannulas and placed in operant chambers where each lever-press response resulted in the injection of a fixed dose of cocaine. The resulting self-injection behavior was viewed as an example of operant conditioning, in which the drug injection served as a reinforcer for responses leading to its presentation. In examining the prominent characteristics of the behavior, Pickens and Thompson found that response rate (injection rate) varied inversely in an almost linear fashion with the size of the injection dose. That is, as the dose was increased, response rate decreased. These changes in response rate that occurred following changes in injection dose resulted in the maintenance of a relatively stable rate of drug intake. That is, while the size of the injection dose was increased over an eightfold range (0.25 to 2.0 mg/kg), drug intake increased only by about 25% (from 5.3 to 7.3 mg/kg/hr).

Even more prominent was their finding that single responses and injections were followed by relatively long, highly uniform periods of time in which no responses occurred (Figure 1). These periods remained relatively constant even when up to 80 responses per injection were required. The duration of these intervals varied directly with the size of the injection dose. For example, at a dose of 0.5 mg/kg, injections were spaced about 7 min apart, while at 1.0 mg/kg, injections occurred about every 11 min. The increases in these intervals with increasing doses therefore explained the decreases in response rate. Similar effects were later obtained in cocaine self-injection in rhesus monkeys.[11,31]

It was apparent from these results that cocaine self-injection behavior had unique temporal

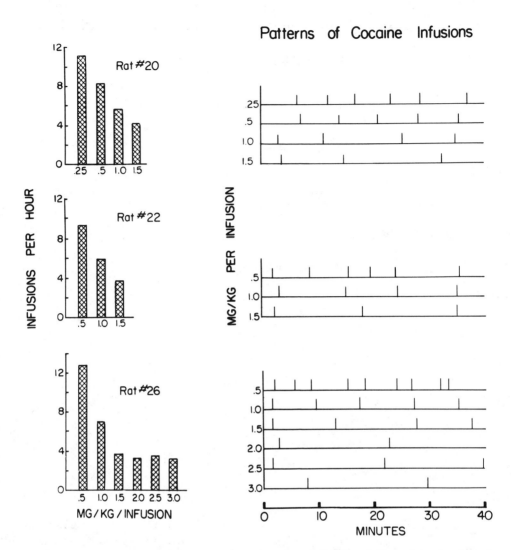

FIGURE 1. Rate and pattern of cocaine self-injections. Left side of figure shows number of injections (infusions) per hour for three rats at several injection doses. Except at the highest doses, there was an inverse relationship between injection dose and injection frequency. The right side illustrates the uniform intervals separating injections and the dependency of the duration of those intervals on the size of the injection dose. Each vertical mark represents a drug injection occurring during a 40-min segment of a longer self-injection session. (From Pickens, R. and Thompson, T., *J. Pharmacol. Exp. Ther.*, 161, 122, 1968. With permission.)

characteristics that could not be explained solely in terms of the reinforcing properties of the drug. Consequently, several hypotheses were advanced which attempted to explain self-injection behavior by reference to other pharmacologic effects of the drug. This avenue of reasoning was further supported by the effects of experimenter-administered doses of cocaine to animals whose lever-pressing responses were reinforced with food pellets. In these animals, cocaine produced dose-dependent pauses in responding that occurred immediately following the drug injection and

which were almost identical in duration to the intervals found during self-injection (Figure 2).

One explanation of the uniformity of the intervals following injections was that the rats were temporarily satiated in a manner analogous to the cessation of responding that occurs in food-reinforced behavior after the delivery of large amounts of food.[19] Another suggestion was that cocaine might produce aversive effects and thereby suppress responding immediately after an injection,[22] or that long intervals might occur because of non-specific disruptive effects of the

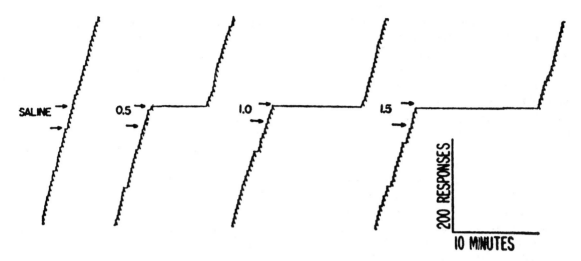

FIGURE 2. Effects of cocaine on the food-reinforced responding. Cumulative records of lever-press responding are depicted, with vertical excursion indicating responses and short diagonal strokes indicating the delivery of a food pellet after the completion of each tenth response (Fixed-Ratio 10 schedule). Intravenous saline (injection started at lower arrow and terminated at upper arrow) had no effect on responding, while cocaine in doses of 0.5, 1.0, and 1.5 mg/kg produced a complete cessation of responding for 6, 10, and 14 min respectively, afterwhich responding abruptly returned to the pre-drug rate. (Pickens, R. and Thompson, T., *J. Pharmacol. Exp. Ther.,* 161, 122, 1968. With permission.)

drug on ongoing responding, perhaps as a result of the stereotyped head and paw movements produced by cocaine.[8,31] On a more pharmacologic level, it was hypothesized that response rate may be adjusted by some mechanism operating to keep drug intake rate or drug plasma levels constant.[31,34]

To learn more about the quantitative and temporal aspects of cocaine self-injection, between 1971 and the present we conducted the series of experiments described in this chapter. Some of the specific questions for which we sought answers included:

1. What is the form of the relationship between injection dose and the ensuing period of nonresponding, and how does the rate of drug intake change when injection dose is varied over a wide range?

2. Are there any systematic changes in self-injection behavior over time?

3. What are the effects of other drugs on the rate and temporal pattern of behavior?

4. Are the uniform intervals which follow injections evident upon first exposure to the drug in naive animals?

Using the data obtained from these studies, we have formulated a systematic account of cocaine self-injection behavior based upon the time course of drug distribution and elimination in the body.

We propose that the temporal pattern of cocaine injections can best be described in terms of known pharmacokinetic processes which characterize the quantitative relationship between the drug and its site(s) of action.

GENERAL METHOD

Subjects — Except where otherwise indicated, the subjects in the following experiments were albino Sprague-Dawley (Holtzman) rats, ranging in age from 120 to 220 days old, with free access to food and water, and maintained at a room temperature of 24°C, in constant illumination.

Drugs — Cocaine hydrochloride powder U.S.P. (Malinkrodt Chemical Co.) was added to sterile physiological saline to make the injection solutions, which were freshly prepared prior to each drug session. Phenobarbital sodium and SKF 525A (diethylaminoethyl diphenylpropylacetate) were both added to sterile water. A stock solution of the former drug was made and used over a period of 4 days, while solutions of the latter drug were prepared just prior to injection. All doses were calculated on the basis of the salts.

Apparatus — Gerbrands Model C operant chambers (23 X 21 X 19 cm deep) were each equipped with two response levers mounted on one wall, small (0.1 W) stimulus lights located above the levers, and a small overhead light for general illumination. The chambers were located within ventilated, sound-attenuating enclosures. Lever-press responses activated electromechanical or solid-state programming equipment (located in an adjoining room) which, in turn, activated the injection pump and illuminated the stimulus lights for the duration of the injection. Responses and interval durations were recorded on digital and print-out counters and on cumulative records. Cocaine injections were delivered into the precava, via an implanted silicone rubber cannula which was attached to a piston-type pump through a flexible harness, leash, and swivel system described in detail elsewhere.[1,20]

Procedure — After cannulation, the rats were attached to the harness and placed in the chambers in which they resided for the duration of each experiment. At least 3 days of recovery were allowed before the introduction of cocaine. To insure cannula patency, noncontingent injections of 0.5-ml heparinized saline were given hourly at times except during cocaine self-injection sessions. Cocaine self-injection was generally restricted to 12-hr sessions conducted approximately every third day, and response levers were operable only during periods of cocaine availability.

Terminology — In most of the experiments discussed below, each lever-press response produced a cocaine injection. In behavioral terminology this is a continuous reinforcement schedule and will be referred to as CRF. Since the period of time separating injections was also a period of time separating responses on CRF schedules, these periods will be referred to as interresponse times or IRTs. The precise definition of pharmacokinetic terms may be found in any standard text.[18]

EFFECTS OF INJECTION DOSE ON IRTs AND DRUG INTAKE RATE

In order to explore the dose-interresponse time (IRT) relationship over a wider range of doses than had previously been used in rats, four rats (T-10, 15, 27, and 28) were allowed to self-inject cocaine at doses of 0.04 to 2.56 mg/kg per injection. Within each drug session, the animal was exposed to three or four injection doses in a random order, with at least 31 consecutive injections obtained at each dose before a new dose was introduced. Except for Rat T-15, each animal was exposed to each dose in three different cocaine sessions. In addition to IRTs, the rate of drug intake in mg/kg/hr was calculated at each dose.

Figure 3 shows that the mean IRT was a direct, linear function of injection dose when plotted on nonlogarithmic coordinates. IRT duration increased by a factor of about 1.8 with each doubling of the dose. A linear regression analysis produced coefficients of determination (r^2) of 0.99 and correlation coefficients (r) of 0.99 in all four rats, and the slopes of the linear functions were similar across all rats.

The injection dose was changed in mid-session by changing the duration of the injection, and this could be accomplished without any indications to the animal. When the dose was changed, the following IRT was immediately adjusted to the appropriate duration without any disruption or transition of the temporal response pattern. For example, when the dose was changed from 1.28 to 0.16 mg/kg, the IRT decreased from about 550 sec to about 100 sec. A nonparametric sign test found no significant differences between the first or second IRT after a dose increase or decrease and the mean IRT at the new dose ($p > 0.05$, N = 19, 28).

Rat T-15 was allowed to self-inject a cocaine dose of 5.12 mg/kg. The first IRT after this dose was about twice as long as the mean IRT at 2.56 mg/kg. Subsequent IRTs were shorter, however, with the rat convulsing after each injection. The rat died after the fourth injection. These convulsions did not reduce responding or decrease drug intake. In fact, after the second injection, drug intake increased before death. This result indicates that any aversive effects that cocaine might produce are not sufficient to prevent the self-injection of lethal amounts of the drug, and they are therefore probably not responsible for the maintenance of uniform IRT durations.

An examination of Figure 4 shows that the rate of drug intake was a rough linear function of log dose, increasing by a factor of two over a range where the dose was doubled six times. This is obviously a consequence of the IRT-dose relationship in which doubling the dose resulted in a 45%, rather than a 50% decrease in injection frequency. This finding is not unusual in that similar intake rate functions are also seen in cocaine self-injection in monkeys,[11,30] and in barbiturate, ethanol, nicotine, and amphetamine self-injection in rats and monkeys.[2,11,32,33]

These findings indicate that a very precise

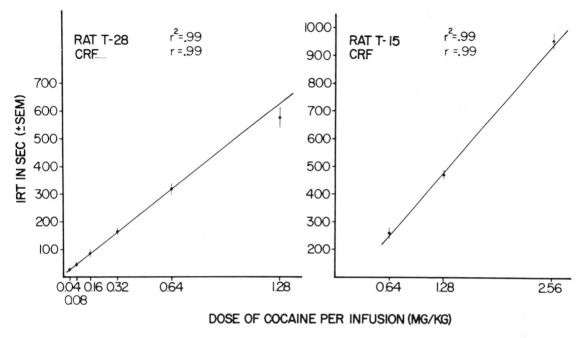

FIGURE 3. Effect of injection dose on IRTs. For Rat T-28, each point is the mean of 90 IRTs collected over several drug sessions. For Rat T-15, the 0.64 mg/kg point represents the mean of 20 IRTs from one session, and the 1.28 and 2.56 mg/kg points were the means of 60 IRTs from three sessions. Rat T-15 died before a full dose-response function could be determined (see text). The injection durations, which ranged from 3 to 50 sec, had no effect on IRTs and were therefore excluded from IRT calculations. The regression line was fitted by visual inspection. The functions for Rats T-10 and T-27 (not shown) were determined over the full dosage range and were identical to that found with Rat T-28.

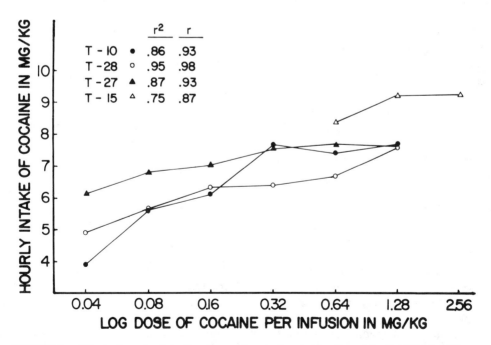

FIGURE 4. Effect of cocaine injection dose on hourly drug intake. Except for Rat T-15 (see Figure 3 legend), each point is the average intake rate in three separate sessions in which cocaine was self-injected according to continuous reinforcement schedule. Hourly intake measure is in real time and therefore includes injection durations. Linear regression analysis coefficients of determination (r^2) and correlation coefficients (r) are listed for each rat.

control over behavior is exerted by some variable associated with the size of the injection dose. The relationship between IRT duration and injection dose was linear over a 64-fold range of doses, with 99% of the variance attributable to the linear functions within animals, and with the slopes of the functions almost identical across animals. Such consistency is remarkable when considered against the variability usually found with behavioral measures of drug effect in more complex situations.

Since the IRT can be regarded as the duration of a behavioral effect of cocaine, the dose-IRT plots can be compared with dose-duration of effect plots typically found in the pharmacological literature. It is commonly found that within the 20 to 80% intensity of effect range, the duration of effect is linear with dose on a log scale.[9,27] The linear functions found between cocaine dose and IRT duration, when plotted on Cartesian coordinates, are therefore quite different, and it is not possible to calculate the exponential half-life of the drug in plasma from the cocaine plots as can be done from log-linear functions.[9] This indicates that either the elimination of cocaine is not exponential (i.e., elimination rate is not directly proportional to the concentration of unchanged drug) or that the relevant intensity of effect is below 20% or above 80% of the maximum. Since it has recently been determined that cocaine is exponentially eliminated from plasma and brain[17] (also see chapter by A. L. Misra), the latter situation is more likely.

The systematic variation in cocaine intake rate with injection dose, while small, suggests that drug intake is not the end point by which response rate is determined. Rather, the data suggest that intake rate and response rate are joint functions of some other variable associated with size of the injection dose. In support of this interpretation are the results from a study of fixed-interval (FI) schedules of cocaine self-injection, where the rate of drug intake can be varied independently of injection dose by varying the minimum period of time between injections.[3] When intake rate was varied between 4.6 and 9.2 mg/kg/hr (FI values of 200 to 480 sec), at an injection dose of 0.64 mg/kg, the mean period of time separating previous injections from the next response remained relatively constant at about 255 sec. Thus, the independence of drug intake rate from the duration of pausing following an injection on

FI schedules further indicates that IRT duration and cocaine self-injection frequency on CRF schedules are not adjusted in order to maintain constant body levels of the drug or a constant rate of drug intake. Rather, IRT duration appears to be an immediate consequence of events occurring subsequent to the previous drug injection.

SYSTEMATIC CHANGES IN IRT DURATION

Although the mean IRT duration at each injection dose remained relatively constant from session to session, there were systematic changes within each period of self-injection. One of these changes consisted of a brief period of very short IRTs (rapid responding) that preceded the appearance of long, uniform IRTs at the beginning of each session. Other changes were cyclical variations in IRT duration that occurred over short periods of time and a gradual lengthening of IRTs over the entire session. A close examination of these changes provides additional information on the variables controlling self-injection behavior.

The durations of the first 32 IRTs in self-injection sessions were recorded in three rats at three injection doses. As can be seen from Figure 5, there were two distinct phases consisting of a period of short IRTs followed by an abrupt (Rat T-24) or relatively gradual (T-27 and 28) change to much longer IRTs characteristic of the remainder of the session. The number of injections before the change to longer IRTs was a function of injection dose, being fewer with higher doses in all three animals. The amount of drug injected during the rapid responding phase did not vary systematically with injection dose but was different across animals. These short IRTs appeared only at the beginning of the session and did not occur when the dose was changed in mid-session (Figures 3 and 4 are based on IRT means which do not include these short IRTs).

The appearance of longer, relatively uniform IRTs after a period of much more rapid responding may reflect the attainment of a pharmacologic steady-state.[18] In terms of drug concentration, steady-state levels reflect the accumulation of drug within the body until the rate of exponential drug elimination rises to equal the rate of drug intake. At steady state, drug concentrations fluctuate between relatively narrow upper and lower limits. The duration of effect,

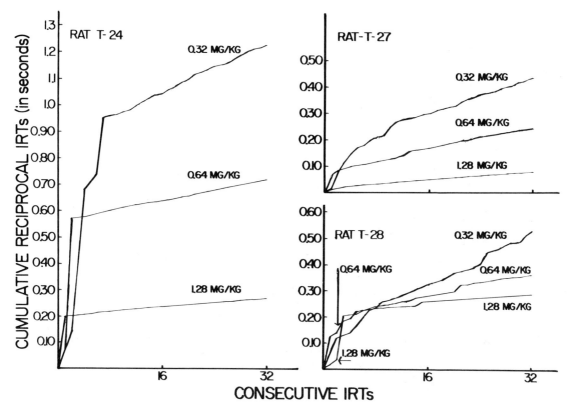

FIGURE 5. Rapid responding at beginning of cocaine session. The durations of the first 32 IRTs in each selected session are plotted as cumulative reciprocals. With a reciprocal transformation of the data, shorter IRT durations are emphasized and the relatively greater variability associated with the much longer durations is minimized, thereby providing a convenient graphical presentation that clearly identifies the transition. All injection durations were 25 sec and were not included in the data analysis.

being proportional to the fluctuations in drug concentration, would also increase and then become stable. Therefore, the duration of cocaine IRTs may increase and become uniform in a similar manner. From these considerations, it also follows that steady state will be attainable faster with higher doses of the drug. The observation that the number of cocaine injections to the appearance of the stable IRT pattern was fewer with higher injection doses may be a reflection of this relationship.

Following the period of rapid responding, IRTs lengthen and fluctuate about a stable modal value. These variations in IRT duration seem to vary in a cyclical manner over short time periods. Figure 6 shows these cyclical variations in one rat at three injection doses. The size of the injection dose had no apparent effect on periodicity, except that responding became irregular at the end of the high-dose session. These variations in IRT duration may reflect a self-adjusting process that is often

seen when the controlling variables of the situation are in part determined by some aspect of behavior (e.g., response pattern on adjusting ratio schedules[23] and shock titration schedules[29]). In cocaine self-injection, a single long IRT may lower drug levels and therefore shorten the duration of effect of the next injection. Shorter IRT durations will then result in progressively higher drug levels which will again produce longer IRTs.

In Figure 6, it appears that the modal IRT duration increases gradually over the session, with the rate of increase being faster at higher injection doses. However, since session length was based on number of IRTs, and not time, the actual rate of increase is obscured. Figure 7 shows that IRT duration actually increased with time independently of injection dose within the range of doses explored. With the exception of the lowest dose for Rat T-27, IRTs increased at about 7% per hour regardless of dose.

There are several possible explanations of these

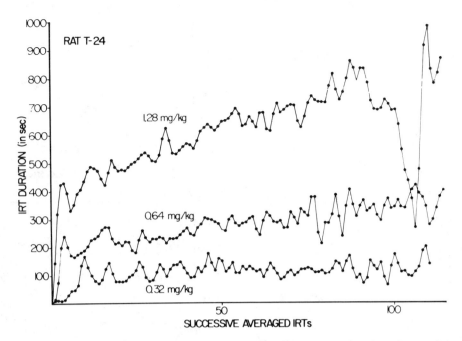

FIGURE 6. Cyclic variation in inter-injection intervals. Graph shows duration of successive IRTs in separate sessions at three injection doses in Rat T-24. Oscillations in IRT duration have been smoothed by the use of a weighted three-term moving average according to the formula: $\bar{x}$ $IRT_j = (IRT_{j-1} + 2IRT_j + IRT_{j+1})/4$ (see Reference 28).

increases in IRTs. Since several investigators have found that successive daily injections of cocaine produced an increased sensitivity to the drug in dogs, rats, and monkeys,[6,7,25] the increases in IRTs may then reflect an increase in physiological sensitivity during the session. More plausible, however, is the possibility that increases in IRT duration reflect the accumulation of less rapidly eliminated active metabolites. It should be noted that in spite of the slow decrease in the rate of cocaine intake within sessions, there was no tendency to either increase or decrease intake across drug sessions.

INDUCTION AND INHIBITION OF COCAINE BIOTRANSFORMATION

The foregoing experiments have suggested that IRT durations are a function of the kinetics of cocaine in the body. Direct evidence for this relationship, in the form of correlations between self-injection behavior and decreases in plasma or brain levels of the drug, is not available. However, the following experiment indirectly explored this relationship by determining changes in IRT duration after phenobarbital induction and SKF 525A inhibition of cocaine biotransformation.

Phenobarbital acts to induce the rate of drug inactivation by enhancing the rate of reactions catalyzed by a collection of nonspecific drug-metabolizing enzymes (the microsomal system) found in the endoplasmic reticulum in cells of the liver and other organs.[10] SKF 525A is widely used to inhibit drug biotransformation and acts primarily by competing with other drugs for microsomal and nonmicrosomal drug-metabolizing enzymes.[15]

Prior to phenobarbital induction, two experienced rats were allowed to self-inject cocaine at 0.64 mg/kg per injection for two 6-hr sessions to provide pretreatment baseline IRT durations. Phenobarbital sodium, 40 mg/kg (as the salt), was then administered i.p. at 5:00 p.m. on 4 successive days. Short, 3-hr cocaine sessions were started at noon on each day following phenobarbital injections in order to observe changes in IRT duration during the development of induction. Starting 2 days after the last injection of phenobarbital, 6-hr cocaine sessions were conducted daily for at least 6 days and then on 2 days 2 weeks later.

Mean IRT duration decreased after the first phenobarbital injection, and it continued to decline after additional injections until reaching a level of 60 to 70% of the pretreatment duration at

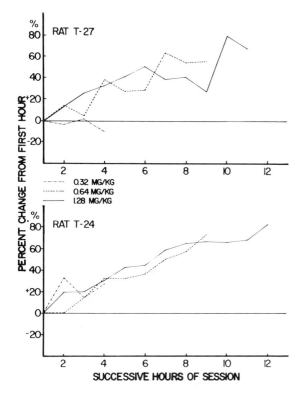

FIGURE 7. Percentage increase in inter-injection intervals within cocaine sessions. The increases are expressed as the mean percent change for each hour of the session relative to the IRT mean in the first hour of stabilized responding (which was the second hour of the session). The first hour of the session was excluded because it contained the initial period of rapid responding. Each session contained from 100 to 120 injections, which accounts for the shorter session lengths at lower injection doses.

48 hr after the last treatment (Figure 8). The mean IRT duration then gradually increased for 4 to 5 days, dropped slightly, and then returned to pretreatment durations 2 weeks later. During induction and recovery the uniformity of the shortened IRTs was not disrupted, but appeared to become even more regular. The time course of IRT duration changes was similar in both rats, and it is almost identical to the time course of stimulation of microsomal N-demethylation and elevation of cytochrome P-450 levels when the same dose, dosage regimen, and strain of rats are used.[24]

Cocaine is a tertiary amine with a methyl group available for N-demethylation by microsomes, a route that has been demonstrated in vitro.[13] This evidence suggests that N-demethylation of cocaine to norcocaine may occur in vivo and may account for up to 25% of the administered dose. This

hypothesis has recently been confirmed by in vivo experiments which have identified norcocaine as a cocaine metabolite in rat brain.[16]

In order to assess the effects of a metabolic inhibitor, SKF 525A in doses of 5.0, 10.0, 20.0, and 40.0 mg/kg (as the salt) was injected i.p. 50 min before the start of 6-hr cocaine sessions scheduled 2 to 3 days apart. Saline control pretreatments were given in the sessions preceding and following each SKF session. Doses of 10.0 mg/kg and above produced dose-dependent increases in cocaine IRT duration in two rats for as long as 10 hr after injection (Figure 9). IRT uniformity after SKF 525A was not systematically different from saline control sessions.

The effect of SKF 525A was also examined on the period of rapid responding occurring at the beginning of each session. SKF 525A produced dose-dependent decreases in the number of injections in this phase. For example, 40.0 mg/kg reduced the number of 0.64 mg/kg cocaine injections to two, as compared with an average of five in sessions following saline pretreatment. This is further support for the suggestion that the appearance of uniform IRTs reflects the attainment of a pharmacologic steady state.

The effects of phenobarbital and SKF 525A on cocaine self-injection are consistent with their known effects on the biotransformation of other drugs. This suggests that IRT duration was decreased by phenobarbital because of an increased rate of cocaine inactivation, and that SKF 525A increased IRT duration by inhibiting cocaine inactivation. Therefore, while it appears that drug interactions unrelated to cocaine's CNS effects may alter quantitative aspects of self-injection behavior, the observation that neither drug affected IRT variability (uniformity) is an indication that the stimulus properties of cocaine and the form of the kinetic relationships were not altered.

Further evidence for IRT durations in intravenous self-injection being determined by cocaine kinetics in the body is obtained from observations of subcutaneous cocaine self-injection behavior. While rats with a history of intravenous cocaine will self-inject via the subcutaneous route, the uniform IRT pattern is not seen. Rather, injections are taken in clusters of 10 to 30 over a period of several minutes and drug intake is much higher. This indicates that rapid onset and offset of drug action are necessary for the maintenance uniform IRTs.

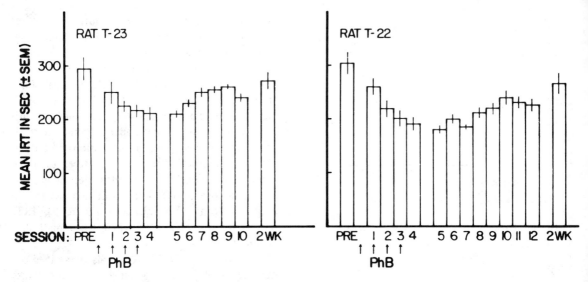

FIGURE 8. Effect of phenobarbital of IRT duration. IRT duration, in seconds, is plotted on vertical axis, with cocaine sessions on the horizontal axis. *PRE* column represents the mean of 100 IRTs collected in two sessions. Arrows indicate 40 mg/kg phenobarbital injections given once daily. Sessions 1 to 4 represent the mean of 20 IRTs from short daily sessions started 19 hr after each phenobarbital injection. Sessions 5 to 10 (Rat T-23) and 5 to 12 (Rat T-22) show the mean of 50 IRTs from daily sessions. *2WK* column is the mean of 100 IRTs from two sessions. A one-tailed t-test was used to compare *PRE* means with the means from Session 5 and *2WK*. The Session 5 means were significantly shorter than *PRE* means for both rats ($p < 0.001$, df = 98), but *2WK* means were not different from *PRE* session values ($0.1 > p > 0.05$, df = 98). (From Dougherty, J. and Pickens, R., Effects of phenobarbital and SKF 525A on cocaine self-administration in rats, in *Drug Addiction, Vol. 3: Neurobiology and Influences on Behavior,* Singh, J. M. and Lal, H., Eds., Symposia Specialists, Miami, 1974. With permission.)

ACQUISITION OF UNIFORM IRTs

If, as is suggested by the previous results, IRT durations are a function of the elimination rate of cocaine in the body, then the behavior of the animal must in some way interact with changes in drug concentration or effect. The immediate appearance of uniform IRTs upon initial exposure of naive animals to cocaine would indicate that this drug-behavior interaction is quite rigidly controlled by the pharmacologic aspects of the drug, i.e., it is analogous to the way in which succinylcholine controls respiratory "behavior." On the other hand, if uniform IRT durations develop gradually with continued exposure to cocaine, then perhaps some process best described in behavioral terms, such as discrimination learning, may also be involved. To evaluate these possibilities, four naive rats (T-23, 24, 27, and 28) were cannulated and placed in the operant chambers for 3 days for recovery. In addition to hourly noncontingent injections of heparinized saline, each lever press during this period produced a 0.5-ml saline injection. This "saline self-injection" period was conducted in order to allow the development of

response topography. On the fourth postoperative day, cocaine was substituted for the saline and the animals were allowed to self-inject cocaine at doses of 0.32 or 0.64 mg/kg (two rats at each dose) until 100 to 120 injections were obtained. At the end of the drug session, the response lever was made inoperative and the hourly saline injections reinstituted until the next period of drug availability. Cocaine sessions were conducted every other day until visual inspection of the records revealed a stable IRT pattern that was similar to that found in experienced animals.

During the recovery period all rats made saline responses, with the average being about 15 per day. In the initial cocaine session, extreme variability in IRT durations was observed (Figure 10), with each animal exhibiting sequences of both very short and very long IRTs. Over the second through fourth sessions, IRT variability decreased to a low level and began to show the gradual increases over the session that are characteristic of stabilized self-injection behavior.

Because of the gradual lengthening of IRT duration within sessions, Figure 10 does not

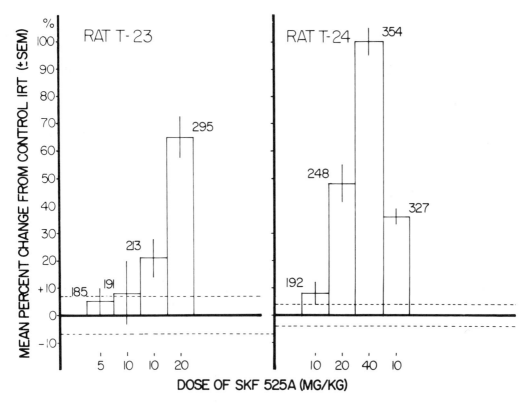

FIGURE 9. Effect of SKF 525A on IRT duration. IRT duration after SKF 525A pretreatment is expressed as mean percent change from previous saline control session. Vertical lines are percent standard errors and numbers adjacent to top of each column indicate mean IRT in seconds. SKF 525A doses are graphed in the sequence in which they were administered. Horizontal dashed lines indicate average percent standard error from all saline control sessions. For Rat T-23, the mean IRT from saline control sessions ranged from 170 to 190 sec and showed no systematic trends. The means of saline control sessions ranged from 182 to 240 sec for Rat T-24 and increased over the experiment. (From Dougherty, J. and Pickens, R., Effects of phenobarbital and SKF 525A on cocaine self-administration in rats, in *Drug Addiction, Vol 3: Neurobiology and Influences on Behavior*, Singh, J. M. and Lal, H., Eds., Symposia Specialists, Miami, 1974. With permission.)

readily reflect IRT uniformity. Therefore, the progressive changes in relative variability of IRTs about the mean (coefficient of variation) are plotted in Figure 11. Because IRT variability is expressed relative to the mean, the systematic increase in mean IRT within sessions does not obscure the development of the stable pattern. The initially high coefficients in the first few sessions reflect a large amount of IRT variability. This variability decreased until the stabilized IRT pattern, as judged from visual inspection of event records, appeared at coefficients of 0.5 or below. The relative variability in the last sessions appears slightly higher for the 0.32 mg/kg rats, but no systematic differences in the number of sessions to stability was seen across doses.

The results indicate that uniform IRTs develop gradually with continued exposure to cocaine and that self-injection of large amounts of the drug in the first session was insufficient to produce the stable pattern. Physiological factors, therefore, do not limit the range of IRT values. Rather, preferences for IRTs of certain durations developed over time. It is likely that internal stimuli related to the intensity of drug effect are discriminable and establish control over lever-pressing behavior. Such an interpretation is supported by the extensive sampling of both high and low drug intake before a stable intermediate rate is finally obtained. Thus, while a variety of drug intake rates and IRTs are possible, both are kept within narrow limits.

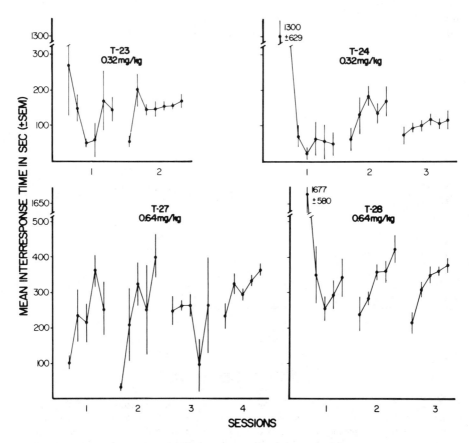

FIGURE 10. Development of uniform IRTs in four naive rats. IRTs are graphed on the horizontal axis for two to four cocaine self-injection sessions. Each point represents the mean and standard error of successive blocks of 20 IRTs over the course of each session. Because IRT durations at 0.64 mg/kg per injection were almost twice as long as at 0.32 mg/kg, session lengths at 0.64 mg/kg were correspondingly longer. (From Dougherty, J. and Pickens, R., *Proc. Am. Psychol. Assoc.*, 81, 1007, 1973. Copyright 1973 by the American Psychological Association. Reprinted by permission.)

PHARMACOKINETICS OF COCAINE SELF-INJECTION

The data obtained thus far indicate that the temporal response pattern, response rate, and drug intake rate in CRF cocaine self-injection can, to a large extent, be accounted for by changes over time in the concentration of the drug at its sites of action, as a result of absorption, distribution, and elimination of the drug. The uniform response pattern appears to be characteristic of a pharmacologic steady state in which IRT durations are determined by the rate of biotransformation and elimination of the drug. Changes in response rate and drug intake rate are apparently secondary to changes in IRT duration.

It is important to distinguish between drug concentration and drug effect when considering dynamic situations such as drug self-injection. Even though the peak effect of a drug is proportional to the concentration, the kinetics of effect differ from the kinetics of drug concentration. Levy[14] has calculated that while drug elimination may proceed exponentially, the decline of intensity of effect will be linear. Linear rates of decline of effect after the administration of exponentially eliminated drugs have been observed with locomotor activity in rats after *d*-amphetamine, and in the impairment of arithmetic performance in humans after LSD.[9,26] In our laboratories, we have observed that the hyperthermia produced by cocaine and morphine also declines at a constant rate.

A recent study on cocaine elimination from brain and plasma has provided information indicating that IRT durations in cocaine self-injection

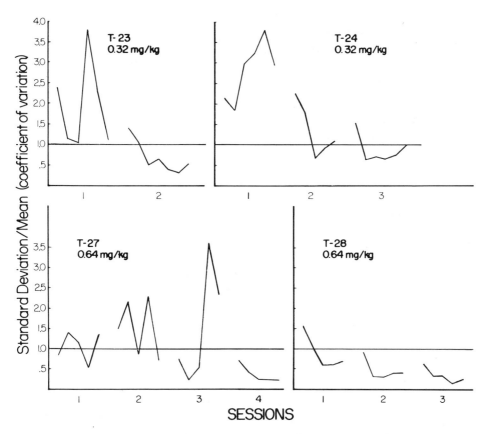

FIGURE 11. Changes in coefficient of variation during development of uniform IRTs. The coefficient of variation is defined as the IRT standard deviation divided by the IRT mean for each of the 20-IRT blocks in Figure 5. It is apparent that the coefficient of variation can provide a convenient numerical index for the assessment of the acquisition of temporal response patterns. (From Dougherty, J. and Pickens, R., *Proc. Am. Psychol. Assoc.*, 81, 1007, 1973. Copyright 1973 by the American Psychological Association. Reprinted by permission.)

are determined by the decline of drug effect rather than drug concentration. Nayak and co-workers[17] (see also chapter by A. L. Misra) measured cocaine concentrations in rats after single i.v. injections. Their data show that cocaine elimination from brain and plasma is not monoexponential but consists of at least two exponential phases. The first phase primarily reflects the distribution from the central kinetic compartment (into which the drug was injected) to a peripheral compartment. The second, slower phase, represents elimination, a combination of biotransformation and excretion. The exponential elimination rate derived from these data was then used to calculate drug levels and to predict IRT durations in cocaine self-injection. We found that while the exponential rate constant did not predict the linear relationship between IRT and injection dose (Figure 3), the use of a linear constant did.

Besides having different kinetics, effect has another property not shared by drug concentration: upper limits. While peak drug concentrations are proportional to the size of the injected dose, the intensity of effect increases with dose until an upper limit of effect is reached. Further increases in dose produce no further increases in effect, resulting in the familiar sigmoid curve relating dose to percent of effect. There is evidence suggesting that in cocaine self-injection the intensity of effect may be fluctuating in the 80 to 100% range. With drugs, such as cocaine, which follow two-compartment kinetics, linear relationships between duration of effect (e.g., IRT) and dose may be found at around the 80% effect intensity level (i.e., the duration of the decline of effect from 100 to 80%), but not at lower intensities where the relationship tends to become linear with log dose. Also, in an experiment now in progress on the effect of cocaine on rectal temperature in rats, we have found that the same peak temperature is reached after injections of 4.0 and 8.0 mg/kg, doses which produce cocaine concentrations in the body in the same range as those occurring at steady state during self-injection.

A study of response duration in cocaine self-injection also suggests that the intensity of effect may be close to 100%. In this experiment, cocaine self-injections were programmed such that the injection continued only for the duration of the lever-press response. In this situation, therefore, the behavior of the animal determined both the size of the injection dose and IRT duration. The behavior on this schedule consisted of short response durations of 200 to 600 msec, and short IRTs. Figure 12 shows cumulative records of this behavior for one rat at three cocaine solution concentrations. Decreases in slope at higher concentrations are because of increases in IRT duration. Response durations remained unchanged across all concentrations, and they were the same as durations found during prior food-reinforced responding and during previous fixed-dose cocaine self-injection within the same animals. Because response durations were unchanged, the mean dose of cocaine obtained per response increased linearly with increases in solution concentration. Similar to fixed-dose self-injection, IRT durations were a direct, linear function of the mean obtained dose per injection.

The absence of differences in response duration indicates that there are no strong preferences for injection doses of a particular size. Perhaps this occurs because of a ceiling on the intensity of effect. A ceiling on the effect of cocaine may also explain why the maximum number of progressive-ratio responses maintained by intravenous cocaine under some conditions increases up to a maximum and then remains constant as injection dose is increased.[12] If the reinforcing properties of cocaine are related to an intensity of cocaine effect, then further increases in dose will not result in higher response rates once the maximal effect has been reached.

After a self-injection of cocaine, the decline of intensity of some pharmacologic effect of the drug to a particular level may be the stimulus condition that determines when a response will be initiated. Likewise, the increase in some intensity of effect to a particular level may be a discriminative stimulus for the cessation of responding. The

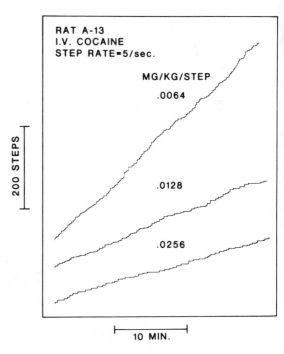

FIGURE 12. Cumulative records of cocaine self-injection. Each curve is a segment of cumulative response records from separate self-injection sessions at different cocaine solution concentrations. Cocaine was delivered only for the duration of the lever-press response. The drug was delivered in 0.01-ml pulses at a rate of five pulses per second while the lever was held down. The cumulative recorder was programmed to step once with each pulse. Therefore, small vertical segments of curves show response durations and number of pulsed injections for each response. For this rat, mean response durations were between 200 to 230 msec at all three solution concentrations. Consequently, the mean amount of drug injected during each response increased from 0.014 to 0.052 mg/kg in a linear fashion as concentration was increased. Differences in the slopes of the cumulative records reflect increases in IRT duration at higher concentrations. Mean IRT durations were 9, 22, and 31 sec at 0.64, 1.28, and 2.56 mg/kg/ml concentrations, respectively. IRT duration was a direct, linear function of the mean amount of drug injected per response.

acquisition of uniform IRT durations over several self-injection sessions in naive animals may reflect the formation of such a discrimination. The absence of uniform IRTs during subcutaneous self-injection in experienced animals supports this interpretation.

CONCLUSIONS

The retrospective application of pharmacokinetic concepts to cocaine self-injection behavior results in our being able to account for many of the dynamic aspects of that behavior in terms of the time course of drug effect. The next step is to validate this approach by finding additional correlations between drug levels and behavior, and by using pharmacokinetic data to predict behavior in new situations. The obvious potential value of the kinetic approach is the well defined mathematical relationships governing the behavior of the drug in the body. To the extent that the behavior of the organism is correlated with drug kinetics, numerical predictions of the probability of behavior in time can then be made.

ACKNOWLEDGMENTS

This research was supported by USPHS Grant MH14112, awarded to the University of Minnesota, and by the Veterans Administration Hospital, Lexington, Kentucky (Project #596-1737-02). We would like to thank Dr. Carol Iglauer for helpful comments on the manuscript.

REFERENCES

1. **Davis, J. D.,** A method for chronic intravenous infusion in freely moving rats, *J. Exp. Anal. Behav.*, 9, 385, 1966.
2. **Deneau, G. and Inoki, R.,** Nicotine self-administration in monkeys, *Ann. N.Y. Acad. Sci.*, 142, 277, 1967.
3. **Dougherty, J. and Pickens, R.,** Fixed-interval schedules of intravenous cocaine presentation in rats, *J. Exp. Anal. Behav.*, 20, 111, 1973.
4. **Dougherty, J. and Pickens, R.,** Development of temporal patterns of cocaine self-administration, *Proc. Am. Psychol. Assoc.*, 81, 1007, 1973.
5. **Dougherty, J. and Pickens, R.,** Effects of phenobarbital and SKF 525A on cocaine self-administration in rats, in *Drug Addiction, Vol. 3: Neurobiology and Influences on Behavior*, Singh, J. M. and Lal, H., Eds., Symposia Specialists, Miami, 1974.
6. **Downs, A. W. and Eddy, N. B.,** The effect of repeated doses of cocaine on the dog, *J. Pharmacol. Exp. Ther.*, 46, 195, 1932.
7. **Downs, A. W. and Eddy, N. B.,** The effect of repeated doses of cocaine on the rat, *J. Pharmacol. Exp. Ther.*, 46, 199, 1932.
8. **Fog, R.,** Sterotyped and non-stereotyped behavior in rats induced by various stimulant drugs, *Psychopharmacologia*, 14, 299, 1969.
9. **Gibaldi, M. and Perrier, D.,** *Pharmacokinetics,* Marcel Dekker, New York, 1975.
10. **Gillette, J. R.,** Factors affecting drug metabolism, *Ann. N.Y. Acad. Sci.*, 179, 43, 1971.
11. **Goldberg, S. R., Hoffmeister, F., Schlichting, U. U., and Wuttke, W.,** A comparison of pentobarbital and cocaine self-administration in rhesus monkeys: Effects of dose and fixed-ratio parameter, *J. Pharmacol. Exp. Ther.*, 179, 277, 1971.
12. **Griffiths, R. G., Snell, J. D., and Brady, J. V.,** Progressive-ratio Performance in Baboons and the Assessment of the Abuse Liability of Drugs: Comparison of Fenfluramine, Chlorphentermine, Diethlpropion, and Cocaine, presented to the Committee on Problems of Drug Dependence, NAS-NRC, Richmond, Virginia, 1976.
13. **Kato, R. and Gillette, J. R.,** Effect of starvation on NADPH-dependent enzymes in liver microsomes of male and female rats, *J. Pharmacol. Exp. Ther.*, 150, 279, 1965.
14. **Levy, G.,** Kinetics of pharmacologic effects, *Clin. Pharmacol. Ther.*, 7, 362, 1966.
15. **Mannering, G. J.,** Inhibition of drug metabolism, in *Handbook of Experimental Pharmacology, Vol. XXVIII, Concepts of Biochemical Pharmacology, Part 2*, Brodie, B. and Gillette, J., Eds., Springer-Verlag, Berlin, 1971.
16. **Misra, A. L., Nayak, P. K., Patel, M. N., Vadlamani, N. L., and Mulé, S. J.,** Identification of norcocaine as a metabolite of (^{3}H) cocaine in rat brain, *Experientia*, 30, 1312, 1974.
17. **Nayak, P. K., Misra, A. L., and Mulé, S. J.,** Physiological disposition and biotransformation of (^{3}H) cocaine in acutely and chronically treated rats, *J. Pharmacol. Exp. Ther.*, 196, 556, 1976.
18. **Notari, R. E.,** *Biopharmaceutics and Pharmacokinetics*, Marcel Dekker, New York, 1971.
19. **Pickens, R., Bloom, W. C., and Thompson, T.,** Effects of reinforcement magnitude and session length of response rate of monkeys, *Proc. Am. Psychol. Assoc.*, 77, 809, 1969.
20. **Pickens, R. and Dougherty, J. A.,** A Method for Chronic Intravenous Infusion of Fluids in Unrestrained Rats, Report No. PR-72-1, Research Laboratories of the Department of Psychiatry, University of Minnesota, 1972.
21. **Pickens, R. and Thompson, T.,** Cocaine-reinforced behavior in rats: Effects of reinforcement magnitude and fixed-ratio size, *J. Pharmacol. Exp. Ther.*, 161, 122, 1968.

22. Schuster, C. R. and Wilson, M. L., The effects of various pharmacological agents on cocaine self-administration by rhesus monkeys, in *Current Concepts on Amphetamine Abuse*, Ellinwood, E. H. and Cohen, S., Eds., Department of Health, Education, and Welfare Publ. No (HSM) 72-9085, U.S.G.P.O., Washington, D.C., 1972.

23. Sidman, M., *Tactics of Scientific Research*, Basic Books, New York, 1960.

24. Sladek, N. E. and Mannering, G. J., Induction of drug metabolism. I. Differences in the mechanisms by which polycyclic hydrocarbons and phenobarbital produce their inductive effects on microsomal N-demethylating systems, *Mol. Pharmacol.*, 5, 174, 1969.

25. Tatum, A. L. and Seevers, M. H., Experimental cocaine addiction, *J. Pharmacol. Exp. Ther.*, 36, 401, 1929.

26. Van Rossum, J. M. and Van Koppen, A. T. J., Kinetics of psychomotor stimulant drug action, *Eur. J. Pharmacol.*, 2, 405, 1968.

27. Wagner, J. G., Kinetics of pharmacologic response. I. Proposed relationships between response and drug concentration in the intact animal and man, *J. Theoret. Biol.*, 20, 173, 1968.

28. Weiss, B., The fine structure of operant behavior during transition states, in *The Theory of Reinforcement Schedules*, Schoenfeld, W. N., Ed., Appleton-Century-Crofts, New York, 1970, chap. 9.

29. Weiss, B. and Laties, V. G., The psychophysics of pain and analgesia in animals, in *Animal Psychophysics*, Stebbins, W. C., Ed., Appleton-Century-Crofts, New York, 1970.

30. Wilson, M. C., Variables Which Influence the Reinforcing Properties of Cocaine in the Rhesus Monkey, Ph.D. thesis, University of Michigan, 1970.

31. Wilson, M. C., Hitomi, M., and Schuster, C. R., Psychomotor stimulant self-administration as a function of dosage per injection in the rhesus monkey, *Psychopharmacologia*, 22, 271, 1971.

32. Winger, G. D. and Woods, J. H., The reinforcing property of ethanol in the rhesus monkey. I. Initiation, maintainance and termination of ethanol-reinforced responding, *Ann. N.Y. Acad. Sci.*, 215, 162, 1973.

33. Yokel, R. A. and Pickens, R., Self-administration of optical isomers of amphetamine and methylamphetamine by rats, *J. Pharmacol. Exp. Ther.*, 187, 27, 1973.

34. Yokel, R. A. and Pickens, R., Drug level of *d*- and *l*-amphetamine during intravenous self-administration, *Psychopharmacologia*, 34, 255, 1974.

Behavior, Psychic, Neuropharmacologic and Physiologic Aspects

The Effects of Cocaine on Aggressive Behavior

THE EFFECTS OF COCAINE ON AGGRESSIVE BEHAVIOR

Ronald R. Hutchinson, Grace S. Emley, and Norman A. Krasnegor

TABLE OF CONTENTS

INTRODUCTION

Cocaine can dramatically influence behavior. Accounts from literature and clinical medicine have described the emotion-altering qualities of cocaine. Though frequently the drug is said to increase feelings of well-being and euphoria, other reports implicate cocaine in the production of negative affect by increasing fear or anger.[1,2]

Our laboratory has been interested for some years in the study of negative affect and particularly in the investigation of the environmental causes of aggressive behavior. Using a variety of techniques with several different species, we have studied the effects of different drugs as they may influence emotional expression.[3-6] Approximately 2 years ago we began studying the effects of cocaine using these methods. The work has produced a body of results that is generally consistent and sheds considerable light on the nature of the influence of cocaine upon aggressive behavior.

In the course of this work, it was necessary to test cocaine's effects on aggressive episodes produced by each of the major classes of environmental causes of aggression and place these findings in context with results obtained earlier in our laboratory with other drugs having certain similarities to cocaine.

WHAT IS AGGRESSION AND HOW TO STUDY IT?

Aggression is a behavioral sequence in which the terminal response causes destruction, dislocation, disfigurement, or other damage, typically to another creature but sometimes to inanimate objects. The causes of aggression are multiple.[7] Strong environmental stimuli can directly trigger immediate and intense episodes of aggressive behavior.[8-11] These powerful environmental stimuli are of two types. First, noxious, painful, startling, or threatening stimuli, sometimes referred to as negative-reinforcement-type stimuli, will by their *onset* produce aggressive episodes directly.[5,8,12-15] A second type of stimulation capable of producing aggression involves the *offset* or termination of positive, beneficial, nutritive, or life-sustaining stimuli, sometimes referred to in learning experiments as positive-reinforcement-type stimuli. The onset of noxious stimuli and the offset of pleasant stimulation are the two major antecedent causes of aggressive behavior in animals[7,16] and man.[17]

Aggressive behavior can also be influenced by stimulus conditions which result as consequences of such behavior, and here also, two major types of environmental stimulation can be identified. The first type of consequent stimulation involves the *offset*, termination, or reduction of painful, destructive, noxious, threatening, or negative-reinforcement-type stimuli. Aggressive behavior causing such stimulus change will, like other escape-avoidance performances, be increased in strength.[16,18] The second type of environmental stimulation capable of strengthening aggressive behavior if it occurs as a consequence to such aggression involves the *onset* or increase in beneficial, life-sustaining, pleasant, or positive-reinforcement-type stimulation. Aggression can be positively reinforced, as is also true with non-aggressive behaviors, and will increase in strength subsequent to such reinforcement.

The two major antecedent causes of aggressive behavior can therefore, by their opposite and reciprocal action following instances of aggression, act also as consequential causes of future aggressive episodes.[7] In our studies of cocaine, it has been necessary to test the drug as it might influence each of these major classes of aggressive behavior.

To study noxious-stimulus-onset-produced attack, squirrel monkeys are restrained at the waist and brief electric pain-shocks are delivered to the shaved tail surface as shown in Figure 1. Situated in front of the subject are several response sensors. At approximately shoulder level, a rubber hose spans the entire width of the chamber. Biting on this hose causes a special air flow switch to be triggered. Grasping, tugging, squeezing, and shaking of the hose with the hands and the arms have no effect on the switch. The intermittent delivery of brief but intense tail shocks results in the subject's grasping the rubber hose, moving toward it, and biting repetitively upon it 20 to 100 times in the 20- to 50-sec period following shock. Following this, the subject does not attack during the period until another shock produces another

series of biting attacks upon the hose. Also suspended on the wall in front of the subject is a small lever connected to a switch. Depression of this lever causes an audible click of a relay mounted on the rear of the intelligence panel. Responses on this lever never have any effect upon shocks or on other conditions of the subject's environment. Subjects depress this lever at a progressively increasing rate up toward the time of next shock delivery, but "freeze" for the last few seconds before shock delivery.

The discovery that repetitive, fixed-time, shock delivery programs would produce the pattern of multiple responses, each following markedly different temporal and topographic patterns, has allowed the investigation of a number of variables including environmental,[3,19] physiologic,[20,21] and pharmacologic influences[4,5] on attack behavior.

EFFECT OF COCAINE ON ANTECEDENT-STIMULUS-PRODUCED ATTACK

To study attack caused by the removal of pleasant-type stimulation, food-deprived pigeons were exposed to recurrent interruptions of the opportunity to receive food after pecking a small translucent key on the side of the chamber as shown in Figure 2. This program of interrupted reinforcement causes the subject to begin attacking a stuffed target pigeon located nearby. Attack responses are recorded automatically by a specially designed trip switch located at the base of the stuffed target bird.

With the pigeon-testing method, a dual response condition also exists, and it is thus possible to observe any differential influence of a drug upon the food-interruption-produced attack behavior and upon the food-acquisition key-pecking behaviors. This method has been useful for elaborating drug influence on "extinction-induced attack."[22]

Using these two testing techniques, cocaine hydrochloride has been administered in a mixed order of dosages on Wednesday of each 5-day testing week with saline administered on Monday, Tuesday, Thursday, and Friday. For squirrel monkeys, drug and control solutions were administered subcutaneously, and for pigeons, the intramuscular route was used. The results of these

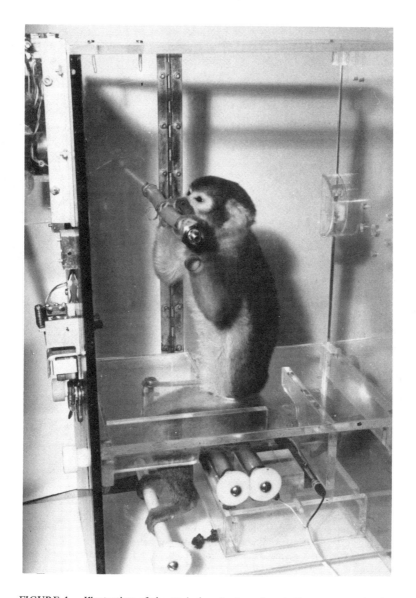

FIGURE 1. Illustration of the typical squirrel monkey testing apparatus for the study of biting attack. The subject is restrained at the waist and the tail is secured in a stockade device. The latex rubber bite hose suspended in front of the subject is connected to an air wave switch for the automatic recording of biting attack. Switch calibration allows detection of biting but not grasping, squeezing, or tugging responses. In different studies, biting attack may be produced by the delivery of brief electric pain shocks (which are delivered through brass electrodes which rest on the tail), interruption of food delivery sequences, or by the reward through escape-avoidance programs or the presentation of food. The response lever, used in certain studies to measure pre-shock manipulative behaviors, is located on the lower portion of the intelligence panel, just above the waist lock.

experiments are shown in Figure 3. Considering first the noxious-stimulus-onset-produced attack, cocaine at increasing doses produced increases in both performances, until at highest drug levels, both responses were reduced. Of greater importance, however, was the discovery that cocaine increased nonattack behaviors more than attack behaviors. The results of cocaine tests with food-interruption-produced attack may be seen by referring to the lower portion of Figure 3. Here also it was found that cocaine differentially affected attack and nonattack behaviors. Non-

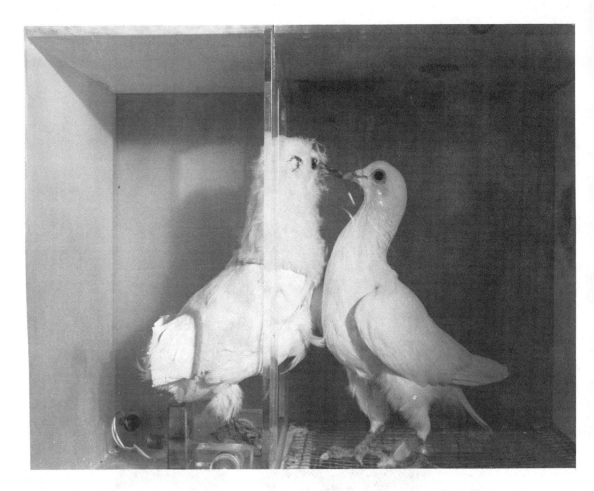

FIGURE 2. Illustration of a typical apparatus for studying attack in the pigeon. A food-deprived pigeon (shown on the right) can peck a plastic translucent disc on the intelligence panel located at the far right to receive periodic deliveries of grain through a solenoid-operated hopper, also mounted on the intelligence panel. Interruptions in food presentation schedules will cause pecking attack against a taxidermically stuffed target pigeon located in the left portion of the test chamber. The target is suspended on a spring-loaded platform connected to a microswitch. Pecking and pulling of the feathers of the target bird are recorded automatically.

attack-type food-acquisition responding was slightly increased at higher doses of cocaine, while attack behavior was actually decreased at higher drug levels.

From both of these testing methods then we found that cocaine certainly did not selectively increase aggressive behavior. Rather the drug, in each instance, caused a relative shift toward nonattack response alternatives.

EFFECT OF COCAINE ON CONSEQUENT-STIMULUS-PRODUCED ATTACK

As described earlier, two major classes of consequent-type stimuli can be influential in the future display of attack. If attack behavior is followed by a reduction in noxious stimulation or by an increase in beneficial or pleasant events, future episodes of attack will be more likely. To investigate the influence of cocaine on attack behavior maintained by these types of conditions, squirrel monkey subjects were trained either to avoid and escape electric shocks by biting on the rubber hose or, in other cases when food-deprived, to procure food on an intermittent schedule by hose biting. These reinforced attack performances then served as baseline conditions for the assessment of the effects of cocaine shown in Figure 4. Looking first at the upper portion of Figure 4, it is seen that cocaine produced a progressive increase in shock-avoidance-maintained biting-attack behavior, except at highest drug doses at which attack was somewhat reduced. The dose-response curve shown here exhibits considerable similarity to that seen in Figure 3 for the nonattack, lever-pressing behavior which occurs prior to shock delivery in free-shock programs. Similar conditions of imminent shock delivery occur in both test situations.

The lower portion of Figure 4 displays results of cocaine administration on a food-reinforced biting-attack response baseline. Here cocaine produces moderate increases in food-acquisition behaviors, just as was noted in earlier experiments described above and illustrated in Figure 3. At higher doses, however, the food-maintained biting attack is actually decreased as compared with nondrug levels.

In these experiments then, we see that cocaine can increase attack behavior if such attack is maintained by either positive or negative reinforcement procedures. The potentiating effect of cocaine upon reinforced nonattack performances has been recurrently demonstrated.[23-26]

WILL COCAINE PRODUCE ATTACK SPONTANEOUSLY?

Up to this point we have described experiments in which cocaine has been administered on baselines of attack behavior maintained by either antecedent or consequent stimulus procedures. To what extent the drug might directly produce spontaneous episodes of aggressive behavior without other provocations or reinforcers was an important issue to investigate. We have administered cocaine to squirrel monkey subjects in an environment containing attack and nonattack response alternatives, where no environmental stimuli were either spontaneously delivered or made contingent upon any performances. The results of drug administration in this "neutral" environment are presented in Figure 5. Here cocaine is seen to increase both attack and nonattack behaviors, but to produce much greater increases in the non-attack response alternative. The similarity in the data of Figure 5 and those presented earlier in

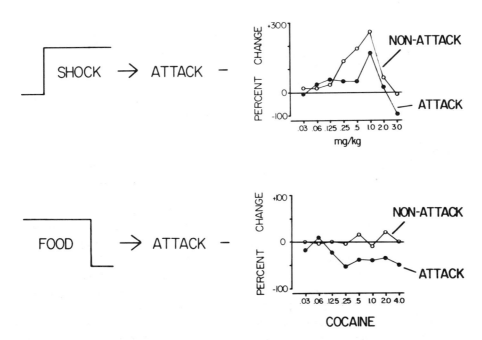

FIGURE 3. The effect of cocaine upon attack and nonattack behaviors generated by two different types of environmental stimulation. For both shock-produced attack and food-interruption-produced attack, cocaine produces a relative shift in performance toward the nonattack alternative.

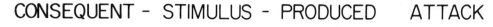

CONSEQUENT - STIMULUS - PRODUCED   ATTACK

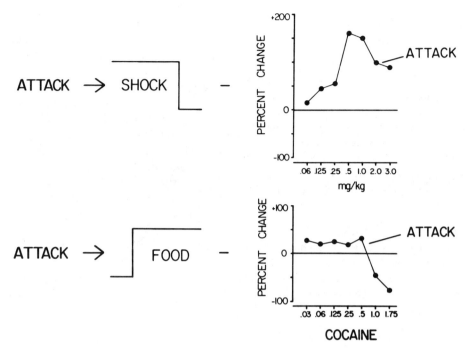

FIGURE 4.   The effect of the administration of cocaine upon two types of rewarded attack performance. Cocaine produces increases in both attack rewarded by the termination of shock and attack rewarded by the onset of and delivery of food.

Figure 3 seems noteworthy. Cocaine generally produces a shift in the relative display of behavior toward nonattack response alternatives, whether aggression is or is not provoked by either of the two major classes of aggression-causing antecedent stimulation.

A COMPARISON OF COCAINE WITH SEVERAL OTHER DRUGS

The findings described thus far can be brought into better perspective by a comparison with the effects of other drugs in similar tests.

We have found that, in general, the stimulant-type drugs increase both aggressive and nonaggressive behaviors, and the sedative or depressant agents in general decrease both aggressive and nonaggressive behaviors, while a third class of compounds referred to as tranquilizers frequently produce the effect of increasing nonattack behaviors while simultaneously decreasing attack behaviors.[3],[4] Cocaine can be compared with other central nervous system stimulants such as *d*-amphetamine, caffeine, and nicotine and a local

analgesic, lidocaine. Figure 6 presents the results of testing each of these compounds in the shock-produced attack paradigm . The effects of cocaine illustrated in the upper portion of Figure 3 which were discussed previously are repeated in Figure 6 for comparison.

When *d*-amphetamine is administered to squirrel monkeys, both attack and nonattack behaviors are elevated in early and intermediate portions of the drug-dose range, while at higher doses both behaviors are considerably reduced. This bitonic pattern of drug influence is similar to that seen for cocaine. However cocaine causes relatively greater increases in nonattack responding; the opposite is true for *d*-amphetamine.

Caffeine administration in this paradigm results in a dose-dependent increase of both attack and nonattack behaviors with relatively greater influence on nonattack behavior, as was also found for cocaine. Within the limits of our studies, we have not found that even higher doses of caffeine are capable of reducing behavior like *d*-amphetamine and cocaine.

Nicotine administration on this dual response

SPONTANEOUS ATTACK

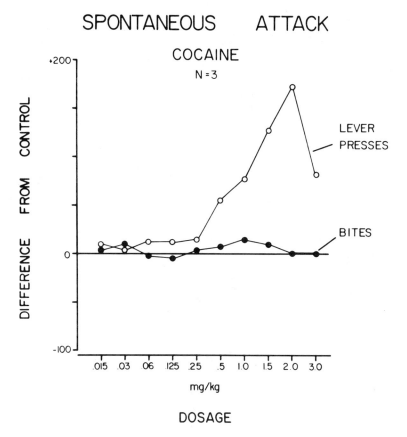

FIGURE 5. The effect of cocaine administration upon the spontaneous occurrence of attack behavior in an environment where neither strong eliciting stimuli nor reinforcing stimuli are present. Cocaine produces differential increases in nonattack-type responding.

baseline of attack and nonattack behaviors results in a dose-dependent increase in nonattack behavior or lever-pressing and biting-attack behavior. This particular drug is interesting because of the dosage range over which a differential increase in non-attack behavior occurs with almost no influence on attack behavior. These low and intermediate dose effects for nicotine are not grossly dissimilar from our findings for chlordiazepoxide and chlorpromazine.[3] Finally, because higher doses of cocaine might produce local analgesic effects, reducing the impact of tail shock and causing some of the response decreases noted, lidocaine has also been tested in this paradigm. Figure 6 shows that lidocaine is essentially ineffective in influencing shock-produced biting-attack or nonattack behaviors.

CONCLUSIONS

We think that these experiments are helpful in understanding the influence of cocaine upon negative affect and particularly upon aggressive behavior. Though it would have been parsimonious to discover that cocaine's influence upon attack remained independent of the nature of aggression-causing stimulation involved, our actual findings are compatible with the fact that aggression results from powerful stimuli often operating in diametrically opposite functional relations to behavior. When attack behavior is produced by powerful antecedent stimuli, whether by the onset of noxious conditions or the offset of pleasant conditions, cocaine causes a relative shift in performance to nonattack alternatives. Conversely, when attack behavior is maintained as other learned responses by reinforcement, it may, just as other learned responses, be increased by cocaine.

Compared with other central nervous system stimulants, our studies show cocaine to be neither more nor less powerful in its absolute ability to produce large changes in negative affect. The

129

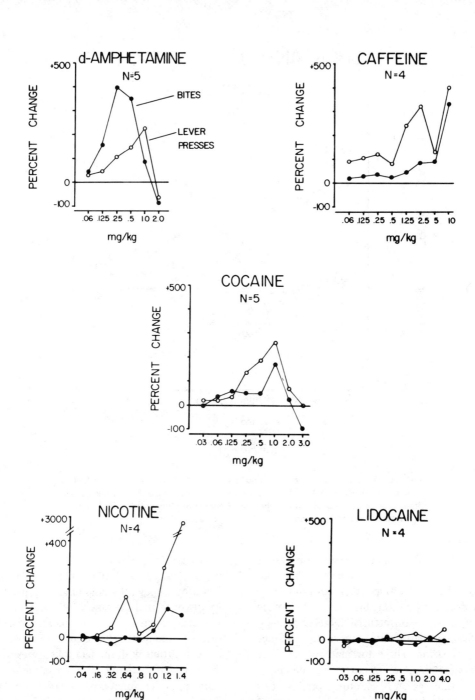

FIGURE 6. The effect of cocaine and several other drugs having certain properties in common with cocaine on shock-produced attack and nonattack-type responding in the squirrel monkey. *d*-Amphetamine, a stimulant, produces increases in both attack and nonattack-type responding, but attack reactions are disproportionately increased. As with cocaine, higher doses of *d*-amphetamine cause both performances to be reduced. Caffeine produces increases in both attack and non-attack behaviors, but as for cocaine, nonattack responding is disproportionately increased. Nicotine also increases both attack and nonattack behaviors, but over a significant portion of the dose-response curve it increases nonattack responding exclusively, and at higher doses though both responses are elevated, nonattack behavior is disproportionately increased. Lidocaine, a local analgesic, produces no effect on attack or nonattack behavior produced by noxious stimulation.

general disruptive effect upon several performances at higher dosages is similar to the effect seen for *d*-amphetamine and may suggest that both are relatively more potent than caffeine or nicotine. From our work this would be no more than speculation. The unique behavioral effects of cocaine, however, seem more closely related to the influences of caffeine and nicotine. Whereas *d*-amphetamine is seen to produce a differential increase in attack-type performances, cocaine, caffeine, and nicotine cause a relative shift toward nonattack alternatives.

ACKNOWLEDGMENTS

The work upon which this publication is based was performed pursuant to Contract No. ADM-45-74-163 and Contract No. 271-75-3075 with the National Institute on Drug Abuse, Alcohol, Drug Abuse, and Mental Health Administration, Department of Health, Education, and Welfare. Our thanks to E. R. Hallin, N. J. Murray, S. H. Crawford, D. Mann, D. Keenan, I. Wing, J. Bushong, D. Santek, K. Dinzik, R. Sewell, and T. Proni for their assistance.

REFERENCES

1. **Jaffe, J. H.,** Drug addiction and drug abuse, in *The Pharmacological Basis of Therapeutics,* 3rd ed., Goodman L. S. and Gilman, A., Eds., Macmillan, Toronto, 1965, 285.
2. **Maurer, D. W. and Vogel, V. H.,** *Narcotics and Narcotic Addiction,* Charles C Thomas, Springfield, 1967.
3. **Hutchinson, R. R. and Emley, G. S.,** Schedule-independent factors contributing to schedule-induced phenomena, in *Schedule Effects: Drugs, Drinking, and Aggression,* Gilbert, R. M. and Keehn, J. D., Eds., University of Toronto Press, Toronto, 1972, 174.
4. **Emley, G. S. and Hutchinson, R. R.,** Basis of behavioral influence of chlorpromazine, *Life Sci.,* 11, 43, 1972.
5. **Hutchinson, R. R. and Emley, G. S.,** Effects of nicotine on avoidance, conditioned suppression and aggression response measures in animals and man, in *Smoking Behavior: Motives and Incentives,* Dunn, W. L., Ed., V. H. Winston, Washington, D. C., 1973, 171.
6. **Hutchinson, R. R., Emley, G. S., and Krasnegor, N. A.,** The effects of cocaine on the aggressive behavior of mice, pigeons and squirrel monkeys, in *Cocaine and Other Stimulants,* Ellinwood, E. H., Ed., Plenum Publishing, New York, in press, 1976.
7. **Hutchinson, R. R.,** The environmental causes of aggression, in *Nebraska Symposium on Motivation, 1972,* Cole, J. K. and Jensen, D. D., Eds., University of Nebraska Press, Lincoln, 1973, 155.
8. **Ulrich, R. E. and Azrin, N. H.,** Reflexive fighting in response to aversive stimulation, *J. exp. Anal. Behav.,* 5, 511, 1962.
9. **Hutchinson, R. R., Azrin, N. H., and Hake, D. F.,** An automatic method for the study of aggression in squirrel monkeys, *J. exp. Anal. Behav.,* 9, 233, 1966.
10. **Azrin, N. H., Hutchinson, R. R., and Hake, D. F.,** Extinction-induced aggression, *J. exp. Anal. Behav.,* 9, 191, 1966.
11. **Hutchinson, R. R., Azrin, N. H., and Hunt, G. M.,** Attack produced by intermittent reinforcement of a concurrent operant response, *J. exp. Anal. Behav.,* 8, 55, 1965.
12. **Azrin, N. H., Hake, D. F., and Hutchinson, R. R.,** Elicitation of aggression by a physical blow, *J. exp. Anal. Behav.,* 8, 55, 1965.
13. **Azrin, N. H., Hutchinson, R. R., and Sallery, R. D.,** Pain-aggression toward inanimate objects, *J. exp. Anal. Behav.,* 7, 223, 1964.
14. **Renfrew, J. W.,** The intensity function and reinforcing properties of brain stimulation that elicits attack, *Physiol. Behav.,* 4, 509, 1969.
15. **Ulrich, R. E., Hutchinson, R. R., and Azrin, N. H.,** Pain-elicited aggression, *Psychol. Rec.,* 15, 111, 1965.
16. **Hutchinson, R. R.,** By-products of aversive control, in *Handbook of Operant Behavior,* Honig, V. and Staddon, J. E. R., Eds., Prentice-Hall, Englewood-Cliffs, New Jersey, in press, 1976.
17. **Hutchinson, R. R., Pierce, G. E., Emley, G. S., Proni, T. J., and Sauer, R. A.,** The laboratory measurement of human anger, *J. exp. Anal. Behav.,* in press, 1976.
18. **Azrin, N. H., Hutchinson, R. R., and Hake, D. V.,** Attack, avoidance and escape reactions to aversive shock, *J. exp. Anal. Behav.,* 10, 131, 1967.
19. **Hutchinson, R. R., Renfrew, J. W., and Young, G. A.,** Effects of long-term shock and associated stimuli on aggressive and manual responses, *J. exp. Anal. Behav.,* 15, 141, 1971.

20. **DeFrance, J. F. and Hutchinson, R. R.,** Electrographic changes in the amygdala and hippocampus associated with biting attack, *Physiol. Behav.,* 9, 83, 1972.
21. **Bushong, J.,** The Interaction Between Body Weight and Stress in the Squirrel Monkey, Master's thesis, Western Michigan University, Kalamazoo, 1974.
22. **Cherek, D. R. and Thompson, T.,** Effects of Δ'-tetrahydro-cannabinol on schedule-induced aggression in pigeons, *Pharmacol. Biochem. Behav.,* 1, 493, 1973.
23. **Smith, C. B.,** Effects of *d*-amphetamine upon operant behavior of pigeons: enhancement by reserpine, *J. Pharmacol. Exp. Ther.,* 146, 167, 1964.
24. **Kosman, M. E. and Unna, K. R.,** Effects of chronic administration of the amphetamines and other stimulants on behavior, *Clin. Pharmacol. Ther.,* 9, 240, 1968.
25. **Geller, I., Hartmann, R. J., and Blum, K.,** The effects of low-dose combinations of d-amphetamine and cocaine on experimentally induced conflict in the rat, *Curr. Ther. Res.,* 14, 220, 1972.
26. **Scheckel, C. L. and Boff, E.,** Behavioral effects of interacting imipramine and other drugs with d-amphetamine, cocaine, and tetrabenazine, *Psychopharmacologia,* 5, 198, 1964.

Behavior, Psychic, Neuropharmacologic and Physiologic Aspects

Cocaine Dependence: Psychogenic and Physiological Substrates

COCAINE DEPENDENCE: PSYCHOGENIC AND PHYSIOLOGICAL SUBSTRATES

Harold L. Altshuler and Neil R. Burch

TABLE OF CONTENTS

INTRODUCTION

Most of the drugs of abuse have been the subject of extensive research, and a great deal has been learned about the psychopharmacological basis of the abuse of the opiates, barbiturates, hallucinogens, and many others. It is surprising that cocaine, one of the drugs which has been in Western society the longest, has until recently, been virtually ignored. Most research on cocaine focused on its effects on the peripheral[1] and autonomic nervous systems,[2] although studies of the behavioral effects of the drug documented some of its effects on animal behavior[3-5] and its ability to serve as a reinforcer for certain operant behaviors.[6-8] Relatively few studies examined the acute effects of cocaine on human behavior,[9,10] and those that did were often based on subjective reports of the drug's effects. Even fewer studies examined the effects of chronic cocaine administration and the ability of the drug to produce tolerance or dependence.

Cocaine is derived from *Erythroxylon coca*, a plant that grows on the slopes of the Andes mountains. The plant's leaves were commonly used by the Incas and other Indian peoples of the area as part of their social and religious customs. The Spanish conquerors of Peru changed the use of the drug considerably, at first forbidding its use by the Indians, and later providing it as payment for work.

The drug was brought to Europe from South America by travelers and became available throughout Europe and North America during the 1800s. A number of review articles[11-13] describe the early history of cocaine in Western society, including the colorful addition to our knowledge of cocaine provided by Freud, Kohler, Halsted, and many others. Other chapters in this book review in greater detail the history and the sociological impact of cocaine on society.

Aside from the anecdotal reports of Freud and others, the effects of the chronic administration of cocaine were not explored scientifically until the 1920s. Among the early scientific studies of the effects of chronic cocaine administration are those by Tatum and Seevers[14] and Downs and Eddy.[15,16] Both teams reported that chronic administration of cocaine to dogs, rats, or monkeys did not result in the development of tolerance to the drug's effects, and these authors suggested that cocaine may produce a sensitization which they termed "reverse tolerance." It is surprising that their research was not reexamined until the last few years.

Many investigators used cocaine in behavioral studies as a stimulus or reinforcement.[6-8,17-19] Most of them neither accounted for nor reported any significant change in the effects of the drug concomitant with chronic administration. In one type of behavioral study, the self-administration model of drug abuse,[17,18] monkeys may self-administer cocaine under a variety of operant schedules and for varying periods of time. Generally the animals stabilize their day-to-day intake of cocaine and do not exhibit any apparent tolerance or reverse tolerance.

Recently there has been a flurry of interest in the effects of chronic administration of cocaine on experimental animals. Post[20,21] reported that he produced reverse tolerance to cocaine when the drug was administered chronically to monkeys, using an increased incidence of drug-induced seizures as the measure of drug effect. He speculated that this type of reverse tolerance is analogous to the neurophysiological procedure of "kindling," a term used to describe the repetitive

stimulation of deep brain structures, usually in the limbic system, with subconvulsant stimulation currents until the stimulation results in seizures. Post speculated that the production of seizures by doses of cocaine which had not previously produced seizures was the pharmacological analogy of "kindling." Ellinwood[22,23] performed similar experiments with other psychomotor stimulants such as amphetamine. Although his data are not quite comparable to Post's, he also observed the development of sensitivity to the convulsant properties of psychomotor stimulants and suggested that these may also be analogous to neurophysiological "kindling." These studies questioned cocaine's ability to produce reverse tolerance, and several research teams are actively investigating that possibility. Research in our laboratories[24-26] suggests that some portions of the neurophysiological response to cocaine increase as the result of chronic administration of the drug. These studies have also shown, however, that other portions of the response become attenuated during chronic cocaine administration.

It is generally understood that the chronic administration of cocaine produces a type of dependence called psychogenic dependence, and that this dependence is solely the result of the drug's positive reinforcement properties and not a pharmacological effect of the drug on biological systems.[27,28] Most of the procedures used to evaluate the potential of compounds to produce psychogenic dependence are based solely on user ratings of the pleasurable sensations associated with the drugs. Seevers[29] pointed out that determining the existence of psychological dependence requires arbitrary decisions by the subject who is evaluating the drug. A number of variables affect the degree to which single exposures to a drug may be considered reinforcing or nonreinforcing, such as the size of the reinforcement (dose), and the environmental setting, method, frequency, and duration of drug administration. Seevers categorized the types and usage patterns of drugs believed to produce psychological dependence on a scale ranging from "occasional use" to "compulsive, continuous, chronic use."

Other investigators have stated that psychological dependence on a drug is not necessarily a function of the drug's positive reinforcing properties, but may result from the drug's subjective effects and the ability of those effects to fill psychological needs of the user. Hoffman[30] pointed out that the human drug user is often quite aware of the consequences of the use and abuse of a drug and is not naively taking the drug merely for its positive reinforcing properties. Hoffman suggested that drug-seeking behavior is caused by a number of inappropriate coping mechanisms, and that drug users are seeking to escape from the world in which they live as well as to gain pleasurable experiences. There have been many studies of the psychological characteristics of drug users who become drug dependent.[31-33] Such studies do not provide a truly rigorous analysis of the personality characteristics of people who are prone to drug dependence; however, they suggest that Hoffman is at least partly correct. Unfortunately, such reports do not shed new light on the phenomenon of psychogenic drug dependence, and the psychological reasons for that type of drug use are unclear. There seems to be general agreement that abusers of most drugs share many psychological personality components, and that the predisposition to abuse cocaine in preference to other drugs may not be due to any special characteristics of cocaine abusers.

Gay[11] stated that "cocaine is probably the best example of a substance with which neither tolerance nor physical dependence develops but can lead to a sporadic though profound type of drug abuse." Studies in our laboratory, as well as those of Post and Ellinwood, suggest that statement to be inaccurate. While cocaine does produce a profound type of psychic dependence, it appears that significant changes do occur in the pharmacological effects of the drug after chronic administration. We suggest, therefore, that the psychological effects of cocaine are the result of a combination of its pharmacological effects, that those effects change during chronic drug administration, and that the changes may be too subtle for the user to perceive. Recent studies[23-26] of the neurophysiological changes which accompany chronic cocaine administration suggest that there are changes in the brain which closely conform to the concepts of tolerance or reverse tolerance which may be responsible for the experience of psychogenic dependence. In this chapter we will present an example of such observations, which resulted from studies in our laboratory, and relate those data to our understanding of the basis of psychogenic dependence.

METHODS

Animal Preparation

The animal subjects used in these studies were rhesus monkeys, *Macaca mulatta*, weighing 4 to 6 kg. The animals had been in our primate colony for some time and were in good health. All animals were drug naive at the start of these experiments, having never received psychoactive drugs other than one dose of pentobarbitol sodium (30 mg/kg i.v.) at the time of surgery.

Electrode Placement and Surgical Preparation

The monkeys were prepared for electroencephalographic (EEG) recordings by implanting surgically stainless steel screws into their calvaria. The electrodes were placed stereotaxically in general accordance with the International 10-20 System, allowing recordings from frontal, central, temporal, and occipital areas bilaterally. Stainless steel wires from the screw electrodes were connected to an electrical connector (Amphenol® No. 22-11N31, 222-12N31) and covered with dental acrylic cement (Nuweld® 1264-881104). The electrical connector was seated firmly in a cap of dental acrylic cement.

Postoperative care consisted of daily complete blood counts and antibiotic therapy if elevations of white blood counts occurred.

Electroencephalographic Recordings and Analysis

The electroencephalograms were recorded on a Beckman®Accutrace (Model 16) or Offner® (Type TC) electroencephalograph and subjected to period analysis. Period analysis is a technique of EEG analysis first described by Burch,[34] which has been used extensively in clinical and animal research. The technique requires that the analog electroencephalographic signal be passed through special purpose instruments (period analyzers) which digitize and encode the EEG signal. The period encoded signal is then written on digital tape and subsequently analyzed with a general purpose computer programmed specifically for these studies. The data generated by computer analysis are examined by trained technical personnel and plotted graphically to provide a visual summary of the electroencephalographic events occurring during each experiment. Where the experimental design permitted, the period analytic descriptors obtained from a group of animals treated with the same drug and dosage were combined for statistical analysis of central tendency.

Period analysis depends on the encoding of baseline crosses of the primary EEG signal and its derivatives. The primary baseline cross is called the major period and corresponds closely to the dominant frequency of the EEG. The first derivative of the major period encodes polarity changes of the primary EEG signal and corresponds to the numbers of peaks and valleys in the EEG signal. The second derivative of the major period is called the minor period and corresponds most closely to the amount of low voltage, high-frequency activity present in the primary EEG signal.

Period analysis has been demonstrated to be extremely sensitive to EEG changes which are the result of sleep, drugs, and other alterations in the animals' physiology and environment. The technique is closely related mathematically to power spectrum analysis of the EEG,[35] and both techniques produce reliable descriptions of the effects of a variety of drugs on the electroencephalogram. Our laboratory demonstrated the utility of period analysis for investigating the effects of many psychoactive drugs on the primate electroencephalogram.[36]

Comparison of the Effects of Cocaine and d-Amphetamine on the Primate EEG

Since cocaine and d-amphetamine are considered to have many similar subjective effects and since both drugs are thought to produce psychogenic dependence, a series of acute experiments was conducted to compare the effects of the two drugs on the period analytic descriptors of the primate EEG.

Cocaine hydrochloride (2.5 mg/kg and 5.0 mg/kg) and d-amphetamine sulfate (0.5 mg/kg and 2.5 mg/kg) were administered intravenously weekly. Electroencephalograms were recorded for 30 min before and 90 min after each dose and the resulting period analytic descriptors summarized. Three or more experiments in which saline instead of drug was administered preceded the drug studies.

Chronic Cocaine Administration

After establishing the profile of EEG responses to acute cocaine administration, we began experiments designed to investigate the EEG effects of the chronic administration of cocaine. A different group of drug-naive animals was implanted surgically with skull electrodes and saline control EEG profiles determined. After such control data were obtained, cocaine administration began. Table 1 summarizes the experimental design of the chronic study. In this design the EEG response to the first intravenous dose of cocaine (3 mg/kg) was considered the prototypic response to cocaine, against which all subsequent responses to the "challenge doses" were compared. In addition to the intravenous challenge doses, cocaine was administered subcutaneously three times a day. This "maintenance dose" provided chronic exposure to cocaine and maintained some degree of stability of drug blood levels throughout the study.

The EEG data obtained during the 8-month study were subjected to period analysis, with emphasis on examining changes in EEG profiles resulting from chronic drug administration. Attention was directed to changes in the pre-dose, spontaneous EEG, post-dose EEG response to the challenge dose, and several other EEG parameters. Since changes in pre-dose major period counts during a chronic study make the comparison of successive post-dose changes during the study difficult, it was necessary to reduce the contribution of that source of variability. A procedure known as "normalization" of the pre-dose EEG was performed on the data. In normalization of control data, all pre-dose values are considered fixed, and post-dose changes are computed as percentage change from pre-dose levels. This allows comparisons of the effects of the challenge drug dose uninfluenced by the initial frequency of the pre-dose EEG. The period analytic descriptors generated during the 8-month experiment were plotted graphically to examine EEG changes which resulted from chronic drug administration.

In addition to the EEG evaluations, twice daily behavioral observations of the monkeys were performed. The observations consisted of objective descriptions of the animals' behavior in their home cages, their responses to food, movement of other animals, and investigator-induced distractions, as well as changes in motor activity and general affective and stereotypic behavior.

RESULTS

Comparison of the EEG Effects of Cocaine and d-Amphetamine

Figure 1 summarizes the effects of cocaine and

TABLE 1

Summary of Protocol for Cocaine Study

Species	*Macaca mulatta*
Sex	Male
Weight range	4.5–6.0 kg
Number of animals	3
Duration of experiment	200 days
Frequency of EEG recordings	weekly (approximate)
Number of saline control experiments before Dose 1	3
Protocol for EEG recording experiment	30 min pre-dose spontaneous EEG 90 min post-dose 3 epochs of photic stimulation 3–30 Hz
Challenge dose	Cocaine HCl, 3 mg/kg i.v. (during weekly EEG recording)
Maintenance dose	Cocaine HCl, 3 mg/kg s.c. 3 times/day
Dosage regimen (example, Week 1)	Dose 1 = 3 mg/kg i.v. challenge dose (+EEG) Dose 2–22 = 3 mg/kg s.c. maintenance dose Dose 23 = 3 mg/kg i.v. challenge dose (+EEG)

d-amphetamine on the EEG from the temporal area of the monkey brain. Intravenous doses of *d*-amphetamine produced increases in the major period counts which were at their peak 10 min post-dose and returned to pre-dose levels within 30 min. Note that the temporal area EEG response to intravenous amphetamine exhibited an increase in counts and did not have any frequency-slowing component.

In contrast, cocaine produced changes in the EEG which were bidirectional and consisted of an initial decrease in EEG frequency (major period counts) which occurred 10 min post-dose and was followed by an increase in major period counts. The biphasic nature of the EEG response to cocaine proved to be important in our subsequent studies of the changes in EEG responses to cocaine resulting from the chronic administration of the drug.

The Effects of the Chronic Administration of Cocaine on the Monkey EEG

This study demonstrated that the chronic administration of cocaine to monkeys produced changes in both the pre-dose EEG and EEG response to challenge doses of cocaine.

The Pre-Dose EEG

The major period counts recorded during the pre-dose portion of the experiments decreased progressively during the study. Table 2 summarizes the pre-dose EEG data for two monkeys in the study and demonstrates the different effects observed in each area of the brain.

EEG Responses to Intravenous Cocaine

One of the ways to evaluate the effects of chronic cocaine administration on the primate EEG was the examination of the EEG response to an acute intravenous dose of cocaine (the challenge dose), with the EEG response to cocaine on Day 1 serving as the prototypic response to which all subsequent responses were compared. That response was different in each brain area on Day 1, although there was a qualitative similarity in the biphasic response patterns, which consisted of an initial decrease in major period counts for 10 min following cocaine injection, followed by a gradual

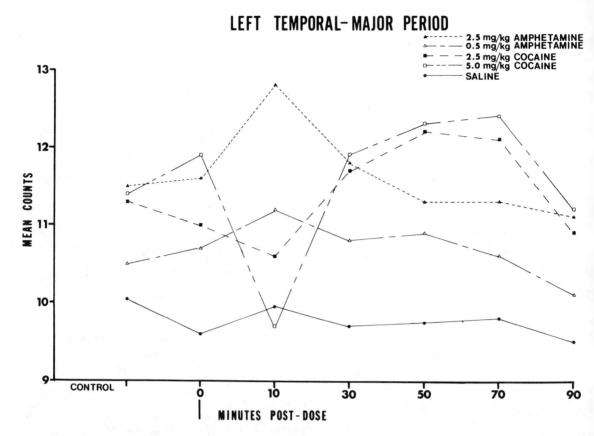

FIGURE 1. Comparative effects of *d*-amphetamine and cocaine HCl on left temporal major period counts. This analysis compares the effects of two behaviorally equivalent doses of *d*-amphetamine and cocaine on the left temporal EEG. Note that the responses occur in a dose-related manner, with the higher doses of each drug producing more pronounced EEG changes than the lower dose. Amphetamine produced an increase in major period counts which is maximal approximately 10 min post-dose. Cocaine produced both a 10 min post-dose decrease in major period counts and a 40 min post-dose increase in counts.

TABLE 2

Changes in Mean Major Period Counts of Pre-Dose, Spontaneous EEG During Chronic Cocaine Study

		Day of experiment				
Brain area	Saline control	1	25	50	100	190
Frontal	12.2	12.4	11.8	12.3	11.6	9.4
Central	13.7	13.6	14.2	13.4	12.9	12.2
Temporal	14.0	14.2	13.6	13.6	13.0	11.0
Occipital	9.9	10.2	10.3	9.8	9.4	8.7

return to pre-dose levels and an increase in major period counts 30 to 40 min post-dose.

Figure 2 summarizes the EEG responses to intravenous cocaine recorded from the temporal area on Days 1, 50, 102, and 193. The first portion of the biphasic EEG response, the decrease

in major period counts during 1 to 10 min post-dose, became progressively more pronounced as the chronic study continued. The second phase of the biphasic EEG response to cocaine, the increase in major period counts occurring approximately 30 to 40 min post-dose, was diminished

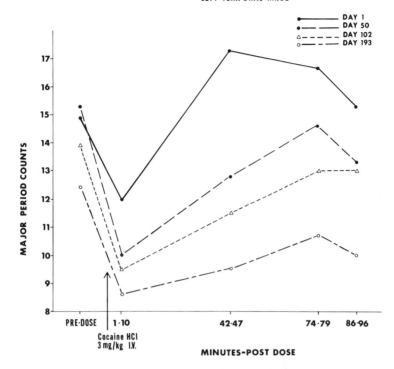

FIGURE 2. The effects of chronic administration of cocaine on temporal area major period counts. This figure illustrates the EEG changes which occur during approximately 200 days of chronic cocaine administration. The Day 1 response is biphasic, consisting of a decrease in major period counts occurring 10 min post-dose and an increase occurring approximately 40 min post-dose. The pre-dose major period counts decreased progressively during the 200 days of drug administration. The decrease in major period counts which occurred 10 min post-dose became greater in an orderly manner during the 200-day experiment, and the increase which occurred 40 min post-dose became reduced. Note that the major period counts never returned to pre-dose levels on Day 193.

substantially during chronic cocaine administration and was absent on Day 193.

Figure 3 summarizes the changes observed in the normalized EEG obtained from the frontal, central, temporal, and occipital areas of one of the monkeys in the study. There were differences in the response patterns of the four brain areas. On Day 1, for example, the frontal area exhibited only the 1 to 10 min post-dose decrease in counts, and the occipital area exhibited only the 30 min post-dose increase in counts. Despite such differences, the changes in the EEG responses from all brain areas produced by chronic cocaine exposure were quite similar to the changes in the temporal area; EEG slowing 10 min post-dose became greater, and EEG acceleration 40 min post-dose became reduced.

Behavioral Measures

Behavioral changes in the monkeys treated chronically with cocaine were unremarkable. The intensity of post-dose stereotyped behavior increased during the first 50 days of the study, then stabilized and did not change substantially for the rest of the study. The animals maintained normal food consumption, weight gains, and health during the entire study, and no convulsions occurred after either the challenge or maintenance cocaine doses.

DISCUSSION

Psychogenic Dependence

Cocaine and several other drugs are believed to produce psychogenic dependence, a concept of drug dependence which differs from physical

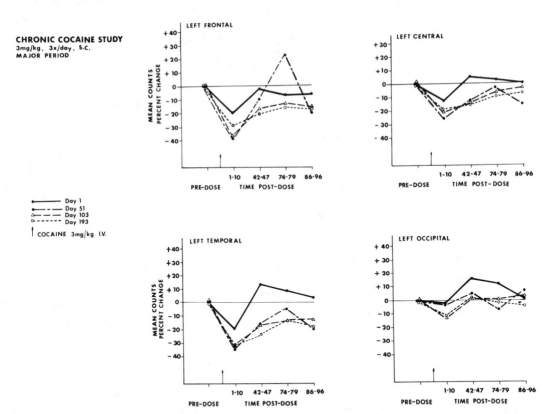

CHRONIC COCAINE STUDY
3mg/kg, 3x/day, S.C.
MAJOR PERIOD

Day 1
Day 51
Day 103
Day 193

COCAINE 3mg/kg I.V.

FIGURE 3. Normalized major period counts recorded from four brain areas during chronic cocaine administration. This figure illustrates changes in major period counts which occurred during chronic cocaine administration when the pre-dose portion of the EEG was normalized and the post-dose responses were considered as percentage changes. Note that the Day 1 response from the left frontal area consisted only of a decrease in major period counts which was maximal 10 min post-dose. That decrease was less pronounced in the central area. The temporal area Day 1 response was bidirectional, consisting of decrease in major period counts 10 min post-dose and an increase of about the same magnitude which occurred 40 min or more post-dose. The drug produced only the 40 min post-dose increase in counts in the occipital area EEG. The changes in the EEG response which resulted from chronic drug administration occurred in a relatively orderly progression, with the 10 min post-dose decrease in counts becoming greater and the 40 min post-dose increase in counts becoming reduced. The 74 to 79 min post-dose increase in counts in the frontal area on Day 51 is probably an artifact.

dependence in a number of ways. Physical dependence is thought to result from biochemical and physiological changes in the drug user that accompany chronic exposure to a drug, making the presence of the drug necessary to maintain a normal state. In psychogenic dependence, on the other hand, no change is believed to occur in the physiology or biochemistry of the drug user, who seeks the drug solely because of its positive reinforcement properties. Withdrawal from drugs like cocaine does not produce a true abstinence syndrome, such as the set of symptoms accompanying the withdrawal from drugs like the opiates, barbiturates, and ethanol. Generally only a psychological depression occurs when users who had been taking high doses of cocaine stop their drug intake. The cause of that depression is unknown and there have been hardly any attempts

to investigate it systematically. In fact, there have been very few attempts to investigate psychogenic dependence in general, despite the fact that we use the term to describe the patterns of drug abuse associated with many drugs. The experiments reported here were designed to investigate one aspect of the physiological basis of psychogenic dependence — the development of neurophysiological changes associated with chronic administration of cocaine.

EEG Effects of Cocaine and d-Amphetamine

Both cocaine and amphetamine are thought to produce psychogenic dependence, and neither is believed to produce physical dependence or tolerance. The drugs have a number of other similarities in behavioral and physiological effects, but despite those similarities, most drug users report quite different qualitative effects associated with each drug. Such statements are difficult to confirm in laboratory studies. The experiment summarized here which found differences in the acute effects of the two drugs on the EEG represents one of the few successful attempts to distinguish the effects of the two drugs in the central nervous system.

One interesting difference between cocaine and amphetamine is that amphetamine principally increases the frequency of the EEG, while cocaine causes bidirectional changes, part of the EEG response being a decrease in EEG frequency and another part being an increase. These observations may explain the subjectively perceived differences between the two drugs and may also reflect differences in their mechanism of action. In addition, these studies suggest that the biphasic EEG response to cocaine may be one of the drug's unique properties, since each phase of the response is affected differently by chronic administration of the drug.

Chronic Cocaine Administration

Several research groups are studying the effects of chronic cocaine administration on animals, and each is approaching the problem differently. The studies reported here were intended to provide a subhuman model of chronic cocaine exposure which simulated human use patterns as closely as possible. Therefore, the dose of the drug used was much lower than the doses used in other laboratories,[20,21,23] and consequently, the observed effects were relatively subtle and less striking than the convulsions and associated phenomena observed by other groups. In addition, in our study animals were maintained on low doses of cocaine for a long time, while other groups used high levels of cocaine for much shorter periods.

The experimental design used in these studies employed two types of cocaine doses, a maintenance dose and a challenge dose. The maintenance dose was administered subcutaneously and served to maintain relatively stable, although low, blood levels of the drug throughout the day. The challenge dose was given intravenously while the animal's EEG was being recorded. That dose was intended to provide a means to measure the changes in the response of the monkey's brain to acute doses of the drug and was also lower than that used elsewhere.

The pre-dose spontaneous EEG reflected primarily changes in the monkey's central nervous system caused by the subcutaneous maintenance doses of cocaine. We observed a progressive slowing in that measure, a surprising finding which differs from the assumptions usually made about the effects of cocaine. The slowing of the pre-dose EEG cannot be explained easily by our understanding of any of the neurochemical or physiological effects of cocaine. It is possible, however, that the slowing pre-dose EEG indicates that chronic cocaine administration may have produced pathological change, possibly in the cerebrovascular system. The possibility that the chronic administration of moderate doses of cocaine may produce neurotoxicity is one of pressing importance and demands an intensive investigation.

The EEG responses to the challenge dose also changed during chronic drug administration. The finding is somewhat surprising, since humans who use cocaine chronically do not report any change in the drug's subjective effects resulting from chronic administration. Since it is unknown which portion of the EEG response to cocaine correlates with its subjective, euphoriant effect, it is difficult to evaluate those subjective reports. It is entirely possible that the user perceives only the combination of the two phases of the biphasic effect of the drug. Since the two phases are directionally opposite, even the changes in response to the drug during chronic exposure may also be imperceptible to the user.

The behavior of the animals treated chronically with cocaine was unremarkable. There were many episodes of hyperactivity and stereotypic behavior, but the changes resulting from chronic treatment were minor. Although monkeys will often exhibit an eagerness for injections of such psychoactive drugs as morphine, this was not observed in these animals during the cocaine study. Post[20,21] and others have reported the development of convulsions associated with chronic cocaine administration, a finding we do not confirm. That difference may be explained by the fact that his doses were considerably higher than ours.

Does Cocaine Produce Tolerance?

The concept of tolerance to a drug's effect was developed to describe the alteration in the effects of the opiates and barbiturates during chronic administration and is a concept which is the cornerstone of our understanding of physical dependence. Tolerance is defined as the diminution of the effects of a fixed dose of a drug as a result of chronic administration so that larger doses of the drug are required to produce the effects of the smaller dose.[27,28] The concept of tolerance cannot be applied easily to such CNS stimulants as cocaine or amphetamine, and humans who use those drugs do not report the development of tolerance. To the contrary, several investigators have suggested that cocaine produces reverse tolerance, and that the response to a given dose of cocaine increases with chronic administration. Our studies of the effects of chronic cocaine administration in subhuman primates show that chronic drug exposure changes the response profile in several ways, and that the responses along some parameters become enhanced, while others are diminished. Such observations, viewed in isolation, could confirm either the development of tolerance or of reverse tolerance. We suggest that those concepts may not be valid or useful to describe the results of the chronic administration of cocaine, and that it would be more appropriate to describe the specific effects of chronic drug administration on each parameter of the spectrum of physiological responses to cocaine. Although it is clear from the research conducted in a number of laboratories, including our own, that chronic exposure to cocaine causes significant alterations in the physiology of the recipient, the clinical significance of those changes is not at all clear. The fact that such changes do occur suggests that the medical and scientific community may need to reexamine the widespread view that the chronic use of cocaine produces a form of dependence resulting only from its psychologically reinforcing properties,

that is, psychogenic dependence. A great deal of accumulating evidence suggests that there are many biological changes which develop during chronic cocaine exposure and that these may play an important role in the development of dependence on the drug.

Conclusion

Cocaine has been used for recreational purposes by several societies for hundreds of years. It is assumed usually that cocaine is a relatively harmless drug which is sought by the user solely for its positively reinforcing properties and that it does not produce physical dependence, but only psychogenic dependence. Several laboratories have reported recently that the chronic administration of cocaine produces significant changes in the central nervous system of the recipient. Such changes, while they do not fit the classical definitions of tolerance, reverse tolerance, or physical dependence, suggest that there may be a biological basis for dependence on cocaine. These findings do not contradict the understanding of psychogenic dependence on cocaine, but they do suggest that it is a more complex phenomenon than has been thought. Furthermore, such findings illustrate that cocaine is unique among the drugs of abuse and that the consequences of its habitual use are poorly understood. The increase in the use of the drug throughout society, especially among groups with little previous exposure to drugs of abuse, mandates an intensive research effort into the pharmacology of cocaine and the nature of the syndrome associated with its abuse.

REFERENCES

1. Ritchie, J. M. and Greengard, P., On the mode of action of local anesthetics, *Ann. Rev. Pharmacol.*, 6, 405, 1966.
2. Kalsner, S. and Nickerson, M., Mechanism of cocaine potentiation of responses to amines, *Br. J. Pharmacol.*, 35, 428, 1969.
3. Castellano, C., Cocaine, pemoline and amphetamine on learning and retention of a discrimination test in mice, *Psychopharmacologia*, 36, 67, 1974.
4. Johansson, J. O. and Jarbe, T. U. C., Antagonism of pentobarbitol induced discrimination in the gerbil, *Psychopharmacologia*, 41, 225, 1975.
5. Fischer, E. and Heller, B., Antagonistic effects of cocaine and adrenaline on the psychomotor activity of mice, *Acta Physiol. Lat. Am.*, 17, 118, 1967.
6. Wilson, M. C. and Schuster, C. R., Interactions between atropine, chlorpromazine and cocaine on food reinforced behavior, *Pharmacol. Biochem. Behav.*, 3, 363, 1975.
7. Geller, I., Hartmann, R. J., and Blum, K., The effects of low dose combinations of d-amphetamine and cocaine on experimentally induced conflict in the rat, *Curr. Ther. Res.*, 14, 220, 1972.
8. Angel, C., Murphree, O. D., and DeLuca, D. C., The effects of chlordiazepoxide, amphetamine, and cocaine on bar press behavior in normal and genetically nervous dogs, *Dis. Nerv. Syst.*, 35, 220, 1974.
9. Post, R. M., Gillin, J. C., White, R. J., and Goodwing, F. K., The effect of orally administered cocaine on sleep of depressed patients, *Psychopharmacologia*, 37, 59, 1974.
10. Isbell, H., General aspects of the treatment of drug dependence relevant to the abuse of amphetamine and amphetamine-like compounds, in *Abuse of Central Stimulants*, Sjoqvist, F. and Tottie, M., Eds., Alqvist and Wilksell, Stockholm, 1969, 15.
11. Gay, G. R., Inaba, D. S., Sheppard, C. W., and Newmeyer, J. A., Cocaine: history, epidemiology, human pharmacology and treatment, a perspective on a new debut for an old girl, *Clin. Toxicol.*, 8, 149, 1975.
12. Woods, J. H. and Downs, D. A., The psychopharmacology of cocaine, in *Drug Use in America: Problem in Perspective*, Technical Papers of the Second Report of the National Commission on Marijuana and Drug Abuse, U.S. Government Printing Office, Washington, D.C., March 1973, 124.
13. Ashley, R., *Cocaine its History, Uses and Effects,* St. Martin's Press, New York, 1975.
14. Tatum, A. L. and Seevers, M. H., Experimental cocaine addiction, *J. Pharmacol. Exp. Ther.*, 36, 401, 1929.
15. Downs, A. W. and Eddy, N. B., The effects of repeat doses of cocaine on the dog, *J. Pharmacol. Exp. Ther.*, 46, 195, 1932.
16. Downs, A. W. and Eddy, N. B., The effect of repeated doses of cocaine on the rat, *J. Pharmacol. Exp. Ther.*, 46, 199, 1932.
17. Deneau, G., Yanagita, T., and Seevers, M. H., Self-administration of psychoactive substances by the monkey, *Psychopharmacologia*, 16, 30, 1969.
18. Schuster, C. R. and Thompson, T., Self-administration of and behavioral dependence on drugs, *Ann. Rev. Pharmacol.*, 9, 483, 1969.
19. Pickens, R. and Thompson, T., Cocaine-reinforced behavior in rats; effects of reinforcement magnitude and fixed-ratio size, *J. Pharmacol. Exp. Ther.*, 16, 122, 1968.
20. Post, R. M. and Kopanda, R. T., Cocaine, kindling and reverse tolerance, *Lancet*, i, 409, 1975.
21. Post, R. M., Comparative psychopharmacology of cocaine and amphetamine, *Psychopharmacol. Bull.*, in press.
22. Ellinwood, E. H., Amphetamine and stimulant drugs, in *Drug Use in America: Problem in Perspective,* Technical Papers of the Second Report of the National Commission on Marijuana and Drug Abuse, U.S. Government Printing Office, Washington, D.C., March 1973, 124.
23. Ellinwood, E. H., Behavioral and electrophysiological correlates of cocaine intoxication: implications for clinical syndromes, *Psychopharmacol. Bull.*, in press.
24. Phillips, P. E., Altshuler, H. L., Sanders, D. W., and Burch, N. R., The effects of chronic cocaine hydrochloride administration on the primate electroencephalogram, *Proc. Soc. Neurosci.*, 1, 284, 1975.
25. Altshuler, H. L., Burch, N. R., and Dossett, R. G., The electroencephalographic effects of long term cocaine administration to rhesus monkeys, *Western Pharmacology Society Proceedings*, 19, in press.
26. Altshuler, H. L. and Burch, N. R., The effects of cocaine on the EEG of the monkey: behavioral and pharmacological correlates, *Psychopharmacol. Bull.*, in press.
27. Martin, W. R., Drug dependence, in *Drills, Pharmacology in Medicine*, 4th ed., Dipalma, J., Ed., McGraw-Hill, New York, 1971, 362.
28. Jaffe, J. H., Drug addiction and drug abuse, in *Pharmacological Basis of Therapeutics*, 5th ed., Goodman, L. S. and Gilman, A., Eds., Macmillan, New York, 1975, 284.
29. Seevers, M. H., Characteristics of dependence on and abuse of psychoactive drugs, in *Chemical and Biological Aspects of Drug Dependence*, Mulé, S. J. and Brill, H., Eds., CRC Press, Cleveland, 1972, 13.
30. Hoffman, F. G., *A Handbook of Drug and Alcohol Abuse*, Oxford University Press, New York, 1975, 49.
31. Stokes, J. P., Personality traits and attitudes and their relationship to student drug using behavior, *Int. J. Addict.*, 9, 267, 1974.
32. Cambell, R. S. and Freeland, J. J., Patterns of drug abuse, *Int. J. Addict.*, 9, 289, 1974.

33. Hoffman, F. G., *A Handbook of Drug and Alcohol Abuse*, Oxford University Press, New York, 1975, 240.
34. Burch, N. R., Nettleton, W. J., Sweeney, J., and Edwards, R. J., Period analysis of the electroencephalogram on a general purpose digital computer, *Ann. N.Y. Acad. Sci.*, 115, 827, 1964.
35. Saltzberg, B. and Burch, N. R., Period analytic estimates of moments of the power spectrum: a simplified EEG time domain procedure, *Electroencephalogr. Clin. Neurophysiol.*, 30, 568, 1971.
36. Altshuler, H. L. and Burch, N. R., Period analysis of the electroencephalogram of subhuman primates, in *Behavior and Brain Electrical Activity*, Burch, N. R. and Altshuler, H. L., Eds., Plenum Press, New York, 1975, 277.

Behavior, Psychic, Neuropharmacologic and Physiologic Aspects

Effects of Cocaine on the Electrical Activity of the Brain and Cardiorespiratory Functions and the Development of Tolerance in the Central Nervous System

EFFECTS OF COCAINE ON THE ELECTRICAL ACTIVITY OF THE BRAIN AND CARDIORESPIRATORY FUNCTIONS AND THE DEVELOPMENT OF TOLERANCE IN THE CENTRAL NERVOUS SYSTEM

Masaji Matsuzaki

TABLE OF CONTENTS

INTRODUCTION

Cocaine is a potent stimulant in the central nervous system (CNS). In high doses, it is capable of producing a high level of euphoric excitement as well as hallucinatory effects. These properties provide a high abuse potential and continued use leads to psychological dependence.[1-3] It has been shown that chronic administration of this drug does not produce tolerance and physiological dependence.[1-14] Reverse tolerance or increasing sensitivity to cocaine with chronic administration has also been reported.[2-15] However, the development of tolerance to this drug has been shown in man[16-18] and in the rat[19] after chronic administration in high doses. Recently, it was reported that repeated daily intravenous injections of cocaine with high doses in the monkey produce tolerance to the convulsant, cardiorespiratory stimulant effects, and the disposition of cocaine.[20,21]

There are a large number of studies on the pharmacology and biochemistry of cocaine,[22] but very little information is available concerning the neuropharmacological and electrophysiological aspects of the CNS action of this compound.[20,21,23,24] In reference to these latter aspects on the CNS action of cocaine, it has been demonstrated that administration of cocaine in high doses produces convulsive discharges localized in the region of the limbic system, which are followed by generalized seizures in the cat[24] and in the monkey.[20,21] Paradoxically, it is capable of blocking cortical seizures evoked by electroshock to the cerebral cortex in nontoxic doses in mice.[25] Recently, it has been shown that cocaine manifests a suppressive effect on the electrical discharges within the limbic system evoked by the electrical stimulation.[20]

This chapter deals with the electrophysiological and neuropharmacological aspects of the CNS action of cocaine in the monkey in acute and chronic states, with a view to gain insight into the central mechanisms underlying the CNS action of this compound in relation to development of tolerance following chronic administration.

METHODS

Subjects and electrode implantation – Rhesus monkeys (*Macaca mulatta*), weighing 3.5 to 4.5 kg, with permanently implanted electrodes in the brain were used as subjects (Ss). For recording electrical activities of the brain (EEGs), bipolar stainless steel electrodes (electrode diameter, 0.2 mm; interelectrode distance, 1.0 mm) were implanted stereotaxically, under pentobarbital anesthesia (45 mg/kg, i.v.), in the subcortical structures including amygdala (basolateral nucleus), hippocampus, thalamus (ventral postero-lateral nucleus), and pontine reticular formation. For recording of the neocortical EEGs, bipolar silver-ball electrodes (ball diameter, 1 mm; ball separation, 5 mm) were placed on the dura in various cortical areas, including the superior and the inferior frontal lobes, and the superior temporal, superior parietal, and occipital lobes. For recording of eye movements, silver-ball electrodes were implanted in the orbital plate. An indifferent electrode was implanted in the bone over the frontal sinus. The electrodes for heart rate recording and a chest-movement transducer for respiratory rate recording were attached to the chest of the Ss. Stereotaxic placement of electrodes and their verifications were based on the atlases of Snider and Lee[26] and Olszewski.[27]

For the injection of drug solution, a silastic catheter (2.2 mm, O.D. and 1.0 mm, I.D.) was chronically inserted in the femoral or jugular vein under the pentobartital anesthesia.

Experimental procedures – The study was carried out in five main parts; the experimental procedures were as follows.

Study I: Effects of Cocaine on the Electrical Activities of the Brain and Behavior

Five Ss were used in this study. They were restrained in a primate chair and placed in an observation chamber (90 × 88 × 75 cm). Polygraphs of EEGs, eye movements, heart rate (H.R.), and respiratory rate (R.R.) were recorded throughout experimental sessions. A 2- to 3-day control experiment was conducted before experimental session of drug administration. Cocaine solution (5.0 mg/ml as free base in 0.9% saline) was injected by a remote control technique through the chronically implanted catheter.

Electrical discharges in the limbic system were evoked by bipolarly delivered electrical stimulation (1 ms pulse width at 50 Hz for 5 to 20 sec) to the hippocampus or the amygdala using the same type of electrodes used for recording. In order to determine a baseline of control limbic discharge threshold, the stimulations were given repeatedly, with as many as necessary to assure a stable baseline of the threshold in each experimental session. This usually occurred after four to six stimulations given at 30- to 40-min intervals. Once control baselines were obtained, cocaine was administered, and data was collected continually on EEG recordings until the experiment was terminated. Only one experimental session of drug administration per week was performed on the same Ss.

Study II: Effects of Cocaine on the Cardio-respiratory Functions

Six Ss were used in this study. They were habituated to the primate chair, and experimentations were carried out by using the same experimental procedures described in Study I. The polygraphs of EEGs, eye movements, H.R., and R.R. were recorded daily throughout an experimental session of drug test. Following a 1- to 2-day period of control experiments, cocaine was administered at doses of 2 to 4 mg/kg i.v. to alert Ss by using the remote-control technique. Mean H.R. and R.R. per min for each subject were determined by ten randomly derived observations from the polygraphic recordings at various times before and after injection of cocaine (5, 10, 30, 60 min and every 0.5 hr thereafter up to 5 to 6 hr after injection).

Study III: Tolerance to the Convulsant Effect of Cocaine

Experimental session consisted of the daily injections of cocaine (once daily) and the polygraphic recordings for 7 to 15 days in the short-term session or for 5 to 6 months in the long-term session.

In the short-term sessions, nine Ss were restrained in the primate chair and placed in the observation chamber. The polygraphic recordings and drug injections were carried out daily throughout a 7- to 15-day period of session. Cocaine solution (5.0 mg/ml) was administered through the venous catheter by a remote-control technique. The minimal convulsant dosage (MCD) of cocaine that produced a minimal grade of convulsions lasting 10 to 30 sec was established by injecting cocaine at a constant infusion rate of 5 mg/ml/10 sec. The injection was terminated as the onset of the convulsive seizures manifested by the EEGs, and at this point the daily MCD was calculated. The MCD of cocaine was given to the Ss daily

while recording the polygraphs. One to two days before the beginning of drug session, the Ss were habituated to the chair and the control experiments were conducted. Following completion of the experimental session of daily cocaine administrations, a 3- to 4-week drug-free period was allowed to the Ss in their home cages until the beginning of the next session.

In the long-term session, two Ss were permanently housed in an open-face cubicle (74 × 71 × 86 cm) and fitted with a monkey jacket (nylon net) connected to a restraining joint-arm attached to the rear wall of the cubicle to allow relatively free movements to the Ss. Cocaine was injected once daily to the Ss at a MCD during recording of the polygraphs, using the same procedures as the short-term session. A complete session consisted of a daily cocaine injection and the polygraphic recordings for 5 consecutive days every week (no drug was given for 2 days over the weekends) over a 5- to 6-month period.

Study IV: Tolerance to Cardiorespiratory Stimulating Effects of Cocaine

Six Ss were used in this study. An experimental session consisted of daily injections of cocaine and polygraphic recordings of EEGs, eye movements, H.R., and R.R. for a period of 7 to 15 days. The Ss were restrained in a primate chair throughout a complete experimental session. Following a 1- to 2-day period of control experiments in which saline was injected and the polygraphs were recorded, an experimental session of drug test was initiated. Cocaine was administered daily at the same subconvulsant doses (2 to 4 mg/kg, i.v.), and the effects of drug on the H.R. and R.R. were determined. Cocaine (5 mg/ml) was injected by the remote-control technique at constant rate of 5 mg/ml/10 sec. Mean H.R. and R.R. per min were determined daily using the same procedures as those in Study I. A 3- to 4-week drug-free period was allowed to the Ss in their home cages following every completion of the experimental session.

Study V: Dispositional Tolerance of Cocaine

Two Ss used in this study were restrained in the primate chair. The blood samples were drawn from the Ss at various times (5, 15, 30, and 60 min, 2, 3, and 4 hr) after i.v. injection of $[^3H]$ cocaine (4.0 mg/kg as free base) while recording polygraphs. $[^3H]$ Cocaine concentration in plasma was determined by the method previously described.[28] Mean half-life (T 1/2) of [³H] cocaine was determined following the [³H] cocaine injection on the first day and on the fourth day following the subsequent two injections (once daily) of the same dose of nonlabeled cocaine (4.0 mg/kg).

EFFECTS OF COCAINE ON THE ELECTRICAL ACTIVITIES OF THE BRAIN AND ANIMAL BEHAVIOR

Excitatory Effects of Cocaine on the Spontaneous EEGs and Animal Behavior

Polygraphs of EEGs, eye movements, and heart and respiratory rates were recorded from the monkey restrained in the primate chair, and the effects of cocaine on these activities were studied. An experimental session of drug administration was conducted following 1 to 2 days of control experiments. A representative pattern of sequential changes in the polygraphic recordings following an i.v. injection of cocaine (4.0 mg/kg) to the monkey was shown in Figure 1. Before injection (Figure 1A), the EEGs showed low-voltage fast wave (LVFW) arousal pattern in the neocortex and the subcortical structures. The animal was behaviorally calm-alert and experienced regular rhythms of respiration, heart rate, and eye movements. Following an injection of cocaine (Figure 1B), the animal showed persistent LVFWs in the EEGs with marked increases in alertness and heart and respiratory rates. Thirty minutes after injection (Figure 1C), high-amplitude spikes appeared in the amygdala and hippocampus, and the animals showed hyper-excitation in their overall behavior accompanied by increases in eye movements and respiratory and heart rates. These arousal patterns in the EEGs and the animal's behavior lasted for 1 to 2 hr (Figure 1D). Four to five hours after the injection (Figure 1E and F), the polygraphic recordings and the animal's behavior returned to the pre-drug control pattern. These results indicate that an injection of cocaine produced an excitatory effect on the EEGs and the animal's behavior with marked increases in the heart and respiratory rates. The intensity and magnitude of the excitatory effects on the EEGs and behavior following the cocaine injection varied depending upon the dosage of the drug; the higher dose produced the higher intensity and longer duration of arousal pattern in the EEGs and behavioral responses.

Convulsant Effect of Cocaine on the EEGs and Animal Behavior

An intravenous injection of cocaine at high doses (4 to 8 mg/kg) in the monkeys produced clonic convulsion with epileptiform seizures in the brain. Figure 2 shows a representative pattern of sequential changes in the polygraphic recordings before and after an i.v. injection of convulsant dose of cocaine in the monkey. An injection of 4.0 mg/kg cocaine was given at a constant injection rate of 5 mg/ml/10 sec through a venous catheter. Immediately after the onset of injection, high-amplitude spike discharges began to appear in the amygdala and hippocampus accompanied by increases in respiration and heart rate. Subsequently, severe convulsive seizures and overt clonic convulsions ensued and lasted for 40 sec (Figure 2B). Following the convulsions (Figure 2B), the epileptiform high-amplitude unitary spike-and-waves persisted to appear predominantly in the frontal lobe of the neocortex and the limbic system structures. Five minutes later (Figure 2C), these spikes disappeared from the neocortex but they still appeared in the limbic system. Subsequently, the LVFWs continued to appear in the neocortex and the limbic system structures (Figure 2D and E). During this period, the heart and respiratory rates and eye movements increased markedly. The animals displayed hyperexcitation in their behavior accompanied by increases in motor activity of extremities with mydriasis and excessive salivation. This post-convulsive behavioral hyperexcitation lasted for 1 hr. Four to five hours after the injection, the heart and respiratory rates returned to the pre-drug control level. Usually, 5 to 6 hr after injection the polygraphic recordings and the animal's behavior returned to the pre-drug control pattern.

The severity and duration of convulsions varied depending upon the dosage of this drug; the higher dosage produced the more severe convulsions and longer duration. Usually, a dose of 4 to 5 mg/kg of cocaine produced a convulsion lasting for 0.5 to 1.0 min, and a dose of 5 to 8 mg/kg produced a convulsion lasting for 1 to 3 min.

Inhibitory Effect of Cocaine on the Electrically Evoked Discharges in the Limbic System

An intravenous injection of cocaine (1 to 4 mg/kg) suppressed the electrical discharges within the limbic system evoked by electrical stimulation, while persisting EEG's and behavioral arousal in

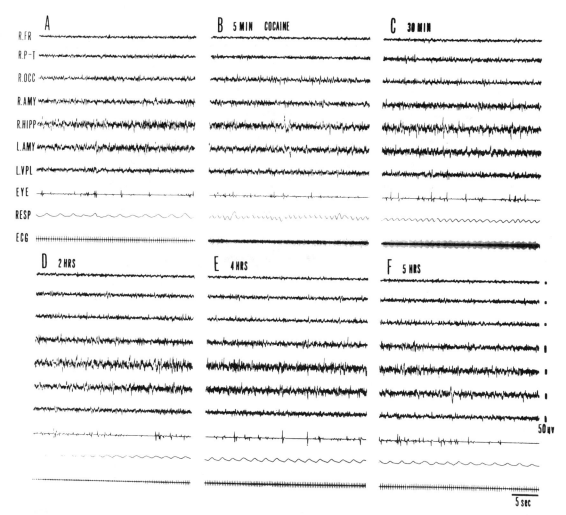

FIGURE 1. Polygraphic recording of EEG activities, eye movements, and respiratory and heart rates before and after an i.v. injection of cocaine (4.0 mg/kg) in the monkey. Recordings represent states before (A), 5 min (B), 30 min (C), 2 hr (D), 4 hr (E), and 5 hr (F) after the injection of drug, respectively. The recordings represent (from top to bottom): EEG of the frontal (R.FR), parietal and temporal (R.P-T), and occipital lobes (R.OCC), amygdala (Basolateral nucleus [R.AMY]), hippocampus (R.HIPP), amygdala (L.AMY), ventral posterolateral nucleus of the thalamus (L.VPL), eye movement (EYE), respiration (RESP), and heart rate (ECG), respectively. R and L incidate right and left side, respectively.

the monkeys. The electrical discharges within the limbic system were evoked by the electrical stimulations of the hippocampus or the amygdala in the monkeys restrained in a primate chair, and an i.v. injection of cocaine was given through the catheter. The representative pattern of the discharges in the limbic system evoked by the electrical stimulation of the hippocampus (4.5 V for 20 sec) in the monkey is shown in Figure 3A. Spike discharges occurred during the electrical stimulation (intrastimulatory discharges, IDs) and after the stimulation (after-discharges, ADs) in the limbic system structures without alteration in the neocortical EEGs. After an injection of cocaine

(4.0 mg/kg, i.v.), the EEGs continued to show LVFWs, and the heart and respiratory rates increased markedly (Figure 3B). Ten minutes after the injection, the same stimulation (4.5 V) failed to evoke the limbic discharges (IDs and ADs). However, an increased intensity of stimulation (5.0, V) was effective in producing the IDs and slight ADs in the ipsilateral amygdala and the IDs in the contralateral hippocampus. Such an effect after 5.0-V stimulation is shown in Figure 3C. One and two hours after the cocaine injection (Figure 3D and E), 7.0 V were required to evoke both IDs and ADs in the same structures. The time course of a typical experiment is shown in Figure 3A to

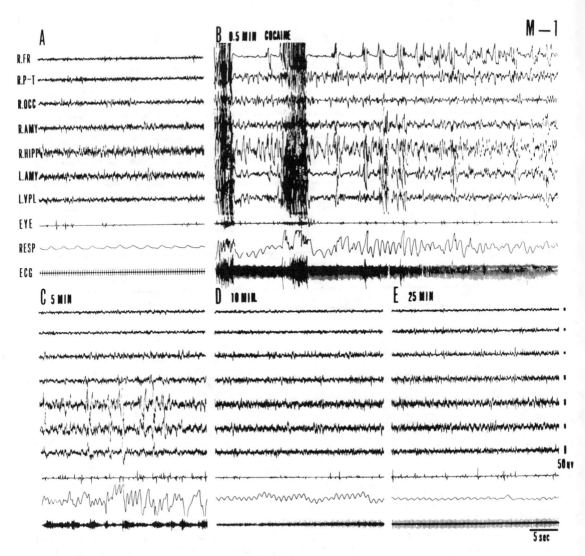

FIGURE 2. Polygraphic recordings of EEG activities, eye movements, and respiratory and heart rates before, during, and after convulsions produced by an injection of cocaine (4.0 mg/kg, i.v.) in the monkey (same monkey used in Figure 1). Recordings represent states before (A), 0.5 min (B), 5 min (C), 10 min (D), and 25 min (E) after cocaine injection, respectively (for abbreviations see legend to Figure 1).

F. Four hours later (Figure 3F), the IDs and ADs began to reappear in the amygdala using the same stimulation as the control (4.5 V), but the ADs in the contralateral hippocampus still did not appear. These results indicated that cocaine suppressed the limbic discharges to the hippocampal stimulation. The same suppressive effect was also seen on the limbic discharges evoked by the amygdaloid stimulation. The IDs' threshold of hippocampal stimulation increased 56% in voltage above the pre-drug control at 1 hr after cocaine injection (4.0 mg/kg) in the monkey, and it returned to the control level within 4 hr after the injection. In the control experiments, an injection of saline (1 ml/kg, i.v.) produced no change in the limbic discharges in the monkeys under the same experimental conditions.

EFFECTS OF COCAINE ON THE CARDIORESPIRATORY FUNCTIONS

As previously shown in the polygraphic recordings (Figures 1 and 2), an injection of cocaine produced marked increases in the heart and respiratory rates in the monkeys. In the control experiments without drug injection using six different monkeys, the mean H.R./min ranged

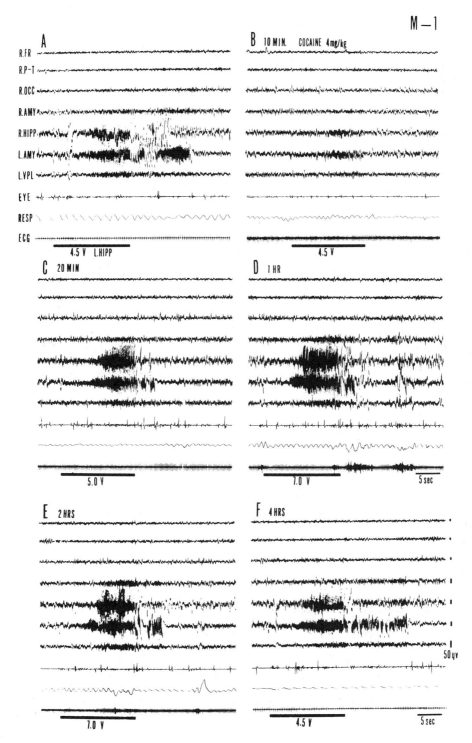

FIGURE 3. Electrical discharges in the interhippocampal-amygdaloid structures elicited by electrical stimulation of the hippocampus in the monkey. Stimulation of the left hippocampus (marked by a horizontal bar at the bottom of the recording) at intensities of 4.5 to 7.0 V (1 ms pulse width at 50 Hz for 20 sec) before and after an injection of the cocaine (4.0 mg/kg, i.v.). A. Intrastimulatory discharges (IDs) and after-discharges (ADs) in the right hippocampus and left amygdala elicited by electrical stimulation of the left hippocampus (4.5 V) before drug injection. B. No IDs and ADs following the same stimulation 10 min after cocaine. C, D, E, and F. Changes in patterns of the IDs and ADs evoked by various intensities of the stimulation at various times following the injection (for abbreviations see legend to Figure 1).

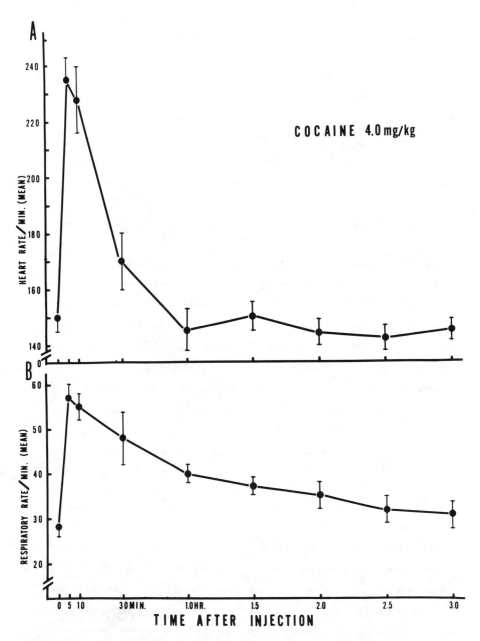

COCAINE 4.0 mg/kg

FIGURE 4. Graphs showing a representative pattern of alterations in heart rate/min (A) and in respiratory rate/min (B) per min. The abscissae represent the time after the injection of drug. Each value represents the mean rate/min ± SD (vertical bar). The means in both heart and respiratory rates were composed of ten randomly derived observations. Both Graphs A and B are the result of simultaneous observation.

from 121 ± 3.5 (SE) to 181 ± 4.0, and the mean R.R./min ranged from 21.7 ± 0.6 (SE) to 30.3 ± 0.6. Figure 4 shows a representative pattern of alterations in the H.R. and R.R. following an injection of cocaine at a subconvulsant dose of 4.0 mg/kg in the monkey. Before injection, the control H.R./min was 150 ± 2.5 (SD) (Figure 4A). Five minutes after injection, the H.R. increased to 238 ± 8.0/min which represents a 58.7% increase above the pre-drug control level. Subsequently, it lowered to a level of 228 ± 12.7 (SD) (+47.5% increase above the pre-drug control) and 168 ± 10.4 (+12.1% increase) at 10 min and 30 min, respectively, after injection. Following this period, the H.R. continued to decline to a level below the pre-drug control (5 to 8% decrease below the control level). Four to five hours after injection, it recovered to the control level.

Simultaneously, as shown in Figure 4B, the R.R. increased an average of 57 ± 3.0 (SD)/min at 5 min after injection. This represents a 100% increase above the pre-drug control level of 28 ± 2.5/min. Subsequently, it lowered to 55 ± 3.1 (SD) (+84% increase above the pre-drug control), 48 ± 7.5 (+61.2% increase), and 40 ± 2.2 (+37.6%

increase) at 10, 30, and 60 min, respectively, after the injection. Four to five hours after injection, it recovered to the pre-drug control level. In the control experiments, an injection of saline (1 to 2 ml/kg) produced no changes in the H.R. and R.R. under the same experimental conditions. These results indicate that cocaine produced marked increases in the heart and respiratory rates in the monkeys.

DEVELOPMENT OF TOLERANCE TO CONVULSANT AND CARDIORESPIRATORY STIMULATING EFFECTS AND DISPOSITION OF COCAINE

Tolerance to the Convulsant Effect of Cocaine

As stated above, an injection of cocaine in high doses produced clonic convulsions, and the severity and duration of the convulsions varied with a dosage of this drug. In this study, monkeys were daily treated with an injection of cocaine at the minimal convulsant dosage for 7 to 15 days in the short-term sessions or for 5 to 6 months in the long-term sessions. With repeated daily injections of cocaine, the MCD of cocaine markedly increased. Typical changes in the MCD of cocaine following repeated daily injections are shown in

Figure 5. An injection of cocaine at a dose of 3.1 mg/kg produced convulsions lasting 30 sec on the first day, but the same dose on the subsequent 3 days did not produce convulsions (Figure 5A). Following 3 days without cocaine injection, an increased dose of 4.7 mg/kg was required to produce a convulsion. The same dose on the subsequent day did not produce a convulsion. In another session using a different subject (Figure 5B), the same dose was given daily over a 2-day span. An injection of 5.4 mg/kg produced a convulsion on the first day but no convulsion on

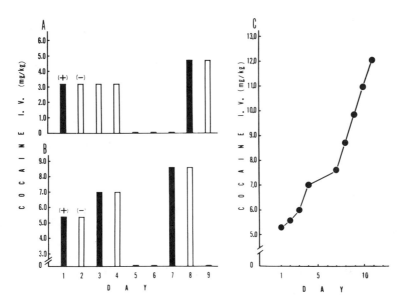

FIGURE 5. Typical pattern of changes in the minimal convulsant dosage (MCD) of cocaine following repeated daily injections in the monkeys. In Graphs A and B, the black bar (+) indicates the MCD and the open bar (−) the dose which did not produce convulsions. No drug was given on the fifth, sixth, and seventh days in Graph A and on the fifth, sixth, and ninth days in Graph B. Different monkeys were used for the data in each of two graphs. In Graph C, values (● - ●) represent daily MCD for 11-day sessions. No drug was given on the fifth and sixth days of drug administration.

the next day. A dose of 7.0 mg/kg produced a convulsion on the third day but no convulsion on the fourth day. Following 2 days without cocaine injection, the MCD increased to 8.6 mg/kg on the seventh day, but this same dose produced no convulsion on the eighth day. These results indicate that a repetition of a daily cocaine injection at the same dose reduced the effect of this drug in producing convulsions. It was necessary to use increased dosages of cocaine to produce its convulsant effect repeatedly following daily injections. Figure 5C is representative of the data indicating daily increases in the MCD of cocaine following repeated daily injections. The MCD on the first day was 5.2 mg/kg, and it rapidly increased to 5.6, 6.0, and 7.0 mg/kg on the second, third, and fourth days respectively.

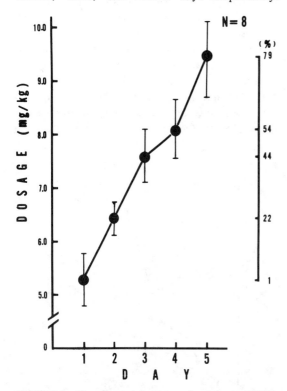

FIGURE 6. The mean minimal convulsant dosage (MCD) of cocaine and the mean percent increases of the MCD above the first MCD for the first 5 days of eight experimental sessions using six different monkeys. Each session consisted of daily injections of cocaine (once daily) for 5 to 10 days. The left ordinate represents i.v. dosage of cocaine and the right ordinate percent increases of the MCD. The abscissa represents days of the experimental sessions. Each value represents the mean ±SE (vertical lines). The mean MCD for the second to fifth days differs significantly from the first MCD (P<0.01) and from each other (P<0.5) using Student's t test. (From Matsuzaki, M., Spingler, P. J., Misra, A. L., and Mulé, S. J., *Life Sci.*, in press, 1976. With permission.)

Following 2 days without a drug injection, the MCD on the seventh day was 7.6 mg/kg and increased continuously to 12.0 mg/kg by the eleventh day of drug administration.

Figure 6 represents the mean MCD of cocaine and the mean percent increase in the MCD from the first dose of cocaine for the first 5 days of eight different experimental sessions using six different monkeys. The mean MCD on the first day was a 5.3 mg/kg, and it increased to a 6.4 mg/kg (+22% increase), 7.6 mg/kg (+44%), and 8.1 mg/kg (+54%) respectively on the second, third, fourth, and fifth days of drug administration. The differences in the mean MCD for each day in comparison to the first MCD and to each other were statistically significant (see Figure 6).

Figure 7 represents a typical pattern of alteration in daily MCD of cocaine during a long-term chronic administration. In the prolonged experimental session, the elevated MCD was maintained by a daily injection of cocaine, and during this period the MCD level migrated between a 50 and 100% increase above the initial MCD. When cocaine was withdrawn after 39 days of chronic administration, the MCD returned to the initial control level (4.1 mg/kg) at 41 days after the discontinuance of cocaine. Following chronic administration and subsequent withdrawal of the drug, the Ss became gentle and inactive, and they were persistently depressed in their overall behavior. Upon withdrawal, the Ss exhibited persistent high-amplitude rhythmic slow-waves (5 to 6 Hz) predominantly in the neocortical EEGs associated with their behavioral depression.

When the animal was reintroduced to chronic administration of cocaine following a 40-day drug-free period (see S2-1 and S2-2 of Figure 7), the MCD rapidly increased by 80% (a dose of 7.7 mg/kg) above the first dose within a 2-week period of daily injection. The MCD gradually lowered from the peak of 80% to a level of 25 to 40% above the control and was maintained at this level for 5 weeks. Subsequently, the MCD elevation stabilized at a 20 to 33% level, and the animals began to have convulsions of a constant intensity and magnitude lasting 20 to 25 sec, as manifested by the EEGs and behavioral responses. The animals displayed post-convulsive hyperexcitation which was also stabilized simultaneously with the convulsions and usually lasted for 2 to 2.5 hr. The animals displayed self-mutilation (biting and chewing of digits of extremities, hands, arms, and

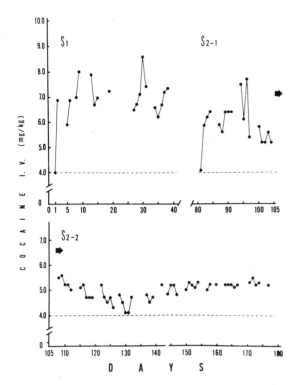

FIGURE 7. Typical pattern of changes in the daily minimal convulsant dosage (MCD) of cocaine during chronic injections in the monkey. In the upper graph S1 represents the daily MCD for the first session (39 days), and S2-1 represents the MCD for the second session which started after 41 days without drug injection following the first session (S1). S2-2 in the lower graph is a continuance of the S2-1 (shown by black arrows). The ordinate represents i.v. dosage of cocaine, and the abscissa, the days of the experimental session. Black dots indicate the daily MCD, and the connecting lines between dots indicate that the daily injections were given on the consecutive days. Usually, a daily injection was given for 4 to 5 consecutive days per week (no drug was given for 2 days over the weekend). The horizontal broken lines in the graph indicate the control MCD level (the first MCD). (From Matsuzaki, M., Spingler, P. J., Misra, A. L., and Mulé, S. J., *Life Sci.,* in press, 1976. With permission.)

legs) during the post-convulsive hyperexcitation. Except during the post-convulsive excitation, the Ss were usually inactive and depressed in their behavior most of the time. At this stage of chronic treatment, the Ss showed hypersensitive excitation following an i.v. injection of cocaine at a subconvulsant low dose, suggesting an increase in sensitivity to the excitatory effect of cocaine. These results indicated that chronic treatment with a daily MCD of cocaine produced a constant intensity of convulsions and post-convulsive excitatory responses, and upon the withdrawal the Ss showed chronic alterations in the EEGs and

behavioral responses suggesting withdrawal syndrome.

These results indicated that the repeated daily administration of cocaine in the monkeys resulted in tolerance to the convulsant effect of cocaine, and this tolerance was maintained by a long-term chronic administration of this drug. Following withdrawal of the drug, the animals showed chronic alterations in the EEGs and their behavioral responses.

Tolerance to the Cardiorespiratory Stimulating Effect of Cocaine

An intravenous injection of cocaine at a subconvulsant dose (2 to 4 mg/kg) as well as a convulsant dose produced marked increases in the heart rate and respiratory rate.[20],[21] However, these effects were reduced by repeated daily injections of cocaine (Figure 8). An injection of cocaine at a subconvulsant dose (4.0 mg/kg, i.v.) produced average increases of 46.1 and 24.0% above the pre-drug control in the H.R. at 10 min and 30 min, respectively, after the injection on the first day (Figure 8A). However, the same dose on the second day produced average increases in the H.R. of only 23.3 and 10.9% at 10 min and 30 min respectively after the injection. Average increases of 18.4 and 10.5% at 10 min and 30 min respectively were observed on the third day. Simultaneously, the R.R. (Figure 8B) increased an average of 65.3 and 46.4% above the pre-drug control at 10 min and 30 min, respectively, after injection on the first day. However, the average increase of R.R. was 40.0 and 24.1% at 10 min and 30 min, respectively, on the second day and 28.2 and 17.8% on the third day. In the control experiments, injections of saline (1 to 2 ml/kg) produced no alterations in the H.R. and R.R. under the same experimental conditions. These results indicated that repeated daily injections of cocaine significantly reduced its stimulating effects on the heart and respiratory rates in the monkeys.

Tolerance to the Physiological Disposition of Cocaine

The repeated daily injections of cocaine (4.0 mg/kg, i.v.) also reduced the biological half-life (T ½) of cocaine in the plasma of monkeys. The mean plasma T ½ of [^{3}H] cocaine on the first day for two monkeys was 93 min, but following the subsequent two daily injections of the same dose of nonlabeled cocaine, it decreased to 48 min on the fourth day, which represented a 48% reduction in T ½. This result suggested development of dispositional tolerance to cocaine following the repeated daily injections at the same dose in the monkeys.

IMPLICATIONS OF ELECTROPHYSIOLOGICAL AND NEUROPHARMACOLOGICAL ASPECTS ON THE CNS ACTION OF COCAINE AND TOLERANCE DEVELOPMENT

Effect of Cocaine on Electrical Activities of the Brain and Cardiorespiratory Functions

This study demonstrated that an i.v. injection of cocaine (2 to 4 mg/kg) produced an excitatory effect on the spontaneous EEGs, as manifested by low-voltage fast-wave arousal pattern in the neocortex and the fast-waves with spikes in the limbic system, accompanied by increases in alertness, motor activities, eye movements, and heart and respiratory rates. The intensity and magnitude of the excitatory responses to cocaine varied depending upon the drug dosage. These results proved the excitatory effects of cocaine on the EEGs and behavioral responses. Furthermore, the stimulant effect on the central sympathetic nervous system was manifested by marked increases in the heart and respiratory rates. With high doses, this drug produced clonic convulsions with seizures in the neocortex and subcortical structures, accompanied by the symptoms of hypersensitive stimulation of the sympathetic nervous system, such as severe tachycardia and hyperventilation, mydriasis, and excessive salivation. The seizures and overt clonic convulsions occurred during or immediately after the i.v. injection of cocaine at a constant infusion rate of 5 mg/ml/10 sec. The severity of convulsions as manifested by the EEGs and behavioral responses was dose-dependent. These results suggest that the convulsant effect of cocaine is due to its direct action on the CNS of the brain.[29-32] The phenomena that the convulsive seizures originated from the amygdala and hippocampus during cocaine injection and that the epileptiform unitary spike-and-waves persisted to appear in these structures and the frontal lobe after convulsions strongly suggest that the limbic system plays an important role in the convulsant effect of this drug.

This study also demonstrated an inhibitory effect of cocaine on the electrically evoked discharges within the limbic system with persistence in the excitatory effect on the spontaneous EEGs and behavior. These results suggest that the limbic system is involved in the mechanisms of the CNS action of cocaine, and the inhibition of the limbic system might be responsible for the excitatory effect on the EEGs and behavioral responses. Therefore, it is conceivable that the excitatory

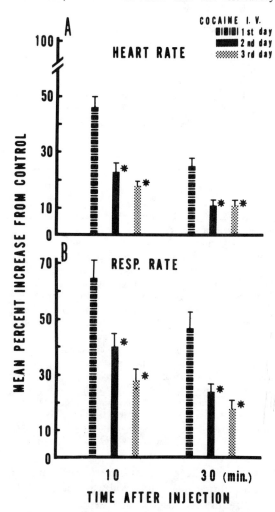

FIGURE 8. Mean percent increase above control in heart rate/min (A) and in respiratory rate/min (B) at 10 min and 30 min, respectively, after the daily i.v. injection of cocaine (4.0 mg/kg) for the first, second, and third days of eight experimental sessions using four different monkeys. Each value represents the mean ± SE (vertical lines). *Values differ significantly from appropriate values observed on the first day (P < 0.01). The differences in values observed on the third, fourth, and fifth days as compared to those on the second day were not statistically significant. (From Matsuzaki, M., Spingler, P. J., Misra, A. L., and Mulé, S. J., Life Sci., in press, 1976. With permission.)

effect of cocaine on the EEGs and behavior is related to its inhibitory action on the inhibitory system of the limbic-reticular activating system. The precise mechanisms of the excitatory and the convulsant effects of this drug remain to be explored.

Potentiation of adrenergic transmission has been postulated repeatedly as the mechanism by which cocaine exerts its peripheral autonomic effects.[33-35] Rothballer[23] has proposed that there is a similar potentiating effect of cocaine at adrenergic receptors in the reticular activating system, and that cocaine exerts its effect on the EEG arousal induced by adrenaline by a mechanism analogous to its peripheral effects. However, the inhibition of the uptake of norepinephrine by cocaine, which causes potentiation of adrenergic receptor, has been confirmed for the peripheral tissues, while brain norepinephrine uptake was unaffected.[29] Other workers[30-32] have suggested that the inhibition of norepinephrine uptake by cocaine may not be an important factor in the hypersensitivity produced by cocaine and that a direct action of this drug on the effector cells leads to hyperresponsiveness.

Development of Tolerance to the Convulsant and Cardiorespiratory Stimulating Effects and Disposition of Cocaine

This study demonstrated the development of tolerance to the convulsant and cardiorespiratory stimulating effects and dispositional tolerance in the monkey. The development of tolerance to the convulsant effects was indicated by a decrease in the effect of this drug in producing convulsions following repeated daily injections at the same dose, and also in the progressive increase of the daily cocaine MCD following chronic administrations. Tolerance to the convulsant effects of cocaine remained for a lengthy period (40 days) following withdrawal of this drug.

A marked reduction in the stimulant effects of cocaine on the heart and the respiratory rates following repeated daily injections of the drug at the same dose provided evidence for the development of tolerance to these effects. A marked reduction in plasma half-life of cocaine following repeated daily injections in the monkeys indicated dispositional tolerance. Thus, these results strongly suggest the development of functional tolerance in the central nervous system in addition to the dispositional tolerance.

Previous studies[1-11] on the chronic administration of cocaine in experimental animals (rats, guinea pigs, rabbits, cats, dogs, and monkeys) have demonstrated no tolerance to the excitatory effects of cocaine and no abstinence syndrome upon abrupt withdrawal.[9,11] Upon repeated daily administration, a pronounced increase in the severity of the behavioral and toxic effects of cocaine occurred.[2-4,7,12,14] In most of these studies, however, the drug was administered in subconvulsant doses either orally, intraperitoneally, or intramuscularly, and the effect of the drug was evaluated by gross visual observations of the animal's responses. Because of very rapid metabolism of cocaine, its effect varied considerably with the route of its administration. In our study, the drug was given intravenously at high doses and high rates of infusion (5 mg/ml/10 sec), and the MCD was determined daily in order to evaluate the drug's effects on the EEGs and behavioral responses. The high infusion rate was a critical factor for producing convulsions during or immediately after intravenous injections. In order to determine the MCD of cocaine, the constant i.v. injection rate (5 mg/ml/10 sec) provided an adequate means for producing convulsions during the injection. The measurement of the MCD of cocaine enabled us to precisely quantitate the development of tolerance to the convulsant effect. In addition, the electrophysiological parameters on the heart and respiratory stimulant effects allowed us to objectify the tolerance development of these activities. These values in conjunction with the EEG activities provide conclusive evidence for cocaine's tolerance development in the sub-human primate.

This study also demonstrated chronic alterations in the EEGs and behavioral responses following chronic cocaine treatment and its withdrawal. The animals became inactive and depressed in their overall behavior accompanied by persistent rhythmic slow-wave (5 to 6 Hz) in the EEGs, suggesting withdrawal syndrome. After reintroduction to chronic administration, the elevated MCD of cocaine gradually lowered and stabilized at a 20 to 30% elevation above control with a constant intensity of convulsion. However, the animal showed the post-convulsive hyperexcitation in addition to the hypersensitive excitation to the subconvulsant dose of cocaine, suggesting an increase in sensitivity to the excitatory effect of this drug. The mechanisms of increasing sensitivity to the excitatory effects of cocaine are presently controversial. It is conceivable that the neuronal mechanisms of convulsions by cocaine may differ from those of the excitatory effects. The central mechanisms underlying the development of tolerance to the convulsant and cardiorespiratory stimulating effects of cocaine remain to be explored.

ACKNOWLEDGMENTS

This work was supported in part by a contract from the U.S. Army Medical Research and Development Command (DADA-17-3080). The author wishes to thank Drs. S. J. Mulé, A. L. Misra, P. J. Spingler, and E. G. Whitlock for their contribution to this work.

REFERENCES

1. Einstein, S., *The Use and Misuse of Drug,* Wadsworth, Belmont, 1970.
2. Deneau, G. A., Yanagita, T., and Seever, M. H., Self-administration of psychoactive substances by the monkey – a measure of psychological dependence, *Psychopharmacologia,* 16, 30, 1969.
3. Seever, M. H., Psychologic dependence defined in terms of individual and social risks, in *Psychic Dependence,* Goldberg, L. and Hoffmeister, F., Eds., Springer-Verlag, Berlin, 1973, 25.
4. Weichowski, W., Über das Schicksal des Cocains and Atropins in Thierkörper *Arch. Exp. Pathol. Pharmakol.,* 46, 155, 1901.
5. Grode, J., Über die Wirkung längerer cocain darreichung bei Tieren, *Arch. Exp. Pathol. Pharmakol.,* 67, 172, 1912.
6. Tatum, A. L. and Seevers, M. H., Experimental cocaine addiction, *J. Pharmacol. Exp. Ther.,* 36, 401, 1929.
7. Downs, A. W. and Eddy, N. B., The effect of repeated doses of cocaine in the dog, *J. Pharmacol. Exp. Ther.,* 46, 195, 1932.
8. Downs, A. W. and Eddy, N. B., The effect of repeated doses of cocaine in the rat, *J. Pharmacol. Exp. Ther.,* 46, 199, 1932.
9. Zapata-Ortiz, V. L., Modificaciones psicologicas y fisiologicas produidas par la coca y la cocaine en los coqueros, *Rev. Med. Exp.,* 3, 132, 1944.
10. Gutierrez-Noriega, C. and Zapata-Ortiz, V., Cocainismo experimental. I. Toxicologia general acostumbra-miento y sensibilization, *Rev. Med. Exp.,* 3, 280, 1944.
11. Gutierrez-Noriega, C. and Zapata-Ortiz, V. L., Intoxicacion cronica por cocaina. I. Effectos sobre el crecimiento y reproduccion de las ratas, *Rev. Med. Exp.,* 5, 68, 1946.
12. Eddy, N. B., Halbach, H., Isbell, H., and Seevers, M. H., Drug dependence, its significance and characteristics, *Bull. WHO,* 32, 721, 1965.
13. Goodman, L. S. and Gilman, A., *The Pharmacological Basis of Therapeutics,* 3rd ed., Macmillan, New York, 1965.
14. Kosman, M. E. and Unna, K. R., Effect of chronic administration of amphetamine and other stimulant drugs on behavior, *Clin. Pharmacol. Ther.,* 9, 240, 1974.
15. Post, R. M. and Kopanda, R. T., Cocaine, kindling and reverse tolerance, *Lancet,* p. 409, February 15, 1975.
16. Sollman, T., *A Manual of Pharmacology,* 8th ed., W. B. Saunders, Philadelphia, 1957, 334.
17. Grollman, A., *Pharmacology and Therapeutics,* Lea & Febiger, Philadelphia, 1962, 436.
18. Caldwell, J. and Sever, P. S., The biochemical pharmacology of abused drugs. I. Amphetamine, cocaine, and LSD, *Clin. Pharmacol. Ther.,* 16, 625, 1974.
19. Mercier, J. and Dessaigne, S., Determination de l'accoutumance experimentale par une methode psychophysiologique. Etude e quelques drogues sympathomimetiques, de la nicotine et de la cocaine, *Ann. Pharm. Fr.,* 18, 502, 1960.
20. Matsuzaki, M., Differential effects of cocaine and pseudococaine on electrical activities in the limbic system of cats and monkeys, *Fed. Proc.,* 34, 781, 1975.
21. Matsuzaki, M., Misra, A. L., and Mulé, S. J., Development of acute tolerance to cardio-respiratory functions and EEG activities of cocaine and pseudococaine in the monkey, *Pharmacologist,* 17, 190, 1975.
22. Phillips, J. L., *A Cocaine Bibliography – nonannotated,* National Institute on Drug Abuse, Rockville, Maryland, 1974.
23. Rothballer, A. B., The effect of phenylephrine, metamphelamine, cocaine and serotonin upon the adrenaline-sensitive component of the reticular activating system, *Electroencephalogr. Clin. Neurophysiol.,* 9, 409, 1957.
24. Eidelberg, E., Lesse, H., and Gault, F. P., An experimental model of temporal lobe epilepsy, studies of the convulsant properties of cocaine, in *EEG and Behavior,* Glaser, G. H., Ed., Basic Books, New York, 1963, 272.

25. Tanaka, K., Anticonvulsant properties of procaine, cocaine, adiphenine and related structures, *Proc. Soc. Exp. Biol. Med.,* 90, 192, 1955.

26. Snider, R. S. and Lee, J. C., *A Stereotaxic Atlas of the Monkey Brain (Macaca Mulatta),* The University of Chicago Press, Chicago, 1961.

27. Olszewski, J., *The Thalamus of the Macaca Mulatta, An Atlas for Use with the Sterotaxic Instrument,* S. Karger, Basel, New York, 1952.

28. Misra, A. L., Nayak, P. K., Patil, M. N., Vadlamani, N. L., and Mulé, S. J., Identification of norcocaine as a metabolite of [^{3}H]-cocaine in rat brain, *Experientia,* 30, 1312, 1974.

29. Glowinski, J. and Axelrod, J., Effect of drugs on the uptake, release and metabolism of [^{3}H] norephinephrine in rat brain, *J. Pharmacol. Exp. Ther.,* 149, 43, 1965.

30. Maxwell, R. A., Wastila, W. B., and Eckhardt, S. B., Some factors determining the response of rabbit aortic strips to dl-norepinephrine-7-3H hydrochloride and influence of cocaine, quanethidine and methyl phenidate on these factors, *J. Pharmacol. Exp. Ther.,* 151, 253, 1966.

31. Kasuya, Y. and Goto, K., The mechanism of supersensitivity to norpinephrine induced by cocaine in rat isolated vas deferens, *Eur. J. Pharmacol.,* 4, 355, 1968.

32. Kalsner, S. and Nickerson, M., Mechanism of cocaine potentiation of response to amines, *Br. J. Pharmacol.,* 35, 428, 1969.

33. Frohlich, A. and Lowei, O., Über eine Steigerrung der Adrenalin-enpfindlichkeit durch Cocaine, *Arch. Exp. Pathol. Pharmakol.,* 62, 158, 1910.

34. Furchgott, R. F., The receptors for epinephrine and norepinephrine (adrenergic receptors), *Pharmacol. Rev.,* 11, 429, 1959.

35. Strömblad, C. B., Effect of denervation and of cocaine on the action of sympathomimetic amines, *Br. J. Pharmacol.,* 15, 328, 1960.

Behavior, Psychic, Neuropharmacologic and Physiologic Aspects

Cocaine: Physiological and Behavioral Effects of Acute and Chronic Administration

COCAINE: PHYSIOLOGICAL AND BEHAVIORAL EFFECTS OF ACUTE AND CHRONIC ADMINISTRATION

Jeffrey S. Stripling and Everett H. Ellinwood, Jr.

TABLE OF CONTENTS

INTRODUCTION

Cocaine has a wide variety of behavioral effects, the exact nature of which is dependent not only upon the species used, but also upon the dose and route of administration. Furthermore, repeated administration of the drug can result in both quantitative and qualitative changes in its behavioral effects. Cocaine has two major pharmacological characteristics which are known — its local anesthetic action and its effects on monoamines. The relationship of these properties to the drug's behavioral effects is at present not fully understood. Most of the research to date has emphasized the involvement of monoamines in the behavioral effects of cocaine. However, the drug's local anesthetic properties also merit consideration. This chapter will selectively review the physiological effects of cocaine, with emphasis on its local anesthetic properties and their possible involvement in certain of the drug's behavioral effects.

PHARMACOLOGICAL PROPERTIES

Cocaine was the first local anesthetic to be discovered, and it was this property of the drug which led to its introduction into medical practice by Koller in 1884.[113] The local anesthetic effect which it and other drugs produce is due to a reversible blockade of action potential conduction in neurons. This is accomplished by a selective blockade of sodium channels in the axonal membrane, thus preventing the transitory increase in sodium conductance which occurs during the action potential. The mechanism by which this occurs is not fully understood.[34,153,154] At concentrations below that required to block conduction completely, local anesthetics reduce the amplitude of the action potential, slow conduction speed, and increase the refractory period of neurons, resulting in a progressive reduction in the ability to follow high frequency stimulation.[34,122] Also, local anesthetics are useful in suppressing certain cardiac arrhythmias, although the mechanism of action responsible for this is uncertain.[170]

Unlike other local anesthetics, cocaine has major effects on monoamines. The best documented of these is the blockade of monoamine uptake at presynaptic terminals. This effect was first demonstrated in the autonomic nervous system, where cocaine blocks the uptake of norepinephrine at various sympathetic effector sites.[41,90,128,192,207] Other local anesthetics do not have this effect.[128,192] In the central nervous system, cocaine blocks the uptake of norepinephrine,[25,156,166] dopamine,[156] and serotonin.[157,158,172]

Since uptake of the monoamines is presumed to play a major role in their inactivation,[91] the effect of cocaine on this process would be expected to potentiate transmission at monoaminergic synapses. However, effects of cocaine related to the monoamines cannot necessarily be ascribed to this mechanism, since cocaine has effects on behavior and catecholamine metabolism not shared by other inhibitors of dopamine or norepinephrine uptake.[164] In addition, cocaine affects measures of monoamine turnover by mechanisms which may or may not be related to its uptake blockade.[21,32,74,169] Furthermore, cocaine's effect on uptake processes is not limited to the catecholamines and serotonin. It also blocks the uptake in brain of tryptophan, a precursor of serotonin[103,118] and of acetylcholine,[112] although this latter effect is present in other local anesthetics as well. Finally, at least at some effector sites in the peripheral nervous system, cocaine appears to have direct post-synaptic effects of functional significance.[96,98,129,149,198]

While the exact nature of cocaine's effects on monoamines may not be clear, there is considerable evidence that these effects are involved in cocaine's behavioral effects. By comparing the effects of cocaine on a certain behavior with those of other local anesthetics on the one hand, and with drugs affecting various monoamines on the other, some information on the source of cocaine's behavioral effects can be obtained.

EFFECTS OF ACUTE COCAINE ADMINISTRATION

Psychomotor Stimulant Effects

Cocaine is classified with the amphetamines and related drugs as a psychomotor stimulant.[194] It shares with these drugs an ability to produce arousal, locomotor activity, and stereotyped behavior, along with several common side effects. Other local anesthetics do not have these properties, and there is considerable evidence to link them to cocaine's effects on monoamines.

Systemic administration of cocaine produces sympathomimetic effects such as vasoconstriction, tachycardia, mydriasis, and hypertension.[65,140, 151,154,189] Other effects which cocaine shares with other psychomotor stimulants include hyperthermia,[32] anorexia,[167,182,196] and suppression of REM sleep.[137] The hyperthermic effect appears at least in part to be an indirect effect of vasoconstriction and drug-induced locomotor activity,[134,154] and may contribute to the toxicity of cocaine.[134] Cocaine is also self-administered[9,93,210,211] and facilitates intracranial self-stimulation.[33] In moderate doses it increases locomotor activity,[32,76,164,176, 178,196,197] while in high doses it produces stereotyped behavior.[66,161,176,203,209]

In the rodent the locomotor and stereotyped effects are somewhat difficult to separate. The locomotor activity which the drug induces has a stereotyped quality, typically consisting of repetitive circling of the cage perimeter. The stereotyped movements include repetitive sniffing, pawing, vertical or horizontal movements of the head, and repetitive rearing. The stereotyped effects can occur admixed with the locomotor activity, but are difficult to obtain in isolation without chronic administration of the drug, which intensifies them (see section on "Effects of Chronic Cocaine Administration"). The stereotyped behavior induced by cocaine is loosely similar to that induced by amphetamine, but does not include the chewing and biting aspects.[164,165]

The pharmacological aspects of these cocaine-induced behaviors in animals have received attention in a number of studies. Although these studies typically attempt to differentiate between the locomotor effects and stereotyped behavior produced by cocaine, this is sometimes difficult, not only because it is difficult to decide when one ends and the other begins, but also because of the nature of the measures used. Studies assessing locomotor activity usually rely on automated activity monitors, typically employing photocells. These monitors can also respond to stereotyped behaviors, thus confounding the two. Consequently, some studies reporting effects on locomotor activity may actually reflect an influence on stereotyped behavior.

The depletion of monoamines by reserpine antagonizes both the locomotor activity[76,104,161,165,176,177,195,197] and stereotyped behavior[203] produced by cocaine. Selective depletion of catecholamines by α-methyl-p-tyrosine weakens cocaine-induced locomotor activity[123,141] and stereotyped behavior,[141,161,203] suggesting primary involvement of the catecholamines in cocaine's effects. However, in comparison with amphetamine, cocaine's effects appear to be relatively more sensitive to reserpine and less sensitive to α-methyl-p-tyrosine.[165,176] This suggests either a greater dependence of cocaine on the reserve storage pool of catecholamines, or a greater involvement of serotonin in the effects of cocaine. With regard to specific catecholamines, there is evidence for the involvement of noradrenergic alpha receptors in the locomotor activity effect of cocaine, since phenoxybenzamine antagonizes this effect.[76,165] Dopamine antagonists also diminish cocaine-induced locomotor activity,[165,176] although this may in part be a reflection of nonspecific depressant effects.[176] Concerning cocaine-induced stereotyped behavior, there is inhibition of this effect by dopamine antagonists,[165,209] while phenoxybenzamine does not reduce it at a dose which strongly antagonizes the locomotor effect.[165]

The evidence for involvement of other neurotransmitters in the psychomotor stimulant effect of cocaine is sparse and often contradictory. Scheel-Krüger et al.[165] reported that a serotonin antagonist or depletion of serotonin by p-chlorophenylalanine produced an augmentation of cocaine-induced locomotor activity. In contrast, others have found no effect of p-chlorophenylalanine on cocaine-induced locomotor activity.[141,176] There are also conflicting reports of augmentation[165] or antagonism[84,141] of cocaine-induced rearing and stereotyped behavior by p-chlorophenylalanine and serotonin antagonists. With regard to acetylcholine, there is some evidence that an acetylcholine mechanism inhibits cocaine-induced psychomotor effects, since physostigmine reduces these effects,[136] while atropine or scopolamine augment or prolong certain of the behavioral effects of cocaine.[85,165]

Electrophysiological Effects of Cocaine

In most areas of the brain the electrophysiological effects of cocaine are those typically associated with behavioral arousal. Thus, moderate to high doses of cocaine produce desynchronization of cortical activity and an increase in multiple unit activity in the reticular formation of the cat[202] and an increase in rhythmical slow activity ("theta") in the hippocampus of the cat and rat.[56]

However, the most prominent electrophysiological effect of cocaine occurs in the olfactory forebrain, where large doses of cocaine produce spindles of high-amplitude sinusoidal activity in the range of 20 to 50 Hz.[47] This effect can be recorded in the olfactory bulb, amygdala, prepyriform cortex, olfactory tubercle, and nucleus accumbens[26,48,55] and has been demonstrated in the rat,[181] cat,[47,48,55,77] and in man.[87] The nature of this effect is illustrated in Figure 1.

The pharmacological mechanism responsible for the cocaine-induced spindles is not entirely clear. Other local anesthetics such as lidocaine produce highly similar effects,[152,199,200] and consequently it would seem that this action of cocaine is responsible. However, amphetamine, which releases catecholamines and blocks their reuptake,[8] has also been reported to produce spindles in the amygdala of the dog,[43] suggesting that cocaine's effects on catecholamines may be involved. The local anesthetic effect would seem to be primarily responsible, however, since in the cat it is much more difficult to produce spindles with amphetamine than with local anesthetics.[51,59]

Since spindling in the olfactory forebrain is the major electrophysiological effect of cocaine, its origin will be explored in some detail. During normal breathing through the nares, spindles of sinusoidal activity (usually in the range of 40 to 60 Hz) can be recorded in the olfactory bulb of a variety of species.[2,124,206] Nasal air flow appears to be essential for the occurrence of olfactory bulb spindles, since blocking the nares[43,78] or artificial respiration via a tracheal tube[77,131] eliminates the spindles. There is one report of olfactory bulb spindles occurring in the absence of nasal air flow in the cat if the animal was aroused.[133] Thus, while it is possible that olfactory bulb spindles occur under certain circumstances without nasal air flow, under normal circumstances the spindles are highly dependent upon it.

There are also central influences upon the olfactory bulb spindle. In the presence of nasal air flow, stimulation of the reticular formation increases the amplitude of the spindle via centrifugal fibers projecting to the olfactory bulb.[131] This is in keeping with studies showing a relationship

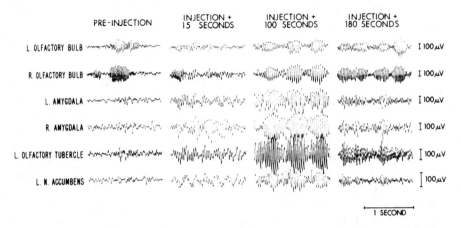

5.0 MG/KG COCAINE HYDROCHLORIDE (I.V.)

FIGURE 1. An illustration of the electrophysiological effect of a rapid intravenous injection of cocaine (5.0 mg/kg) in the cat. All recordings are monopolar with a bone screw as reference. Pre-injection: Normal olfactory spindles are present in the olfactory bulbs at a frequency of 40 Hz. Injection + 15 seconds: Spindle activity begins to appear in the amygdala, olfactory tubercle, and nucleus accumbens at a frequency of 25 to 30 Hz. Note that the right olfactory bulb exhibits activity both at this frequency and at a higher frequency similar to that present before injection. Injection + 100 seconds: The spindle response has reached its maximum amplitude. The frequency in all leads is approximately 25 Hz. Injection + 180 seconds: The drug effect is declining. The frequency in all leads has increased to approximately 35 Hz.[26]

between the olfactory bulb spindle and behavioral arousal.[51,88,108]

The olfactory bulb projects directly to the anterior olfactory nucleus, the olfactory tubercle, the corticomedial amygdala, and the prepyriform cortex.[22,162,163] The prepyriform cortex projects in turn to the basolateral amygdala.[107] Olfactory spindles have been recorded from a number of these areas in drug-free laboratory animals, including the prepyriform cortex[68,70,155,213] and both the basolateral and corticomedial amygdala.[43,78,110,132] Similar spindles have also been reported in man.[87,150] In some studies the spindles occurred regularly and in conjunction with nasal air flow,[43,155,213] while in other studies spontaneous spindling was less often seen in these areas while it was clearly present in the olfactory bulb[26,55,77] (see Figure 1). This discrepancy may be due in part to varying amounts of odors in the air, since this has been shown to influence amygdaloid spindles in the rat.[24] The arousal level of the animal may also be a factor. Several studies have found a strong relationship between arousal level or "emotional" behavior and the appearance of spindles in the amygdala or prepyriform cortex.[62,69,110,132] Cain[23] has suggested that the spindle in this area may be a reflection of a forebrain arousal system.

It is uncertain which structures in addition to the olfactory bulb can generate the spindles,[49,68,70] but it is clear that they can be recorded from the amygdala and prepyriform cortex. Spindles in these areas are dependent upon input via the olfactory bulb, since they can be blocked by prevention of nasal air flow[43,78] or olfactory bulb ablation.[10] However, the spindles in these areas are not merely a passive projection of olfactory bulb activity, because they can occur at lower frequencies than those simultaneously present in the olfactory bulb[69] (see Figure 1). The manner in which the spindles are generated in the olfactory bulb and other structures has been investigated in detail by Freeman[68,70,71] and Shepherd.[173-175]

The cocaine-induced spindles are not simply an augmentation of naturally occurring activity. While cocaine can augment spindle activity in the olfactory bulb, its effects are much more pronounced in the amygdala, where it produces very large spindles at sites that may exhibit no spindle activity at all in the absence of cocaine (see Figure 1). Often an initial depression of spindle amplitude in the olfactory bulb is seen following cocaine injection, while simultaneously a pronounced increase in spindling is evident in the amygdala.[55] Furthermore, cocaine causes a marked slowing of the sinusoidal activity contained in the spindles, often to a frequency one half (or less) that of the activity occurring in the absence of the drug in the olfactory bulb or amygdala[26,55,77] (see Figure 1). Thus cocaine appears to be acting to potentiate selectively the spindles in the amygdala and other central structures in comparison to the olfactory bulb.

The role of nasal air flow in the effect of cocaine is of interest. Just as in the case of spontaneous spindles, prevention of nasal air flow blocks amygdaloid spindles induced by cocaine,[27] as well as those induced by lidocaine[152,200] and amphetamine.[43] This raises the possibility that the drug-induced spindles may simply be a reflection of stimulation of respiration by the drug, thereby increasing nasal air flow. This would seem particularly plausible in the case of cocaine and amphetamine, both of which produce stereotyped sniffing as one of their major behavioral effects in some species. Furthermore, Domino and Ueki[43] found that a respiratory stimulant, trans-π-oxocamphor, also augmented amygdaloid spindles.

However, while effects on respiration may be a contributing factor, cocaine appears to produce spindling by a direct central effect. Several factors suggest that this is so. First, as previously mentioned, cocaine has a greater effect on spindles in the amygdala than in the olfactory bulb. Secondly, lidocaine produces an electrophysiological effect similar to that of cocaine in the amygdala, yet it does not cause stereotyped sniffing or stimulate respiration. Finally, Gault and Coustan[77] found that cocaine produced amygdaloid spindling in acute cats which were paralyzed, artificially respirated, and received nasal air flow at a constant rate. Thus, although nasal air flow appears to be necessary to the cocaine-induced spindles, the drug would appear to achieve its effect via a direct central mechanism. Riblet and Tuttle[152] reached a similar conclusion with respect to lidocaine. There do not appear to be any data on whether the effect reported for amphetamine is due to alteration of respiration or not.

It should be noted that the studies cited to this point do not prove that spindles can never occur without nasal air flow; in fact, one study has reported such an occurrence.[133] Furthermore, the injection of epinephrine directly into the olfactory bulb[133] or the injection of hypertonic saline via the carotid artery[183] can produce sinusoidal activity in the olfactory bulb without the presence of nasal air flow. While the pharmacological relevance of these effects to that of cocaine is unclear, they do suggest that under some circumstances the cocaine spindle in the olfactory forebrain might become independent of olfactory input. However, in our experience, the block of the cocaine-induced spindles in the cat by interruption of nasal air flow is dramatic and complete even with convulsant doses of cocaine.[27]

Another factor to consider in the effect of cocaine is the role of the reticular formation. As previously noted, stimulation of the reticular formation augments spindles in the undrugged animal.[131] There are apparently no data on the involvement of the reticular formation in the cocaine-induced spindle, but Riblet and Tuttle[152] found that lidocaine produced spindling in the intact cat or in a midbrain deafferented preparation, but not in a cerveau isolé preparation. This suggests that input from the reticular formation is necessary for the lidocaine effect and presumably for that of cocaine as well. It is doubtful that the drugs act at this site, however, since lidocaine does not produce behavioral arousal.

In summary, then, cocaine in large doses produces spindling in the olfactory forebrain which appears dependent upon nasal air flow and probably on reticular formation input, but does not appear to act at these sites. Presumably it acts either at the sites from which the activity is recorded or upon structures which project to those sites. The effect is similar if not identical to that produced by other local anesthetics.

Effects of Cocaine on Seizure Susceptibility

Cocaine has a biphasic effect on seizure susceptibility. In moderate doses it is an anticonvulsant, while in high doses it produces convulsions. Its anticonvulsive effects in laboratory animals include elevation of the electroconvulsive shock threshold,[184] prevention of the tonic phase of electroconvulsive shock- or pentylenetetrazol-induced convulsions,[186] reversal of the reserpine potentiation of pentylenetetrazol- or caffeine-induced convulsions,[29] prevention of audiogenic seizures,[17] prevention of seizures induced by hyperbaric oxygen,[106] and blockade of afterdischarges produced by electrical stimulation of the amygdala or hippocampus.[121] The convulsant properties of cocaine were discovered early in its clinical use and have been repeatedly demonstrated in laboratory animals.[26,47,51,141,182]

There are data implicating both the local anesthetic and monoamine effects of cocaine in these phenomena.

Lidocaine, procaine, and other commonly used local anesthetics have also been found to have anticonvulsant activity in laboratory animals. This anticonvulsant effect is active against a variety of experimentally induced convulsions or epileptiform activity, including penicillin-induced epileptiform activity in the cortex,[95] cortical afterdischarges elicited by electrical stimulation,[11,13,14,72] electroconvulsive shock-induced seizures,[15,64,72,186] audiogenic seizures,[63] pentylenetetrazol convulsions,[15,186] convulsions induced by hyperbaric oxygen,[106] and ethanol withdrawal seizures.[73] Furthermore, local anesthetics have been shown to have anticonvulsive effects in man with respect to both electroconvulsive shock-induced seizures[208] and epilepsy.[12,19] On the basis of these data, the anticonvulsant effect of local anesthetics seems quite potent.

Local anesthetics also produce behavioral convulsions at high doses which are similar to those induced by cocaine. This has been demonstrated in the mouse,[39,114,160] rat,[16,139] rabbit,[199,200] cat,[40,191,199-201] dog,[119] monkey,[126,127] and in man.[3,193]

The mechanism by which local anesthetics produce both convulsive and anticonvulsive effects is not established. It is difficult to explain both effects via a single mechanism. It has been suggested that local anesthetics produce only inhibitory effects on neurons, and that the convulsant effect of these drugs is due to a selective depression of inhibitory neurons.[67] This is supported by electrophysiological studies which indicate that local anesthetics selectively block inhibitory processes in the neocortex in high doses.[86,187,204] Such an action could be due to the tendency of local anesthetics to block conduction selectively in small-diameter axons.[34] However, with this model it is difficult to explain the anticonvulsant effect of local anesthetics.

The convulsant and anticonvulsant effects of these drugs may be differentially localized within the brain. In particular, a number of studies suggest that the convulsant effect of cocaine and other local anesthetics originates in the olfactory forebrain where their electrophysiological effects are most prominent. As previously indicated, these drugs in large doses produce high-amplitude spindles localized in this area. In convulsive doses,

these drugs have been reported to produce spike discharges in the amygdala which develop into a generalized electrographic and behavioral convulsion.[199,200] Furthermore, they can activate preexisting seizure foci in the amygdala or other limbic structures.[37,143,180] Finally, bilateral ablation of the amygdala in the rat has been reported to prevent cocaine convulsions.[49]

Diazepam is a potent antagonist of cocaine and other local anesthetic-induced seizures,[35,36,48] and it also antagonizes spindle activity in the amygdala.[48] Wale and Jenkins[201] found that diazepam did not prevent lidocaine convulsions in the cat when injected into the amygdala, but prevented the seizures when injected into the reticular formation. This suggests that diazepam may prevent the convulsions by blocking the reticular formation mechanism necessary to the electrophysiological effects of local anesthetics.[152] In contrast to diazepam, cocaine and other local anesthetics do not appear to act at the reticular formation. Jolly and Steinhaus[94] injected drugs into either the internal carotid or vertebral arteries following ligation of the basilar artery, thus permitting selective administration of drugs to either the forebrain or brainstem. They found that cocaine produced convulsions when administered via the internal carotid but not vertebral artery, indicating that its site of action in producing convulsions is rostral to the brainstem. Furthermore, this differential effect of cocaine was not seen in any of the other stimulants tested (pentylenetetrazol, nikethamide, and picrotoxin). emphasizing the rostral site of cocaine's convulsive action. Tuttle and Elliott[191] found that localized infusion of local anesthetics into the amygdala or hippocampus of the cat via chronically implanted cannulae produced high-voltage discharges in these sites, but that injection into the reticular formation was without effect. Infusion into the hippocampus was of particular interest because it induced synchronous activity in the amygdala and pyriform cortex which was reported to be similar to that seen following systemic administration of the drugs.

Further evidence of the localized nature of the convulsant effect of cocaine and other local anesthetics comes from consideration of their anticonvulsant effects. If these drugs produced convulsions by causing a generalized excitation of the central nervous system, then one would expect that their anticonvulsive effect would gradually shift to a proconvulsive effect as the dose is increased. However, available evidence indicates that local anesthetics continue to antagonize seizures induced by electroconvulsive shock and cortical afterdischarges elicited by electrical stimulation even when administered in doses near or above the convulsive threshold.[14,72,184,208]

An explanation for this is suggested by the work of Racine et al.[148] They found that procaine in a moderate or high dose augmented afterdischarges elicited by electrical stimulation of the amygdala in the rat, while the high dose (but not the moderate dose) blocked afterdischarges elicited by neocortical stimulation. Procaine also facilitated the development of behavioral convulsions to daily stimulation of the amygdala (kindling). Thus, in high doses, local anesthetics appear to exert anticonvulsive effects in the cortex while exerting proconvulsive effects in the area of the amygdala, which is also the site of the spindles produced by these drugs. The difference between brain areas does not seem to be entirely a qualitative one, since local anesthetics can evoke discharges when applied directly to the cortex in the appropriate concentration,[179] and cocaine and lidocaine have been reported to block afterdischarges in the amygdala in the proper dose.[121,185] Rather, there may be a difference in sensitivity to the drugs, with both the anticonvulsant and convulsant effects occurring at a lower dosage in the basal forebrain than in the cortex. This is supported by the fact that the amygdala and prepyriform cortex are among the most seizure-susceptible areas in the brain.[80]

Nothing which has been presented conclusively demonstrates that the amygdala or neighboring areas is the source of cocaine and local anesthetic convulsions, but available evidence points in this direction. It should be noted that the drug-induced spindles originating in the vicinity of the amygdala are not themselves the cause of the convulsions, since cats with their nares blocked have cocaine-induced behavioral convulsions without the appearance of any spindles in the amygdala.[27] Whether or not the spindles contribute to the convulsive effect is difficult to assess. The convulsive threshold to these drugs seems to be elevated in animals that are paralyzed and artificially respirated, but in this situation the elimination of the spindles is confounded with the effects of neuromuscular blocking agents.[77,127,131]

There is also evidence that factors other than the local anesthetic effect of cocaine are involved in its effects on seizure susceptibility. Matsuzaki[121] reported that cocaine in moderate doses suppressed afterdischarges in the amygdala and hippocampus produced by electrical stimulation, but pseudocaine, an isomer with cocaine's local anesthetic but not its psychomotor stimulant effects, did not. This suggests that the effects of cocaine on monoamines may contribute to its anticonvulsive action.

An examination of the data on monoamines and convulsions does indicate that they have an anticonvulsive effect. Thus, depletion of monoamines by reserpine increases susceptibility to electroconvulsive shock,[42,159,205] pentylenetetrazol convulsions,[159] and audiogenic seizures[109] and increases the rate of seizure development due to repeated electrical stimulation of the amygdala (kindling).[6] A number of studies indicate that specific depletion of catecholamines has a potentiating effect on convulsions due to electroconvulsive shock,[159,205] pentylenetetrazol,[31] and audiogenic seizures[20,109] and facilitates the rate of kindling due to amygdala stimulation.[6,31] In addition, amphetamine, which releases catecholamines, has an anticonvulsant action in epilepsy,[168] electroconvulsive shock,[42,159,184] audiogenic seizures,[81,109] and convulsions elicited by electrical stimulation of the amygdala.[185] The majority of studies concerning the relative contribution of dopamine and norepinephrine to this anticonvulsant effect implicates norepinephrine.[59,115,159,205]

There is also evidence for an anticonvulsive effect of serotonin.[18,28] Depletion of serotonin by p-chlorophenylalanine produces increased seizure susceptibility to electroconvulsive shock,[205] pentylenetetrazol,[4,38,159] and audiogenic seizures.[109] It is not certain what the net influence on seizure susceptibility might be of the combined effects of cocaine on all the monoamines, but it is plausible that the result might be a greater anticonvulsive effect for cocaine than for other local anesthetics, as suggested by the findings of Matsuzaki[121] (see above).

While depletion of monoamines with reserpine creates an increased seizure susceptibility in the case of standard convulsive agents, reserpine protects against the convulsions induced by cocaine.[47,160] The data are inconclusive as to which monoamine is critical to this effect. Eidelberg et al.[47] reported that dibenamine, a noradrenergic alpha blocking agent, or chlorpromazine, which has anti-catecholaminergic effects, prevented cocaine convulsions. Sanders[160] substantiated the finding with chlorpromazine but not with dibenamine. On the other hand, de Oliveira et al.[39,40] have presented evidence that serotonin is important in local anesthetic-induced convulsions, since depletion of serotonin with p-chlorophenylalanine raises the convulsive threshold, while the serotonin precursor 5-hydroxytryptophan lowers it.

These data do not resolve the extent to which cocaine's convulsive and anticonvulsive effects are related to its effects on monoamines, nor do they indicate the relative contribution of the various monoamines. The effects of monoamines on cocaine's convulsant and anticonvulsant properties may reflect their general involvement in convulsive phenomena rather than a specific action as the mediator of cocaine's effects. This possibility is reinforced by the evidence of de Oliveira et al.[39,40] that serotonin has effects on convulsions induced by local anesthetics other than cocaine. In any case it is puzzling why monoamines appear to have opposing effects on convulsions induced by cocaine versus those produced by other agents. This is not an entirely anomalous finding, since decapitation convulsions and certain aspects of electroconvulsive shock convulsions are also antagonized by depletion of the monoamines or catecholamines.[75,97] However, the opposing effects on cocaine's convulsive and anticonvulsive properties may be indicative of different anatomical sites for the two effects, as some of the local anesthetic data suggest (see above).

EFFECTS OF CHRONIC COCAINE ADMINISTRATION

Reports indicating that certain effects of cocaine become augmented with repeated use have existed for some time.[105] A number of studies indicate that repeated administration of cocaine can result in a potentiation of its convulsant effects. This has been shown in three different ways. First, the repeated daily administration of a subconvulsive dose of cocaine can eventually result in a convulsion. This has been demonstrated in the rat[46,135] and monkey.[188] While with a high dose the seizures develop rapidly,[46] this effect can also occur over a period of several months with a lower dose.[188] This effect is somewhat difficult to interpret due to the confounding effects of aging

and body weight changes. Furthermore, there is evidence that even daily handling or chronic administration of saline produces enhanced seizure susceptibility.[92]

The second method of demonstrating sensitization to cocaine's convulsant effect is to examine the number of days between successive drug-induced convulsions when a constant dose of cocaine is administered once daily. Using this method, the frequency of seizures in monkeys was found to increase during chronic administration of cocaine.[135] However, this measure requires that repeated convulsions be elicited in each animal, and thus the increasing seizure frequency may be due to the previous convulsions rather than to the effect of cocaine per se. Evidence indicates that convulsions induced by a number of commonly used agents produce increased seizure susceptibility.[1,120,142]

The third method of examining the effects of cocaine on seizure susceptibility is to administer chronically either a subconvulsive dose of cocaine or saline and then test for the convulsive threshold to cocaine. Since a control group is used and no convulsions are induced in the initial treatment, the effect of cocaine can be reliably assessed. Using this method, Stripling and Ellinwood[182] found that chronic cocaine treatment lowered the convulsive threshold in the rat. Furthermore, this effect persisted for at least 9 days after termination of cocaine administration.

A second effect of cocaine which shows potentiation with chronic administration is the drug-induced locomotor activity and stereotyped behavior. For some time there have been reports of increasing stimulant effects of cocaine on behavior as a result of chronic administration.[46,188] Furthermore, this increased sensitivity has been reported to persist for at least 10 days after the termination of chronic administration of cocaine.[188] Recently this effect has been studied in a more quantitative fashion. Using activity meters which would be expected to respond to the stereotyped behavior as well as locomotor activity, Post[135] reported that the amount of drug-induced activity increased over several weeks of chronic administration of a moderate dose of cocaine in rats. Ho et al.,[89] using similar methods in rats, found a similar increase for the first 7 days of chronic cocaine administration, but beyond that point the effect declined. This conflict is puzzling, since the same dose of cocaine was used in the two studies. Post[135] also found that chronic cocaine administration in monkeys produced an increasing amount of stereotyped behavior (as assessed by a rating scale) for several weeks, followed by a decline in the effect. Using a rating scale which incorporates both locomotor activity and stereotyped behavior, studies in our laboratory have found increased effects of cocaine in rats with chronic administration of either moderate or high doses over a period of 10 to 14 days.[99,181,182] Furthermore, this increased responsiveness to cocaine also appears to persist beyond termination of the chronic injection series for a period of weeks or more.[99,181,182] Effects similar to this have also been reported with amphetamine.[99,102,116,171]

A third effect of cocaine which is augmented by chronic administration is the drug-induced spindle activity in the olfactory forebrain. Stripling and Ellinwood[181] found that chronic administration of a high dose of cocaine for 13 days produced a progressively greater electrophysiological response in the amygdala to the drug. This sensitization appeared to persist for at least several weeks beyond the termination of chronic administration of cocaine.

Thus quantitative increases in three of the major effects of cocaine have been shown to occur with chronic administration. Each of these increases has been reported to persist for a period of a week or more. No study has yet clearly demonstrated the full extent of this persistence.

The sensitization to cocaine which has been demonstrated under laboratory conditions is of interest because of its possible relationship to the effects in man which chronic usage of cocaine and other psychomotor stimulants has been reported to have. Chronic amphetamine usage in man can produce a syndrome which progresses from compulsive inquisitiveness to a paranoid psychosis.[30,58,61] Cocaine has been reported to have similar effects, although the only clinical data available on this point are quite old (e.g., Lewin[111] and Maier[117]). Ellinwood et al.[58,60] have documented an animal model of psychomotor stimulant psychosis using chronic administration of increasing doses of methamphetamine in the cat. This chronic treatment resulted in an evolution of the behavioral response to the drug from stereotyped investigatory behavior to a reactive stage in which the animals exhibited enhanced startle reactions to real or nonexistent stimuli, and eventually to certain catatonic or cataleptic effects.

These changes appear qualitative rather than quantitative in nature, and it would seem that the quantitative changes described earlier are not sufficient to account for them. There is relatively little information on qualitative changes with cocaine in a laboratory setting. In a pilot study using chronic administration of a constant dose of cocaine in the cat for more than 1 year, we have seen the slow development of pronounced hyperreactive behaviors over time.[53] Chronic administration of cocaine has also been reported to produce cataleptic effects in the monkey[135,138] and dog.[83] The monkey data indicated a gradual shift in the effect of cocaine from stereotyped behavior to catalepsy over a period of several months. We have not yet seen this effect in the cat after a year of administration.

Thus, while there is not much information on qualitative changes with cocaine, available data show parallels with those for the amphetamines. It is of interest that most of the data on quantitative changes produced by chronic cocaine come from experiments with rats, while most data showing qualitative changes come from higher animals. It is not clear to what extent this is due to species differences as opposed to differences in the type of experiments performed with the various species. It should be noted that experiments with rats using rating scales[99,181,182] show some qualitative changes with chronic treatment, such as from locomotor activity to stereotyped behavior. This type of effect may be a true change in the nature of the drug effect, but it might also be due to quantitative changes in the intensity of competing responses.

The mechanism(s) responsible for these changes in the effects of cocaine with chronic administration is not known. There are a number of possibilities to be considered. In general there are few data which bear on the situation, because most studies have dealt with a single administration of cocaine. Some of the possibilities are listed below.

Metabolic changes — The most straightforward explanation of cocaine's enhanced effects with chronic administration is that it either accumulates in the body with repeated administration or that metabolic changes occur which result in its being inactivated more slowly, resulting in a more prolonged and possibly a more intense effect. Although long-term persistence of cocaine or its metabolites in rat brain has been reported after chronic administration by subcutaneous injection,[125] the residual amount was very small (0.5% of the amount present 2 hr after injection). It is doubtful that this small amount could significantly alter the response to subsequent administration of cocaine. The half-life of cocaine in the monkey is unchanged after chronic treatment,[135] while that in the rat and dog is shorter.[89,125,130] Thus changes in the metabolic rate would not seem to be responsible for the effects of chronic cocaine.

Absorption and distribution changes – There is some evidence to suggest that cocaine enters the blood and brain more readily with chronic administration. Ho et al.[89] reported that blood and brain levels of cocaine were higher 5 min following intraperitoneal injection in chronically treated rats than in naive ones, and that this change correlated with an increase in the locomotor activity induced by the drug. This new and important finding will require further exploration to determine its relationship to the augmented effects of cocaine with chronic administration.

A previous experiment by Angel and Roberts[5] contributes to this line of thought. They found that repeated administration of electroconvulsive shock or tricyclic antidepressants in rats increased the amount of cocaine in rat brain by 50 to 95% 20 min following an intraperitoneal injection. While the mechanism underlying this effect is unclear, the result is striking. The effect of electroconvulsive shock may reflect a general effect of convulsions on blood-brain barrier permeability or other factors affecting brain levels, which could explain the increasing frequency of convulsions to repeated high doses of cocaine.[46,135] The effect of the tricyclic antidepressants is even more interesting, since they share with cocaine the effect of blocking the uptake of norepinephrine. If the increase in brain levels of cocaine which they cause is due to this action, then chronic cocaine administration might reasonably have the same effect. The heuristic value of this experiment is limited, however, by the short interval between the last administration of tricyclic antidepressants (2 hr) or the last electroconvulsive shock (6 hr) and the administration of cocaine. Since sensitization to cocaine is persistent after chronic cocaine administration, it would be of interest to know the duration of the effects demonstrated in this experiment.

Miscellaneous effects of high doses – The chronic administration of high (but not moderate) doses of cocaine results in autonomic signs of stress in rats, including hypertrophy of the adrenal cortex (but not medulla).[101] Furthermore, toxic effects such as liver damage have been reported following chronic administration of high doses of cocaine.[83] Also, the hyperthermia and hypertension caused by high doses of cocaine might produce damage to the nervous system or its blood supply. The extent to which these effects actually occur at the high doses which some behavioral studies have used, and the extent to which they would alter the behavioral response to cocaine if they were present remain to be determined. Some of the behavioral changes reported with chronic administration of cocaine occur at moderate doses where such effects would not be prominent (e.g., Ho et al.,[89] Kilbey and Ellinwood,[99] and Post[135]).

Neurotransmitter effects – Chronic cocaine administration may result in alterations in the effect cocaine has on monoamines. For example, Gunne and Jonsson[82] found that chronic administration of a high dose of cocaine in rats resulted in a progressive elevation of the daily urinary excretion of norepinephrine, which returned to normal gradually over a period of 2 weeks or so after termination of the injections. This effect, indicative of an enhanced turnover of norepinephrine, is of particular interest because of its persistence similar to that of the sensitization to the behavioral effects of cocaine.

With respect to levels of monoamines, acute administration of cocaine has been found to lower brain levels of norepinephrine,[164] and Ho et al.[89] found reduced levels of norepinephrine and serotonin in rat brain after chronic administration of a moderate dose. In contrast, Gunne and Jonsson[82] found no significant change in norepinephrine levels after either acute or chronic treatment with a high dose of cocaine. Even if these results did not conflict, it is difficult to relate brain levels of neurotransmitters with the potency of cocaine, since neurons with low levels of neurotransmitter may still function normally.

Receptor sensitivity changes – Chronic administration of cocaine may result in the alteration of receptor sensitivity, as appears to occur for dopamine receptor sensitivity with chronic amphetamine treatment.[102] Ongoing research in our laboratory has thus far indicated that chronic administration of a high dose of cocaine in the rat results in an enhanced behavioral response to the dopamine agonist apomorphine.[100]

Conditioning — Under proper conditions, the response to a psychomotor stimulant can increase with repeated administration due to a conditioning process.[50,190] Explanations originally suggested include both classical conditioning, in which stimuli associated with the experimental procedure are paired with the behavioral effects of the drug, and instrumental conditioning, in which the behavior elicited by the drug is reinforced by the rewarding properties of the drug. While these factors undoubtedly influence the response to the drug,[54,57] it is difficult to assess the extent to which they are responsible for the sensitization to cocaine. In some experiments certain possibilities can be eliminated. Post[135] found no response to saline test injections, indicating that the sensitization which he found was not due to a conditioned response to the injection procedure. Experiments which gathered data in the animals' home cages indicate that a conditioned response to a novel test environment is not necessary to obtain sensitization.[99,182] Other possibilities remain in these experiments, such as a conditioned response to the stimulus properties of cocaine, or reinforcement of drug-induced behavior by the rewarding properties of cocaine.

Long-term neuronal reorganization — The evidence which has been provided thus far supports the possible involvement of several mechanisms in the behavioral changes seen with chronic cocaine administration. However, some of these mechanisms, such as changes in absorption or distribution of the drug, are only capable of accounting for the quantitative changes in cocaine effects. There remain what appear to be qualitative changes in both man and animals (see above). While localized and specific changes in cocaine's effects on neurotransmitters or changes in receptor sensitivity are adequate to explain these qualitative effects of chronic cocaine, other changes of a fundamental nature also merit consideration. Ellinwood[52] and Post and Kopanda[138] have previously proposed that the chronic administration of cocaine may produce effects similar to that of the kindling phenomenon first described systematically by Goddard and his colleagues.

Goddard[79] found that in certain areas of the brain, brief daily unilateral low-intensity electrical stimulation which was initially without behavioral effect produced a progressively larger effect each day, until eventually a behavioral convulsion was produced. Subsequent study[80] demonstrated that this "kindling effect" was most easily elicited in the amygdala; it could also be produced in other olfactory and limbic areas with a greater number of daily stimulations, but in other areas of the brain it was difficult to produce. Racine[144,145] found that kindling in the amygdala resulted from two apparently independent processes. First there was a presumably localized reorganization within the amygdala being stimulated, resulting in the development of afterdischarges at the site of stimulation. Secondly there was a progressive augmentation of the propagation of these afterdischarges to other areas of the limbic system, accompanied by a similar augmentation of the behavioral effects of the stimulation from localized myoclonic effects to a full bilateral clonic convulsion. The number of afterdischarges at the site of stimulation seemed to be the critical variable for the development of behavioral seizures, and repeated stimulations which did not produce such afterdischarges did not alter the number of afterdischarges subsequently needed to produce a behavioral convulsion.

Thus the kindling phenomenon seems to reflect a general ability of areas of the limbic system, and particularly the amygdala, to: (a) respond with increasing excitability to daily electrical stimulation and (b) propagate this excitability to other areas of the brain with greater and greater efficiency. These changes are gradual and can be monitored both electrophysiologically and behaviorally, and they are not restricted to epileptiform activity, since kindling facilitates the propagation of evoked potentials along the kindled pathways.[44,147] Also, the effects of kindling are relatively permanent, persisting for at least several months after the last stimulation with little or no deterioration.[80] These characteristics of the kindling phenomenon are quite similar to the development of seizure activity with chronic cocaine treatment. Furthermore, first-time seizure activity can be elicited by prolonged electrical stimulation of the amygdala,[146] in parallel with the seizure activity seen after a single high dose of cocaine.

It is in the area of the brain most sensitive to kindling that the electrophysiological effects of cocaine appear to originate. If the drug produces excitatory effects in this area it may be able to induce changes in some ways analogous to the kindling phenomenon. Although the kindling process involves the generation of epileptiform afterdischarges at the site of stimulation, which cocaine does not do except at near convulsant doses, a major part of the kindling phenomenon is an increased responsiveness of the areas to which the site of stimulation projects as a result of increased neural activity at the site of stimulation.[145] This suggests that other causes of periodic large increases in neural activity at a site such as the amygdala might produce a similar effect. In fact, potentiation of evoked potential propagation has been observed to occur in a kindling paradigm even in the absence of an afterdischarge at the site of stimulation.[44] Furthermore, there is evidence that chronic cocaine administration in cats can result in the development of spontaneous spike discharges in the amygdala.[55] Also, a local anesthetic has been shown to facilitate kindling produced by stimulation of the amygdala.[148]

Additional evidence in support of a similarity between the effects of chronic cocaine and kindling comes from their similar response to pharmacological manipulations. As previously noted, the benzodiazepines such as diazepam are very effective in suppressing seizures induced by cocaine and other local anesthetics, as well as in the selective suppression of the olfactory spindle in the amygdala and other forebrain areas.[48] Diazepam also prevents the occurrence of kindling to electrical stimulation of the amygdala.[148,212] Furthermore, diazepam and chlordiazepoxide depress the expression of previously kindled seizures.[7,185] In contrast, diphenylhydantoin, a standard anticonvulsant, is ineffective against kindling to amygdaloid stimulation[148] and against cocaine seizures.[47]

If cocaine does produce a kindling-like phenomenon, it could explain not only the augmentation of the effects of cocaine with chronic administration, and the persistence of this augmentation, but also the qualitative changes in the effects of the drug, due to the facilitation of neural pathways from areas of drug-induced activity. Such a model could serve as a general explanation of the chronic effects of other drugs as well. It could, for example, explain the develop-

ment of seizures with chronic administration of lidocaine,[139] something which cannot be explained by mechanisms related to the monoamine effects of cocaine. The difference in the behavioral effects of chronic lidocaine and cocaine demonstrates that a local anesthetic "kindling" effect is not sufficient to produce the major chronic effects of cocaine on behavior, but it may help shape and channel the psychomotor stimulant effect of cocaine in the direction of the chronic effects, as well as providing a means for their augmentation. In this respect it would be interesting to determine if chronic administration of a local anesthetic produces alterations in the response to cocaine. A kindling-like action may serve as an explanation of some of the chronic effects of other psychomotor stimulants as well, due to effects as yet poorly understood (e.g., Ellinwood et al.[59]).

More than one of the mechanisms listed here are probably important to the chronic effects of cocaine, and many of them may be involved to some extent. Hopefully this listing points out the complexity of the effects of this drug and the importance of pursuing diverse lines of inquiry.

CONCLUSION

The purpose of this chapter was to overview some of the effects of cocaine with an emphasis on its local anesthetic action, which does not normally receive attention with respect to the drug's behavioral effects. The electrophysiological effects of the drug appear to be primarily of local anesthetic origin, and while their behavioral significance has yet to be established, they may play an important role in the long-term effects of cocaine.

ACKNOWLEDGMENT

Supported in part by NIDA Grants DA-00057 and DA-01665, and by NIMH Grant MH-08394.

REFERENCES

1. **Adler, M. W., Sagel, S., Kitagawa, S., Segawa, T., and Maynert, E. W.,** The effects of repeated flurothyl-induced seizures on convulsive thresholds and brain monoamines in rats, *Arch. Int. Pharmacodyn. Ther.,* 170, 12, 1967.

2. **Adrian, E. D.,** Olfactory reactions in the brain of the hedgehog, *J. Physiol.* (London), 100, 459, 1942.

3. **Adriani, J. and Campbell, D.,** Fatalities following topical application of local anesthetics to mucous membranes, *JAMA,* 162, 1527, 1956.

4. **Alexander, G. T. and Kopeloff, L. M.,** Metrazol seizures in rats: Effect of *p*-chlorophenylalanine, *Brain Res.,* 22, 231, 1970.

5. **Angel, C. and Roberts, A. J.,** Effect of electroshock and antidepressant drugs on cerebrovascular permeability to cocaine in the rat, *J. Nerv. Ment. Dis.,* 142, 376, 1966.

6. **Arnold, P. S., Racine, R. J., and Wise, R. A.,** Effects of atropine, reserpine, 6-hydroxydopamine, and handling on seizure development in the rat, *Exp. Neurol.,* 40, 457, 1973.

7. **Babington, R. G. and Wedeking, P. W.,** The pharmacology of seizures induced by sensitization with low intensity brain stimulation, *Pharmacol. Biochem. Behav.,* 1, 461, 1973.

8. **Baldessarini, R. J.,** Release of catecholamines, in *Handbook of Psychopharmacology,* Section I, Volume 3, Iversen, L. L., Iversen, S. D., and Snyder, S. H., Eds., Plenum Press, New York, 1975.

9. **Balster, R. L., Kilbey, M. M., and Ellinwood, E. H., Jr.,** Methamphetamine self-administration in the cat, *Psychopharmacologia,* in press, 1976.

10. **Becker, C. J. and Freeman, W. J.,** Prepyriform electrical activity after loss of peripheral or central input, or both, *Physiol. Behav.,* 3, 597, 1968.

11. **Bernhard, C. G. and Bohm, E.,** The action of local anesthetics on experimental epilepsy in cats and monkeys, *Br. J. Pharmacol.,* 10, 288, 1955.

12. **Bernhard, C. G. and Bohm, E.,** *Local Anesthetics as Anticonvulsants: A Study on Experimental and Clinical Epilepsy,* Almqvist & Wiksell, Stockholm, 1965.

13. **Bernhard, C. G., Bohm, E., Kirstein, L., and Wiesel, T.,** The difference in action on normal and convulsive cortical activity between a local anaesthetic (lidocaine) and barbiturates, *Arch. Int. Pharmacodyn. Ther.,* 108, 408, 1956.

14. **Bernhard, C. G., Bohm, E., and Wiesel, T.,** On the evaluation of the anticonvulsant effect of different local anaesthetics, *Arch. Int. Pharmacodyn. Ther.,* 108, 392, 1956.

15. **Berry, C. A., Sanner, J. H., and Keasling, H. H.,** A comparison of the anticonvulsant activity of mepivacaine and lidocaine, *J. Pharmacol. Exp. Ther.,* 133, 357, 1961.

16. **Blumer, J., Strong, J. M., and Atkinson, A. J., Jr.,** The convulsant potency of lidocaine and its *n*-dealkylated metabolites, *J. Pharmacol. Exp. Ther.,* 186, 31, 1973.

17. **Boggan, W. O.,** Psychoactive compounds and audiogenic seizure susceptibility, *Life Sci.,* 13, 151, 1973.

18. **Boggan, W. O.,** Serotonin and convulsions, in *Serotonin and Behavior,* Barchas, J. and Usdin, E., Eds., Academic Press, New York, 1973.

19. **Bohm, E., Flodmark, S., and Petersen, I.,** Effects of lidocaine (Xylocaine®) on seizure and interseizure electroencephalograms in epileptics, *AMA Arch. Neurol. Psychiatry.,* 81, 550, 1959.

20. **Bourn, W. M., Chin, L., and Picchioni, A. L.,** Enhancement of audiogenic seizure by 6-hydroxydopamine, *J. Pharm. Pharmacol.,* 24, 913, 1972.

21. **Bralet, J. and Lallemant, A. M.,** Influence du traitement par la cocaine sur la synthese et la liberation de la noradrenaline cerebrale, *Arch. Int. Pharmacodyn. Ther.,* 217, 332, 1975.

22. **Broadwell, R. D.,** Olfactory relationships of the telencephalon and diencephalon in the rabbit, *J. Comp. Neurol.,* 163, 329, 1975.

23. **Cain, D. P.,** The role of the olfactory bulb in limbic mechanisms, *Psychol. Bull.,* 81, 654, 1974.

24. **Cain, D. P. and Bindra, D.,** Responses of amygdala single units to odors in the rat, *Exp. Neurol.,* 35, 98, 1972.

25. **Carmichael, F. J. and Israel, Y.,** *In vitro* inhibitory effects of narcotic analgesics and other psychotropic drugs on the active uptake of norepinephrine in mouse brain tissue, *J. Pharmacol. Exp. Ther.,* 186, 253, 1973.

26. **Castellani, S., Ellinwood, E. H., Jr., and Petrie, W. M.,** Cocaine-induced olfactory-limbic spindling and seizures: EEG, behavior, and effects of dopaminergic and cholinergic agents, in preparation.

27. **Castellani, S., Kilbey, M. M., and Ellinwood, E. H., Jr.,** unpublished observations.

28. **Chase, T. N. and Murphy, D. L.,** Serotonin and central nervous system function, *Ann. Rev. Pharmacol.,* 13, 181, 1973.

29. **Chen, G. and Bohner, B.,** The anti-reserpine effects of certain centrally-acting agents, *J. Pharmacol. Exp. Ther.,* 131, 179, 1961.

30. **Connell, P. H.,** *Amphetamine Psychosis,* Oxford University Press, London, 1958.

31. **Corcoran, M. E., Fibiger, H. C., McCaughran, J. A., Jr., and Wada, J. A.,** Potentiation of amygdaloid kindling and Metrazol-induced seizures by 6-hydroxy-dopamine in rats, *Exp. Neurol.,* 45, 118, 1974.

32. **Costa, E., Groppetti, A., and Naimzada, M. K.,** Effects of amphetamine on the turnover rate of brain catecholamines and motor activity, *Br. J. Pharmacol.,* 44, 742, 1972.

33. **Crow, T. J.,** Enhancement by cocaine of intra-cranial self-stimulation in the rat, *Life Sci.,* 9, Part 1, 375, 1970.

34. **de Jong, R. H.,** *Physiology and Pharmacology of Local Anesthesia,* Charles C Thomas, Springfield, Illinois, 1970.

35. **de Jong, R. H. and Heavner, J. E.,** Diazepam prevents local anesthetic seizures, *Anesthesiology,* 34, 523, 1971.

179

36. **de Jong, R. H. and Heavner, J. E.,** Diazepam and lidocaine-induced cardiovascular changes, *Anesthesiology,* 39, 633, 1973.
37. **de Jong, R. H. and Walts, L. F.,** Lidocaine-induced psychomotor seizures in man, *Acta Anesthesiol. Scand.,* Suppl. 23, 598, 1966.
38. **De La Torre, J. C., Kawanaga, H. M., and Mullan, S.,** Seizure susceptibility after manipulation of brain serotonin, *Arch. Int. Pharmacodyn. Ther.,* 188, 298, 1970.
39. **de Oliveira, L. F. and Bretas, A. D.,** Effects of 5-hydroxytryptophan, iproniazid, and *p*-chlorophenylalanine on lidocaine seizure threshold of mice, *Eur. J. Pharmacol.,* 29, 5, 1974.
40. **de Oliveira, L. F., Heavner, J. E., and de Jong, R. H.,** 5-Hydroxytryptophan intensifies local anesthetic-induced convulsions, *Arch. Int. Pharmacodyn. Ther.,* 207, 333, 1974.
41. **Dengler, H. J., Spiegel, H. E., and Titus, E. O.,** Effects of drugs on uptake of isotopic norepinephrine by cat tissues, *Nature,* 191, 816, 1961.
42. **De Schaepdryver, A. F., Piette, Y., and Delaunois, A. L.,** Brain amines and electroshock threshold, *Arch. Int. Pharmacodyn. Ther.,* 140, 358, 1962.
43. **Domino, E. F. and Ueki, S.,** An analysis of the electrical burst phenomenon in some rhinencephalic structures of the dog and monkey, *Electroencephalogr. Clin. Neurophysiol.,* 12, 635, 1960.
44. **Douglas, R. M. and Goddard, G. V.,** Long-term potentiation of the perforant path-granule cell synapse in the rat hippocampus, *Brain Res.,* 86, 205, 1975.
45. **Downs, A. W. and Eddy, N. B.,** The effect of repeated doses of cocaine on the dog, *J. Pharmacol. Exp. Ther.,* 46, 195, 1932.
46. **Downs, A. W. and Eddy, N. B.,** The effect of repeated doses of cocaine on the rat, *J. Pharmacol. Exp. Ther.,* 46, 199, 1932.
47. **Eidelberg, E., Lesse, H., and Gault, F. P.,** An experimental model of temporal lobe epilepsy: Studies of the convulsant properties of cocaine, in *EEG and Behavior,* Glaser, G. H., Ed., Basic Books, New York, 1963, 272.
48. **Eidelberg, E., Neer, H. M., and Miller, M. K.,** Anticonvulsant properties of some benzodiazepine derivatives, *Neurology,* 15, 223, 1965.
49. **Eidelberg, E. and Woodbury, C. M.,** Electrical activity in the amygdala and its modification by drugs. Possible nature of synaptic transmitters. A review, in *The Neurobiology of the Amygdala,* Eleftheriou, B. E., Ed., Plenum Press, New York, 1972, 609.
50. **Ellinwood, E. H., Jr.,** "Accidental conditioning" with chronic methamphetamine intoxication: Implications for a theory of drug habituation, *Psychopharmacologia,* 21, 131, 1971.
51. **Ellinwood, E. H., Jr.,** Behavioral and EEG changes in the amphetamine model of psychosis, in *Neuropsychopharmacology of Monoamines and Their Regulatory Enzymes,* Usdin, E., Ed., Raven Press, New York, 1974, 281.
52. **Ellinwood, E. H., Jr.,** Physiological Effects of Cocaine, presented at NIDA conference on cocaine research, Washington, D.C., September 1974.
53. **Ellinwood, E. H., Jr.,** unpublished observations.
54. **Ellinwood, E. H., Jr. and Kilbey, M. M.,** Amphetamine stereotypy: The influence of environmental factors and prepotent behavioral patterns on its topography and development, *Biol. Psychiatry,* 10, 3, 1975.
55. **Ellinwood, E. H., Jr., Kilbey, M. M., Castellani, S., and Khoury, C.,** Amygdala hyperspindling and seizures induced by cocaine, in *Cocaine and Other Stimulants,* Ellinwood, E. H., Jr. and Kilbey, M. M., Eds., Plenum Press, New York, in press, 1976.
56. **Ellinwood, E. H., Jr. and Stripling, J. S.,** unpublished observations.
57. **Ellinwood, E. H., Jr., Stripling, J. S., and Kilbey, M. M.,** Chronic changes with amphetamine intoxication: Underlying processes, in *Neuroregulators and Hypotheses of Psychiatric Disorders,* Usdin, E. and Barchas, J., Eds., Oxford University Press, London, in press, 1976.
58. **Ellinwood, E. H., Jr. and Sudilovsky, A.,** Chronic amphetamine intoxication: Behavioral model of psychoses, in *Psychopathology and Psychopharmacology,* Cole, J. O., Freedman, A. M., and Friedhoff, A. J., Eds., Johns Hopkins University Press, Baltimore, 1973, 51.
59. **Ellinwood, E. H., Jr., Sudilovsky, A., and Grabowy, R.,** Olfactory forebrain seizures induced by methamphetamine and disulfiram, *Biol. Psychiatry,* 7, 89, 1973.
60. **Ellinwood, E. H., Jr., Sudilovsky, A., and Nelson, L.,** Behavioral analysis of chronic amphetamine intoxication, *Biol. Psychiatry,* 4, 215, 1972.
61. **Ellinwood, E. H., Jr., Sudilovsky, A., and Nelson, L. M.,** Evolving behavior in the clinical and experimental amphetamine (model) psychosis, *Am. J. Psychiatry,* 130, 1088, 1973.
62. **Ellinwood, E. H., Jr., Sudilovsky, A., and Nelson, L. M.,** Behavior and EEG analysis of chronic amphetamine effect, *Biol. Psychiatry,* 8, 169, 1974.
63. **Essman, W. B.,** Anticonvulsive properties of Xylocaine in mice susceptible to audiogenic seizures, *Arch. Int. Pharmacodyn. Ther.,* 164, 376, 1966.
64. **Essman, W. B.,** Prilocaine as an anticonvulsant: Protective effects against electroshock-induced convulsions in mice, *Arch. Int. Pharmacodyn. Ther.,* 171, 159, 1968.
65. **Fischman, M. W. and Schuster, C. R.,** Physiological and behavioral effects of intravenous cocaine in man, in *Cocaine and Other Stimulants,* Ellinwood, E. H. and Kilbey, M. M., Eds., Plenum Press, New York, in press, 1976.
66. **Fog, R.,** Stereotyped and non-stereotyped behavior in rats induced by various stimulant drugs, *Psychopharmacologia,* 14, 299, 1969.

67. **Frank, G. B. and Sanders, H. D.,** A proposed common mechanism of action for general and local anaesthetics in the central nervous system, *Br. J. Pharmacol.,* 21, 1, 1963.

68. **Freeman, W. J.,** Distribution in time and space of prepyriform electrical activity, *J. Neurophysiol.,* 22, 644, 1959.

69. **Freeman, W. J.,** Correlation of electrical activity of prepyriform cortex and behavior in cat, *J. Neurophysiol.,* 23, 111, 1960.

70. **Freeman, W. J.,** The electrical activity of a primary sensory cortex: Analysis of EEG waves, *Int. Rev. Neurobiol.,* 5, 53, 1963.

71. **Freeman, W. J.,** Average transmission distance from mitral-tufted to granule cells in olfactory bulb, *Electroencephalogr. Clin. Neurophysiol.,* 36, 609, 1974.

72. **French, J. D., Livingston, R. B., Konigsmark, B., and Richland, K. J.,** Experimental observations on the prevention of seizures by intravenous procaine injections, *J. Neurosurg.,* 14, 43, 1957.

73. **Freund, G.,** The prevention of ethanol withdrawal seizures in mice by lidocaine, *Neurology,* 23, 91, 1973.

74. **Friedman, E., Gershon, S., and Rotrosen, J.,** Effects of acute cocaine treatment on the turnover of 5-hydroxytryptamine in the rat brain, *Br. J. Pharmacol.,* 54, 61, 1975.

75. **Fukuda, T., Araki, Y., and Suenaga, N.,** Inhibitory effects of 6-hydroxydopamine on the clonic convulsions induced by electroshock and decapitation, *Neuropharmacology,* 14, 579, 1975.

76. **Galambos, E., Pfeifer, A. K., Gyorgy, L., and Molnar, J.,** Study on the excitation induced by amphetamine, cocaine and alpha-methyltryptamine, *Psychopharmacologia,* 11, 122, 1967.

77. **Gault, F. P. and Coustan, D. R.,** Nasal air flow and rhinencephalic activity, *Electroencephalogr. Clin. Neurophysiol.,* 18, 617, 1965.

78. **Gault, F. P. and Leaton, R. N.,** Electrical activity of the olfactory system, *Electroencephalogr. Clin. Neurophysiol.,* 15, 299, 1963.

79. **Goddard, G. V.,** Development of epileptic seizures through brain stimulation at low intensity, *Nature,* 214, 1020, 1967.

80. **Goddard, G. V., McIntyre, D. C., and Leech, C. K.,** A permanent change in brain function resulting from daily electrical stimulation, *Exp. Neurol.,* 25, 295, 1969.

81. **Graham, J. M., Jr., Schreiber, R. A., and Zemp, J. W.,** Effect of *d*-amphetamine sulfate on susceptibility to audiogenic seizures in DBA/2J mice, *Behav. Biol.,* 10, 183, 1974.

82. **Gunne, L.-M. and Jonsson, J.,** Effects of cocaine administration on brain, adrenal and urinary adrenaline and noradrenaline in rats, *Psychopharmacologia,* 6, 125, 1964.

83. **Gutierrez-Noriega, C.,** Inhibition central nervous system produced by chronic cocaine intoxication, *Fed. Proc.,* 9, 280, 1950.

84. **Hatch, R. C.,** Cocaine-elicited behavior and toxicity in dogs pretreated with methiothepin or *p*-chlorophenylalanine, *Pharmacol. Res. Commun.,* 5, 321, 1973.

85. **Hatch, R. C. and Fischer, R.,** Cocaine-elicited behavior and toxicity in dogs pretreated with synaptic blocking agents, morphine, or diphenylhydrantoin, *Pharmacol. Res. Commun.,* 4, 383, 1972.

86. **Hazra, J.,** Disinhibition of the inhibitory effect of darkness on optic evoked potentials by lidocaine, *Fed. Proc.,* 29, 252, 1970.

87. **Heath, R. G. and Gallant, D. M.,** Activity of the human brain during emotional thought, in *The Role of Pleasure in Behavior,* Heath, R. G., Ed., Harper & Row, New York, 1964, 83.

88. **Hernandez-Peon, R., Lavin, A., Alcocer-Cuaron, C., and Marcelin, J. P.,** Electrical activity of the olfactory bulb during wakefulness and sleep, *Electroencephalogr. Clin. Neurophysiol.,* 12, 41, 1960.

89. **Ho, B. T., Taylor, D. L., Estevez, V. S., Englert, L. F., and McKenna, M. L.,** Behavioral effects of cocaine — metabolic and neurochemical approach, in *Cocaine and Other Stimulants,* Ellinwood, E. H. and Kilbey, M. M., Eds., Plenum Press, New York, in press, 1976.

90. **Iversen, L. L.,** *The Uptake and Storage of Noradrenaline in Sympathetic Nerves,* Cambridge University Press, London, 1967.

91. **Iversen, L. L.,** Uptake processes for biogenic amines, in *Handbook of Psychopharmacology,* Section I, Vol. 3, Iversen, L. L., Iversen, S. D., and Snyder, S. H., Eds., Plenum Press, New York, 1975.

92. **Izquierdo, I., Fernandes, J., Oliveira, R., and Settineri, F.,** Effect of daily saline, drug, or blank injections on the susceptibility to the convulsant effect of drugs, *Pharmacol. Biochem. Behav.,* 3, 721, 1975.

93. **Johanson, C. E. and Schuster, C. R.,** A choice procedure for drug reinforcers: Cocaine and methylphenidate in the rhesus monkey, *J. Pharmacol. Exp. Ther.,* 193, 676, 1975.

94. **Jolly, E. R. and Steinhaus, J. E.,** The effect of drugs injected into limited portions of the cerebral circulation, *J. Pharmacol. Exp. Ther.,* 116, 273, 1956.

95. **Julien, R. M.,** Lidocaine in experimental epilepsy: Correlations of anticonvulsant effect with blood concentrations, *Electroencephalogr. Clin. Neurophysiol.,* 34, 639, 1973.

96. **Kalsner, S. and Nickerson, M.,** Mechanism of cocaine potentiation of responses to amines, *Br. J. Pharmacol.,* 35, 428, 1969.

97. **Kamat, U. G. and Sheth, U. K.,** The role of central monoamines in decapitation convulsions of mice, *Neuropharmacology,* 10, 571, 1971.

98. **Kasuya, Y. and Goto, K.,** The mechanism of supersensitivity to norepinephrine induced by cocaine in rat isolated vas deferens, *Eur. J. Pharmacol.,* 4, 355, 1968.

99. Kilbey, M. M. and Ellinwood, E. H., Jr., Chronic administration of stimulant drugs: Tolerance and response potentiation, in *Cocaine and Other Stimulants*, Ellinwood, E. H. and Kilbey, M. M., Eds., Plenum Press, New York, in press, 1976.

100. Kilbey, M. M. and Ellinwood, E. H., Jr., unpublished observations.

101. Kirkby, R. J. and Petchkovsky, L., Chronic administration of cocaine: Effects on defaecation and adrenal hypertrophy in the rat, *Neuropharmacology*, 12, 1001, 1973.

102. Klawans, H. L., Crossett, P., and Dana, N., Effect of chronic amphetamine exposure on stereotyped behavior: Implications for pathogenesis of 1-DOPA-induced dyskinesias, in *Advances in Neurology*, Vol. 9, Calne, D. B., Chase, T. N., and Barbeau, A., Eds., Raven Press, New York, 1975.

103. Knapp, S. and Mandell, A. J., Narcotic drugs: Effects on the serotonin biosynthetic systems of the brain, *Science*, 177, 1209, 1972.

104. Kobinger, W., Differentiation between the sedative actions of 5-hydroxytryptamine and reserpine in mice by means of two stimulating substances, *Acta Pharmacol. Toxicol.*, 14, 138, 1958.

105. Kosman, M. E. and Unna, K. R., Effects of chronic administration of the amphetamines and other stimulants on behavior, *Clin. Pharmacol. Ther.*, 9, 240, 1968.

106. Krenis, L. J., Liu, P. L., and Ngai, S. H., The effect of local anesthetics on the central nervous system toxicity of hyperbaric oxygen, *Neuropharmacology*, 10, 637, 1971.

107. Lammers, H. J., The neural connections of the amygdaloid complex in mammals, in *The Neurobiology of the Amygdala*, Eleftheriou, B. E., Ed., Plenum Press, New York, 1972, 123.

108. Lavin , A., Alcocer-Cuaron, C., and Hernandez-Peon, R., Centrifugal arousal in the olfactory bulb, *Science*, 129, 332, 1959.

109. Lehmann, A. G., Psychopharmacology of the response to noise, with special reference to audiogenic seizure in mice, in *Physiological Effects of Noise*, Welch, B. and Welch, A., Eds., Plenum Press, New York, 1970.

110. Lesse, H., Rhinencephalic electrophysiological activity during "emotional behavior" in cats, *Psychiatr. Res. Rep.*, 12, 224, 1960.

111. Lewin, L., *Phantastica. Narcotic and Stimulating Drugs,* translated by P. H. A. Wirth, E. P. Dutton, New York, 1931.

112. Liang, C. C. and Quastel, J. H., Effects of drugs on the uptake of acetylcholine in rat brain cortex slices, *Biochem. Pharmacol.*, 18, 1187, 1969.

113. Liljestrand, G., The historical development of local anesthesia, in *International Encyclopedia of Pharmacology and Therapeutics*, Section 8, Vol. 1, Lechat, P., Ed., Pergamon Press, New York, 1971, 1.

114. Lutsch, E. F. and Morris, R. W., Circadian periodicity in susceptibility to lidocaine hydrochloride, *Science*, 156, 100, 1967.

115. McKenzie, G. M. and Soroko, F. E., Inhibition of the anticonvulsant activity of 1-dopa by FLA-63, a dopamine-beta-hydroxylase inhibitor, *J. Pharm. Pharmacol.*, 25, 76, 1973.

116. Magos, L., Persistence of the effect of amphetamine on stereotyped activity in rats, *Eur. J. Pharmacol.*, 6, 200, 1969.

117. Maier, H. W., *Der Kokainismus*, Verlag, Leipzig, 1926.

118. Mandell, A. J. and Knapp, S., Neurobiological antagonism of cocaine by lithium, in *Cocaine and Other Stimulants*, Ellinwood, E. H. and Kilbey, M. M., Eds., Plenum Press, New York, in press, 1976.

119. Mark, L. C., Brand, L., and Goldensohn, E. S., Recovery after procaine-induced seizures in dogs, *Electroencephalogr. Clin. Neurophysiol.*, 16, 280, 1964.

120. Mason, C. R. and Cooper, R. M., A permanent change in convulsive threshold in normal and brain-damaged rats with repeated small doses of pentylenetetrazol, *Epilepsia*, 13, 663, 1972.

121. Matsuzaki, M., Differential effects of cocaine and pseudococaine on electrical activities in the limbic systems of cats and monkeys, *Fed. Proc.*, 34, 781, 1975.

122. Matthews, P. B. C. and Rushworth, G., The relative sensitivity of muscle nerve fibers to procaine, *J. Physiol.* (London), 135, 263, 1957.

123. Menon, M. K., Dandiya, P. C., and Bapna, J. S., Modification of the effect of some central stimulants in mice pretreated with alpha-methyl-1-tyrosine, *Psychopharmacologia*, 10, 437, 1967.

124. Moulton, D. G. and Tucker, D., Electrophysiology of the olfactory system, *Ann. N. Y. Acad. Sci.*, 116, 380, 1964.

125. Mulé, S. J. and Misra, A. L., Physiological disposition and biotransformation of ^{3}H-cocaine in acute and chronically-treated animals, in *Cocaine and Other Stimulants*, Ellinwood, E. H. and Kilbey, M. M., Eds., Plenum Press, New York, in press, 1976.

126. Munson, E. S., Martucci, R. W., and Wagman, I. H., Bupivacaine and lignocaine induced seizures in rhesus monkeys, *Br. J. Anaesth.*, 44, 1025, 1972.

127. Munson, E. S. and Wagman, I. H., Elevation of lidocaine seizure threshold by gallamine, *Arch. Neurol.*, 28, 329, 1973.

128. Muscholl, E., Effect of cocaine and related drugs on the uptake of noradrenaline by heart and spleen, *Br. J. Pharmacol.*, 16, 352, 1961.

129. Nakatsu, K. and Reiffenstein, R. J., Increased receptor utilization: Mechanism of cocaine potentiation, *Nature*, 217, 1276, 1968.

130. Nayak, P. K., Misra, A. L., and Mulé, S. J., Physiological disposition and biotransformation of (^{3}H) cocaine in acute and chronically treated rats, *Fed. Proc.*, 34, 781, 1975.

131. **Pagano, R. R.,** The effects of central stimulation and nasal air flow on induced activity of olfactory structures, *Electroencephalogr. Clin. Neurophysiol.*, 21, 269, 1966.

132. **Pagano, R. R. and Gault, F. P.,** Amygdala activity: A central measure of arousal, *Electroencephalogr. Clin. Neurophysiol.*, 17, 255, 1964.

133. **Penaloza-Rojas, J. H. and Alcocer-Cuaron, C.,** The electrical activity of the olfactory bulb in cats with nasal and tracheal breathing, *Electroencephalogr. Clin. Neurophysiol.*, 22, 468, 1967.

134. **Peterson, D. I. and Hardinge, M. G.,** The effect of various environmental factors on cocaine and ephedrine toxicity, *J. Pharm. Pharmacol.*, 19, 810, 1967.

135. **Post, R. M.,** Progressive changes in behavior and seizures following chronic cocaine administration: Relationship to kindling and psychosis, in *Cocaine and Other Stimulants*, Ellinwood, E. H. and Kilbey, M. M., Eds., Plenum Press, New York, in press, 1976.

136. **Post, R. M., Davenport, S., and Squillace, K.,** Antagonism of cocaine effects by physostigmine, in preparation.

137. **Post, R. M., Gillin, J. C., Wyatt, R. J., and Goodwin, F. K.,** The effect of orally administered cocaine on sleep of depressed patients, *Psychopharmacologia*, 37, 59, 1974.

138. **Post, R. M. and Kopanda, R. T.,** Cocaine, kindling, and reverse tolerance, *Lancet, i*, 409, 1975.

139. **Post, R. M., Kopanda, R. T., and Lee, A.,** Progressive behavioral changes during chronic lidocaine administration: Relationship to kindling, *Life Sci.*, 17, 943, 1975.

140. **Post, R. M., Kotin, J., and Goodwin, F. K.,** The effects of cocaine on depressed patients, *Am. J. Psychiatry,* 131, 511, 1974.

141. **Post, R. M., Sanadi, C., and Reichenbach, L.,** Cocaine hyperactivity, stereotypy, and seizures: Aminergic mechanisms, in preparation.

142. **Prichard, J. W., Gallagher, B. B., and Glaser, G. H.,** Experimental seizure-threshold testing with flurothyl, *J. Pharmacol. Exp. Ther.*, 166, 170, 1969.

143. **Prince, D. A. and Wagman, I. H.,** Activation of limbic system epileptogenic foci with intravenous lidocaine, *Electroencephalogr. Clin. Neurophysiol.*, 21, 416, 1966.

144. **Racine, R. J.,** Modification of seizure activity by electrical stimulation. I. Afterdischarge threshold, *Electroencephalogr. Clin. Neurophysiol.*, 32, 269, 1972.

145. **Racine, R. J.,** Modification of seizure activity by electrical stimulation. II. Motor seizure, *Electroencephalogr. Clin. Neurophysiol.*, 32, 281, 1972.

146. **Racine, R. J., Burnham, W. M., and Gartner, J. G.,** First trial motor seizures triggered by amygdaloid stimulation in the rat, *Electroencephalogr. Clin. Neurophysiol.*, 35, 487, 1973.

147. **Racine, R. J., Gartner, J. G., and Burnham, W. M.,** Epileptiform activity and neural plasticity in limbic structures, *Brain Res.*, 47, 262, 1972.

148. **Racine, R., Livingston, K., and Joaquin, A.,** Effects of procaine hydrochloride, diazepam, and diphenylhydantoin on seizure development in cortical and subcortical structures in rats, *Electroencephalogr. Clin. Neurophysiol.*, 38, 355, 1975.

149. **Reiffenstein, R. J.,** Effects of cocaine on the rate of contraction to noradrenaline in the cat spleen strip: Mode of action by cocaine, *Br. J. Pharmacol. Chemother.*, 32, 591, 1968.

150. **Reite, M.,** Non-invasive recording of limbic spindles in man, *Electroencephalogr. Clin. Neurophysiol.*, 38, 539, 1975.

151. **Resnick, R. B., Kestenbaum, R. S., and Schwartz, L. K.,** Acute systemic effects of cocaine in man: A controlled study by intranasal and intravenous routes of administration, in *Cocaine and Other Stimulants,* Ellinwood, E. H. and Kilbey, M. M., Eds., Plenum Press, New York, in press, 1976.

152. **Riblet, L. A. and Tuttle, W. W.,** Investigation of the amygdaloid and olfactory electrographic response in the cat after toxic dosage of lidocaine, *Electroencephalogr. Clin. Neurophysiol.*, 28, 601, 1970.

153. **Ritchie, J. M.,** The mechanism of action of local anesthetic agents, in *International Encyclopedia of Pharmacology and Therapeutics,* Section 8, Vol. 1, Lechat, P., Ed., Pergamon Press, New York, 1971, 131.

154. **Ritchie, J. M., Cohen, P. J., and Dripps, R. D.,** Cocaine: Procaine and other synthetic local anesthetics, in *The Pharmacological Basis of Therapeutics,* Goodman, L. S. and Gilman, A., Eds., Macmillan, New York, 1970, 371.

155. **Rosenthal, F. and Timiras, P. S.,** Prepyriform electrical activity after 250 r whole-body X-irradiation in rats, *Am. J. Physiol.*, 204, 63, 1963.

156. **Ross, S. B. and Renyi, A. L.,** Inhibition of the uptake of tritiated catecholamines by antidepressant and related agents, *Eur. J. Pharmacol.*, 2, 181, 1967.

157. **Ross, S. B. and Renyi, A. L.,** Accumulation of tritiated 5-hydroxytryptamine in brain slices, *Life Sci.*, 6, 1407, 1967.

158. **Ross, S. B. and Renyi, A. L.,** Inhibition of the uptake of 5-hydroxytryptamine in brain tissue, *Eur. J. Pharmacol.*, 7, 270, 1969.

159. **Rudzik, A. D. and Johnson, G. A.,** Effect of amphetamine and amphetamine analogues on convulsive thresholds, in *Amphetamines and Related Compounds,* Costa, E. and Garattini, S., Eds., Raven Press, New York, 1970.

160. **Sanders, H. D.,** A comparison of the convulsant activity of procaine and pentylenetetrazol, *Arch. Int. Pharmacodyn. Ther.*, 170, 165, 1967.

161. **Sayers, A. C. and Handley, S. L.,** A study of the role of catecholamines in the response to various central stimulants, *Eur. J. Pharmacol.*, 23, 47, 1973.

162. **Scalia, F.**, A review of recent experimental studies on the distribution of the olfactory tracts in mammals, *Brain Behav. Evol.*, 1, 101, 1968.

163. **Scalia, F. and Winans, S.**, The differential projections of the olfactory bulb and accessory olfactory bulb in mammals, *J. Comp. Neurol.*, 161, 31, 1975.

164. **Scheel-Krüger, J.**, Behavioral and biochemical comparison of amphetamine derivatives, cocaine, benztropine, and tricyclic anti-depressant drugs, *Eur. J. Pharmacol.*, 18, 63, 1972.

165. **Scheel-Krüger, J., Braestrup, C., Nielsen, M., Golembiowska, K., and Mogilnicka, E.**, Cocaine: Discussion on the role of dopamine in the biochemical mechanism of action, in *Cocaine and Other Stimulants*, Ellinwood, E. H. and Kilbey, M. M., Eds., Plenum Press, New York, in press, 1976.

166. **Schildkraut, J. J., Schanberg, S. M., Breese, G. R., and Kopin, I. J.**, Norepinephrine metabolism and drugs used in the affective disorders: A possible mechanism of action, *Am. J. Psychiatry*, 124, 600, 1967.

167. **Schmidt, G.**, Anorexigene wirkung des cocains, *Arch. Int. Pharmacodyn. Ther.*, 156, 87, 1965.

168. **Schmidt, R. P. and Wilder, B. J.**, *Epilepsy*, F. A. Davis, Philadelphia, 1968.

169. **Schubert, J., Fyro, B., Nyback, H., and Sedvall, G.**, Effects of cocaine and amphetamine on the metabolism of tryptophan and 5-hydroxytryptamine in mouse brain *in vivo*, *J. Pharm. Pharmacol.*, 22, 860, 1970.

170. **Scott, D. B. and Julian, D. G., Eds.**, *Lidocaine in the Treatment of Ventricular Arrhythmias*, Livingstone, Edinburgh, 1971.

171. **Segal, D. S. and Mandell, A. J.**, Long-term administration of *d*-amphetamine: Progressive augmentation of motor activity and stereotypy, *Pharmacol. Biochem. Behav.*, 2, 249, 1974.

172. **Segawa, T. and Kuruma, I.**, The influences of drugs on the uptake of 5-hydroxytryptamine by nerve-ending particles of rabbit brain stem, *J. Pharm. Pharmacol.*, 20, 320, 1968.

173. **Shepherd, G. M.**, The olfactory bulb as a simple cortical system: Experimental analysis and functional implications, in *The Neurosciences. Second Study Program*, Schmitt, F. O., Ed., Rockefeller University Press, New York, 1970, 539.

174. **Shepherd, G. M.**, Synaptic organization of the mammalian olfactory bulb, *Physiol. Rev.*, 52, 864, 1972.

175. **Shepherd, G. M.**, *The Synaptic Organization of the Brain*, Oxford University Press, London, 1974.

176. **Simon, P., Sultan, Z., Chermat, R., and Boissier, J.**, La cocaine, une substance amphetaminique? Un probleme de psychopharmacologie experimentale, *J. Pharmacol.* (Paris), 3, 129, 1972.

177. **Smith, C. B.**, Enhancement by reserpine and a-methyl dopa of the effects of *d*-amphetamine upon the locomotor activity of mice, *J. Pharmacol. Exp. Ther.*, 142, 343, 1963.

178. **Smith, C. B.**, Effects of *d*-amphetamine upon brain amine content and locomotor activity in mice, *J. Pharmacol. Exp. Ther.*, 147, 96, 1965.

179. **Sorel, L. and Lejeune, R.**, Modifications of l'EEG du lapin sous l'action de divers succedanes de la cocaine injectes par voie intraveineuse, *Arch. Int. Pharmacodyn. Ther.*, 102, 314, 1955.

180. **Stevens, J. R., Mark, V. H., Erwin, F., Pacheco, P., and Suematsu, K.**, Deep temporal stimulation in man, *Arch. Neurol.*, 21, 157, 1969.

181. **Stripling, J. S. and Ellinwood, E. H., Jr.**, Augmentation of the behavioral and electrophysiological response to cocaine by chronic administration in the rat, submitted for publication.

182. **Stripling, J. S. and Ellinwood, E. H., Jr.**, Potentiation of the behavioral and convulsive effects of cocaine by chronic administration in the rat, submitted for publication.

183. **Sundsten, J. W. and Sawyer, C. H.**, Electroencephalographic evidence of osmosensitive elements in olfactory bulb of dog brain, *Proc. Soc. Exp. Biol. Med.*, 101, 524, 1959.

184. **Tainter, M. L., Tainter, E. G., Lawrence, W. S., Neuru, E. N., Lackey, R. W., Luduena, F. P., Kirtland, H. B., Jr., and Gonzalez, R. I.**, Influence of various drugs on the threshold for electrical convulsions, *J. Pharmacol. Exp. Ther.*, 79, 42, 1943.

185. **Tanaka, A.**, Progressive changes in behavioral and electroencephalographic responses to daily amygdaloid stimulations in rabbits, *Fukuoka Acta Medica*, 63, 152, 1972.

186. **Tanaka, K.**, Anticonvulsant properties of procaine, cocaine, adiphenine, and related structures, *Proc. Soc. Exp. Biol. Med.*, 90, 192, 1955.

187. **Tanaka, K. and Yamasaki, M.**, Blocking of cortical inhibitory synapses by intravenous lidocaine, *Nature*, 209, 207, 1966.

188. **Tatum, A. L. and Seevers, M. H.**, Experimental cocaine addiction, *J. Pharmacol. Exp. Ther.*, 36, 401, 1929.

189. **Teeters, W. R., Koppanyi, T., and Cowan, F. F.**, Cocaine tachyphylaxis, *Life Sci.*, 7, 509, 1963.

190. **Tilson, H. A. and Rech, R. H.**, Conditioned drug effects and absence of tolerance to *d*-amphetamine induced motor activity, *Pharmacol. Biochem. Behav.*, 1, 149, 1973.

191. **Tuttle, W. W. and Elliott, H. W.**, Electrographic and behavioral study of convulsants in the cat, *Anesthesiology*, 30, 48, 1969.

192. **Trendelenburg, U.**, Mechanisms of supersensitivity and subsensitivity to sympathomimetic amines, *Pharmacol. Rev.*, 18, 629, 1966.

193. **Usubiaga, J. E., Wikinski, J., Ferrero, R., Usubiaga, L. E., and Wikinski, R.**, Local anesthetic-induced convulsions in man – an electroencephalographic study, *Anesth. Analg.* (Paris), 45, 611, 1966.

194. **van Rossum, J. M.**, Mode of action of psychomotor stimulant drugs, *Int. Rev. Neurobiol.*, 12, 307, 1970.

195. **van Rossum, J. M. and Hurkmans, J. A. T. M.**, Mechanism of action of psychomotor stimulant drugs, *Int. J. Neuropharmacol.*, 3, 227, 1964.

196. **van Rossum, J. M. and Simons, F.,** Locomotor activity and anorexigenic action, *Psychopharmacologia,* 14, 248, 1969.
197. **van Rossum, J. M., van der Schoot, J. B., and Hurkmans, J. A. T. M.,** Mechanism of action of cocaine and amphetamine in the brain, *Experientia,* 18, 229, 1962.
198. **Varma, D. R. and McCullough, H. N.,** Dissociation of the supersensitivity to norepinephrine caused by cocaine from inhibition of H^3-norepinephrine uptake in cold-stored smooth muscle, *J. Pharmacol. Exp. Ther.,* 166, 26, 1969.
199. **Wagman, I. H., de Jong, R. H., and Prince, D. A.,** Effects of lidocaine on the central nervous system, *Anesthesiology,* 28, 155, 1967.
200. **Wagman, I. H., de Jong, R. H., and Prince, D. A.,** Effects of lidocaine on spontaneous cortical and subcortical electrical activity, *Arch. Neurol.,* 18, 277, 1968.
201. **Wale, N. and Jenkins, L. C.,** Site of action of diazepam in the prevention of lidocaine induced seizure activity in cats, *Canad. Anaesth. Soc. J.,* 20, 146, 1973.
202. **Wallach, M. B. and Gershon, S.,** A neuropsychopharmacological comparison of *d*-amphetamine, 1-DOPA, and cocaine, *Neuropharmacology,* 10, 743, 1971.
203. **Wallach, M. B. and Gershon, S.,** The induction and antagonism of central nervous system stimulant-induced stereotyped behavior in the cat, *Eur. J. Pharmacol.,* 18, 22, 1972.
204. **Warnick, J. E., Kee, R. D., and Yim, G. K. W.,** The effects of lidocaine on inhibition in the cerebral cortex, *Anesthesiology,* 34, 327, 1971.
205. **Wenger, G. R., Stitzel, R. E., and Craig, C. R.,** The role of biogenic amines in the reserpine-induced alteration of minimal electroshock seizure thresholds in the mouse, *Neuropharmacology,* 12, 693, 1973.
206. **Wenzel, B. M. and Sieck, M. H.,** Olfaction, *Annu. Rev. Physiol.,* 28, 381, 1966.
207. **Whitby, L. G., Hertting, G., and Axelrod, J.,** Effect of cocaine on the disposition of noradrenaline labelled with tritium, *Nature,* 187, 604, 1960.
208. **Wikinski, J. A., Usubiaga, J. E., Morales, R. L., Torrieri, A., and Usubiaga, L. E.,** Mechanism of convulsions elicited by local anesthetic agents. I. Local anesthetic depression of electrically induced seizures in man, *Anesth. Analg.* (Paris), 49, 504, 1970.
209. **Willner, J. H., Samach, M., Angrist, B. M., Wallach, M. B., and Gershon, S.,** Drug-induced stereotyped behavior and its antagonism in dogs, *Commun. Behav. Biol.,* 5, 135, 1970.
210. **Wilson, M. C., Hitomi, M., and Schuster, C. R.,** Psychomotor stimulant self administration as a function of dosage per injection in the rhesus monkey, *Psychopharmacologia,* 22, 271, 1971.
211. **Wilson, M. C. and Schuster, C. R.,** Aminergic influences on intravenous cocaine self-administration by rhesus monkeys, *Pharmacol. Biochem. Behav.,* 2, 563, 1974.
212. **Wise, R. A. and Chinerman, J.,** Effects of diazepam and phenobarbital on electrically-induced amygdaloid seizures and seizure development, *Exp. Neurol.,* 45, 355, 1974.
213. **Woolley, D. E. and Timiras, P. S.,** Prepyriform electrical activity in the rat during high altitude exposure, *Electroencephalogr. Clin. Neurophysiol.,* 18, 680, 1965.

Behavior, Psychic, Neuropharmacologic and Physiologic Aspects

Physiological Aspects of Cocaine Usage

PHYSIOLOGICAL ASPECTS OF COCAINE USAGE

John Caldwell

TABLE OF CONTENTS

INTRODUCTION

Cocaine, or benzoylmethylecgonine, which is a tropane-type alkaloid present in the leaves of the bushes of the *Erythroxylon* species, has a variety of interesting pharmacological effects. It was the first local anesthetic to be discovered, and like all local anesthetics, it is able to block nerve conduction in all parts of the nervous system when applied locally. Additionally, it is able to interfere with the conduction of impulses in other systems where this is important, such as the heart and within the central nervous system. As well as exhibiting these general effects of local anesthetics, cocaine is unique among such drugs in having a very powerful stimulant action on the central nervous system and in its potent effects on the sympathetic nervous system. These latter actions originate in the ability of cocaine to block the reuptake of noradrenaline into its nerve endings. It is the powerful central stimulant action which is the basis of the abuse of cocaine. This chapter will review the pharmacology of cocaine, the effects of chronic administration, evidence for and against tolerance, and the toxicity of cocaine.

BLOCKADE OF NERVE CONDUCTION

The action of cocaine in blocking the conduction of electrical impulses in nerves has been known for many years, and the effects resulting from this blockade have been thoroughly documented. However, the mechanism underlying this blockade has proved hard to elucidate. It now seems clear that the action is at the level of the nerve cell membrane and that the permeability of this membrane to sodium and potassium ions is altered by the drug. When applied in sufficient concentrations, cocaine will block nerve conduction in all types of nerves, both within the CNS and in the periphery. This action is completely reversible, and it is noteworthy that small non-myelinated fibers are blocked more easily than larger myelinated fibers.

The block of nerve conduction brought about by cocaine arises at the cell membrane of the nerve fiber by the prevention of the normal generation and conduction of electrical impulses.[1] Normally, a slight depolarization of the nerve causes a transient permeability of the membrane to Na^+,

and the entry of Na^+ into the nerve results in the appearance of the action potential. It is this transient permeability to Na^+ which is prevented by cocaine[1] and, as cocaine anesthesia develops, the threshold of the nerve for electrical excitability increases, which results in the blockade of the conduction of impulses.

Cocaine does not influence the normal resting potential across the nerve membrane even though the passage of impulses is blocked,[2] and this indicates that the permeability of the neuronal membrane towards K^+ is reduced as well as that towards Na^+. It is thought that calcium has a controlling influence on the permeability of the nerve membrane to ions and that cocaine apparently acts by competing for Ca^{++} at its receptors in the membrane.[3] The mechanisms involved in the changes of membrane permeability caused by cocaine are still obscure.[4]

Based on these findings, it has been suggested that cocaine influences membrane permeability in general, and this has certainly been observed in muscle fibers which swell in solutions with a high K^+ concentration due to K^+ entering the fiber. Such swelling can be inhibited by cocaine.[5]

Small nonmyelinated fibers are blocked more easily than large myelinated nerves, and this differential sensitivity of the fibers has been used to explain the well-known definite order in which sensation is lost. When cocaine is applied, the first sensation to be lost is that of pain, followed by cold, heat, and deep pressure in that order. It is very likely that these sensations are conducted through nerve fibers of increasing size, and that the progressive blockade of larger and larger fibers is responsible for the well-defined way in which sensation is lost.[6]

Much work has been performed in an attempt to show whether or not the cocaine molecule must be in an ionized form to exert its local anesthetic action. It has been suggested that it must be unionized, since the action of cocaine, a weak base, may be potentiated when it is applied in alkaline solution[7] in which it exists in the molecular form. This potentiation of cocaine is most marked in tissues where the buffering capacity is limited. Despite this, it is likely that the cation is the active form at the nerve cell membrane[8] and that the role of the free base is to enable the drug to diffuse through connective tissue and cell membranes to reach its site of action.

CENTRAL NERVOUS SYSTEM

All local anesthetics affect conduction within the central nervous system, resulting in stimulation which may lead to convulsions. This stimulation is characteristically followed by CNS depression and, in overdose death, is generally due to respiratory depression, which is typically the result of excessive CNS stimulation. Although this appears to be a biphasic action on the CNS, it does in fact have only one mechanism, since it appears that the origin of the two phases lies in depression of neuronal activity.[9] The initial stimulation is due to an inhibition of inhibitory neurones, while the later depression is due to inhibition of excitatory pathways.

Cocaine is alone among the local anesthetics in having a powerful stimulant action on the cerebral cortex, and CNS stimulation proceeds from above downwards.[4] In animals, the initial result of the administration of cocaine is a hyperactivity, while in man there occurs an elevation of mood, restlessness, and garrulousness. The performance of simple mental tasks may be enhanced and fatigue is reduced. This apparent reduction in fatigue may well result in an increased capacity for muscular work (see Reference 10).

Following cortical stimulation, there is a progressive action on the lower brain centers. This results in incoordinated movements and tremor, and convulsions can ensue. Spinal cord reflex activity increases and tonic-clonic convulsions occur. It is apparently paradoxical that nontoxic doses of cocaine prevent the tonic-clonic component of electroshock-induced seizures;[11] but if, as has been suggested, cocaine has a single depressant action on neuronal activity,[9] this would explain the anticonvulsant action of small doses of cocaine. Cocaine also inhibits seizures induced by pentylenetetrazol, but at higher doses there can be synergism with the convulsant, which can be fatal.[11]

Stimulation of the medulla results in an increase in respiratory rate. At first, the depth of respiration is unaffected, but it is soon reduced.[12] The application of cocaine to the floor of the fourth ventricle results in apnea and death from paralysis of the central control of respiration. This procedure also depresses the characteristic response to the intratracheal administration of carbon dioxide.[13] Emesis frequently occurs as a consequence of the stimulation of the vomiting center; the vasomotor center is also affected and this has a variety of cardiovascular effects, which will be described later.

The heat-regulating centers are stimulated, and this contributes towards the pyrexia which is a result of the use of cocaine.

After the initial stimulation, the higher centers are very easily depressed, and this may occur as the lower centers are being stimulated. Finally, the lower centers also become depressed and death may ensue from respiratory depression.

BODY TEMPERATURE

Cocaine is a very potent hyperthermic agent in animals and man, and the so-called "cocaine fever" contributes significantly to the toxic effects of this drug. The fever is frequently preceded by a chill, which is thought to be due to a direct action of cocaine on the heat-regulating centers; the chill results when the body temperature adjusts to an elevated level. Three mechanisms are involved in the hyperthermia,[4] one of which is the central action referred to previously. In addition, cocaine causes an increase in physical activity which raises heat production, and vasoconstriction (q.v.), again of central origin, decreases heat loss. It is interesting to note that Barbour and Marshall[14] found that in the rabbit pyretic doses of cocaine cause a water loss from the blood, which is accompanied by an increase in the water content of the liver. This redistribution of water is complete within 30 min of the administration of cocaine, and the liver thus plays an important role in the cocaine hyperthermia by storing water at a time when it is required for the purposes of heat exchange.

CARDIOVASCULAR SYSTEM

Local anesthetics have many actions on the cardiovascular system, but in general, these are only seen when high concentrations of the drug are present in the body. There are actions direct on the myocardium and also on the vasculature. The electrical excitability, conduction rate, and force of contraction are all reduced by cocaine, and these effects are prevented by digitalis[15] which is thus able to protect animals against the toxic effects of cocaine. The depression of the myocardium may be so marked as to cause asystole.[16] In addition to this, there is a centrally mediated vasoconstriction.

The action of cocaine on the heart muscle has been studied using suitable preparations of isolated atria and ventricles and has been shown to be quinidine-like, since the refractory period is lengthened, the stimulation threshold is raised, and there is a prolongation of the conduction time. These actions lead to the characteristic effects of local anesthetics on the electrocardiogram. The QRS complex widens and there may be, less frequently, lengthening of the P-R and Q-T intervals and alteration of the T waves (see Reference 17).

Small amounts of cocaine can slow the heart since they cause vagal stimulation, but larger quantities will cause tachycardia. This is not due to vagal paralysis, since electrical stimulation will still slow the heart, but probably results from the marked central and peripheral effects of cocaine on the sympathetic nervous system.[4]

Cocaine has very marked pressor effects which originate from the tachycardia and a centrally mediated vasoconstriction, and the latter may be prevented by section of the spinal cord.[12] Large doses of cocaine can cause death from cardiovascular collapse, and this is discussed separately.

MUSCLE

The powerful antifatigue action of cocaine has been referred to earlier, and it has frequently been suggested that there is a real increase in the force of muscular contractions in man and animals after small doses of cocaine. However, this has not been proven in definitive experiments.[13] Cocaine can inhibit contractions in smooth muscle, both in isolated strips and in the whole animal. Salant and Parkins[18] have examined the effect of cocaine on the motility of the isolated intestine of cat, rabbit, and rat at various pH values of the cocaine solution. In cat and rabbit intestine, the depression is maximal at pH 7.8, but in rat intestine, the depression is unaffected by pH. Crohn, Olson, and Necheles[19] studied the influence of cocaine on the intestinal hypermotility produced by the inflation of balloons *in situ* in man. They found a marked spasmolytic action, which is due both to the abolition of local reflexes and to depression of sensory receptors in the intestine. Cocaine decreases the synthesis of creatine in the gastrocnemius muscle of the rat, but the activity of phosphorylase is increased,[20] and this is similar to the effects of denervation.

SYMPATHETIC NERVOUS SYSTEM

Cocaine has a number of important actions on the sympathetic nervous system. It sensitizes the sympathetically innervated organs to noradrenaline, sympathetic nerve stimulation, and indirect-acting sympathomimetic amines. This was first seen in the early years of this century by Frölich and Loewi, and has been repeated many times since then. This sensitization is dependent on the presence of a functioning nerve supply, since denervated tissues do not show any response to cocaine. Many explanations have been put forward to account for this supersensitivity to the sympathetic transmitter, involving changes in receptor sensitivity and inhibition of monoamine oxidase. Over the last 15 years, it has become clear that cocaine is a potent inhibitor of the reuptake of catecholamine neurotransmitters by their nerve terminals,[21] and this results in the amines remaining in the vicinity of their receptors for longer than normal. There is thus an exaggerated response to exogenously applied amines as well as to sympathetic nerve stimulation.

The supersensitivity caused to electrical stimulation is only seen with weak submaximal nerve stimulation, since the maximal responses to supramaximal stimulation are unaffected by cocaine.[22] The responses of the nictitating membrane of the cat to noradrenaline and submaximal stimulation are unaffected by cocaine; and similarly, the volume change of the spleen caused by noradrenaline and nerve stimulation is increased by cocaine, but the output of noradrenaline on nerve stimulation is unchanged. In the cat, the rise in blood pressure caused by noradrenaline is directly related to the plasma level of this transmitter, and although cocaine potentiates the pressor effects of noradrenaline, this relationship is unchanged. This shows that the supersensitivity has its origin in the ability of cocaine to prolong the half-life of noradrenaline in the body, thus delaying its disappearance from the vicinity of its receptors.[22]

This potentiation of noradrenaline has a profound effect on the cardiovascular system, and Graham, Abboud, and Eckstein[23] have shown that the effects of cocaine are due to its potentiation of the actions of noradrenaline on the vasculature, rather than to effects on the cardiac output. In the intact dog, stimulation of the cardiac nerves in the presence of cocaine produces increases in both peripheral resistance and cardiac output, without affecting the heart rate or venous pressure significantly. The action of cocaine in potentiating the effects of weak submaximal nerve stimulation is not universal, since the stimulation of some sympathetically innervated preparations (such as the vasculature of the rabbit ear and the dog foreleg) is not potentiated by cocaine (see Reference 23).

Unlike other local anesthetics, cocaine causes vasoconstriction and mydriasis, and this is almost certainly due to the blockade of noradrenaline uptake.[4] During tonic sympathetic activity in the presence of cocaine, less of the neurotransmitter is inactivated by neuronal reuptake than normal, and the contraction of smooth muscle in these organs is therefore potentiated, giving the characteristic effects of cocaine on these tissues.

EYE

In the past, cocaine found great application in ophthalmology as a local anesthetic. When applied locally, the cornea is anesthetized, there is local vasoconstriction which blanches the sclera, and there is marked mydriasis.[12] These latter effects originate from the potentiation of noradrenaline released during normal nerve activity as described above, and the marked mydriasis is also seen after the systemic administration of cocaine.

Because of the mechanism by which cocaine dilates the pupil, it will still contract to light and when cholinergic drugs are applied. Further mydriasis can be produced by anticholinergics such as atropine, and the atropinized eye still shows dilatation of the pupil when cocaine is applied.[4] It is clear, then, that cocaine does not paralyze the sphincter of the iris, but as described, potentiates the effects of normal sympathetic stimulation of the radial muscle of the iris. At high doses, cocaine can cause cycloplegia, but normally any loss of accommodation is small.

Generally, the vasoconstriction produced by cocaine causes a reduction in the intraocular pressure, but the mydriasis can block drainage from the anterior chamber of the eye, which can be so marked as to precipitate attacks of glaucoma.[12]

If applied locally, cocaine damages the cornea, with clouding, pitting, and ulceration all resulting. This is aided by the inhibition of the blink reflexes, which reduces tear flow and impairs the normal protection of the cornea.

MUCOUS MEMBRANES AND THE SKIN

Cocaine in solution is able to anesthetize the mucous membranes when applied locally in all regions of the body, including the pharynx, larynx, esophagus, stomach, rectum, urethra, bladder, vagina, nose, and eye. This property is the basis of the only application of cocaine given by the oral route — that is its use as an analgesic in inoperable carcinoma of the stomach, since it also alleviates nausea and vomiting.[12] Cocaine is a cytotoxic drug,[12] and this is presumably the reason for the very marked scarring seen at injection sites.[7]

METABOLIC EFFECTS

As might be expected of a drug with such a profound action on the sympathetic nervous system, cocaine has a number of effects on the metabolism. An increase in blood sugar occurs in experimental animals, but this is not always seen in man. There is a remarkable increase in the basal metabolic rate in animals and man,[10] and cocaine increases both oxygen consumption and blood lactic acid levels in the rabbit.[24] It will also potentiate the effects of noradrenaline on these two parameters.

COCAINE POISONING AND ITS TREATMENT

There is a considerable inter-individual variation in the susceptibility to cocaine, and as a result, episodes of acute poisoning occur not infrequently. This is referred to in another section (see "Idiosyncrasy"). The minimum fatal dose is generally stated to be 1.2 g, but in some circumstances as little as 20 mg has proved fatal, death being due to cardiovascular collapse.[25] The symptoms of cocaine intoxication are extensions of the effects of the drug seen when given in normal doses. The subject first becomes excited, anxious, and confused, with enhanced reflexes and, usually, headaches. The pulse is accelerated and there may be a chill, which precedes a sudden and dramatic temperature rise. Vomiting occurs only rarely, but there is exophthalmos and, of course, pupillary dilatation.[26] The respiration is affected, becoming rapid and shallow, and Cheyne-Stokes breathing can occur later in the course of poisoning. The reflexes are more easily elicited and there is tremor and slight convulsive movements. There are two forms of cocaine poisoning which differ in the susceptibility of the cardiovascular and respiratory systems to cocaine.[12,26] In the first, delirium occurs, followed by convulsions during which there is extreme acceleration of the heart with rapid and dyspneic breathing; respiratory arrest may occur during a convulsion. More frequently, convulsions do not occur, and fainting and collapse result. The skin is cyanosed and cold, and the heart slow and weak, with respiration much depressed. Death occurs from respiratory failure. The course of cocaine poisoning is in general a rapid one, but in some cases death may be almost immediate, and this is particularly associated with the intravenous injection of large doses of cocaine (see "Idiosyncrasy").

TREATMENT

Experimental cocaine poisoning in animals is marked by rapid irregular respiration and convulsions, and this led Tatum, Atkinson, and Collins[27] to examine the possible use of barbital to counter these effects. They found that the minimum lethal dose of cocaine was increased severalfold in animals treated with barbital, but although this procedure was adopted clinically, it was of doubtful efficacy. Steinhaus and Tatum[28] found that the dose of pentobarbital required for effective prophylaxis against cocaine poisoning was one half of the anesthetic dose, while the sedative dose gave little protection. They concluded that the use of barbiturates in the treatment of cocaine poisoning is limited to the control of convulsion, and larger doses than those required for this purpose greatly increased the risk of respiratory collapse. When high plasma levels of cocaine are attained rapidly, cocaine can produce serious cardiovascular depression and the incidence of this increases when barbiturates are given also. The depression of the heart can be effectively countered by the use of adrenaline or other pressor amines, especially those with a marked positive inotropic effect,[7] and artificial respiration may be required (see below). A tourniquet may aid in preventing the absorption of the drug from a systemic site, while gastric lavage may be of help if the drug has been taken orally. Evacuation of the bladder has been recommended to help prevent reabsorption of the drug from the urine.[12]

The major aim of the therapy of cocaine intoxication must be the prevention of convulsion and cardiovascular collapse. It is essential that cerebral hypoxia be avoided, since convulsions will increase the oxygen consumption of the brain to a point where demand exceeds supply, and thereby impair respiration.[4] Convulsions can be prevented by a short-acting barbiturate, and succinylcholine has been used with success to control the peripheral muscle spasms occurring during convulsion.[29] The latter is useful in relaxing the musculature to aid artificial respiration, which may require an endotracheal tube, but does not influence the cerebral hypoxia. It is essential that oxygenation be maintained after clearing the mouth and pharynx if required, either by mouth-to-mouth resuscitation or with a ventilator. The head must be stretched back as far as possible to keep the tongue from blocking the airway. Hypotension should be treated with intravenous fluids and with pressor amines, if it is severe. If the heart has stopped, closed-chest cardiac massage must be commenced. The legs should be raised and intravenous fluids given rapidly. Hypoxia may give rise to a metabolic acidosis, which should be treated with the intravenous infusion of sodium bicarbonate (50 to 300 meq).[4] Although somewhat draconian, these measures are frequently successful in the management of cocaine intoxication.[4,7]

IDIOSYNCRASY

It has been stated that a small number of people exhibit a hypersensitivity to cocaine, which may give rise to an allergic dermatitis or an asthmatic attack.[4] There may be oedema, including glottal oedema, and pruritis, with the possibility of an anaphylactic reaction.[29] It is interesting to note that there may be a cross-sensitization with food dyes, some sulphonamides, and p-phenylenediamine.[29] Some people show an idiosyncrasy towards cocaine which manifests itself as a dramatically increased toxicity of the drug.[25] Adriani and Campbell[16] have noted that these deaths generally occur in situations where resuscitation equipment is not available and the subjects have frequently received a barbiturate even though they show marked respiratory depression. The parallels between this and the illicit use of cocaine are obvious. This form of toxic reaction is extremely rapid in onset, with syncope and cardiovascular collapse as the first signs. Convulsions do not occur, and at post-mortem, no cause of death is apparent, which leads to such deaths being ascribed to allergy or abnormal sensitivity to the drug, even though there is no real reason for such a conclusion. Adriani and Campbell[16] suggest that the cause of death in these cases is an extremely rapid absorption of the drug with the appearance of transient, very high plasma levels. This leads to myocardial depression, giving asystole, and a marked vasodilatation which together result in extreme hypotension. If this circulatory collapse is accompanied by respiratory failure, which is a frequent result of cocaine poisoning, the outcome will be fatal. This analysis led Adriani and Campbell[16] to conclude that there is no hypersensitivity to the drug, such as the anaphylactic shock mentioned above, but that the marked toxicity seen in a small number of cases under particular circumstances is entirely explicable in terms of the pharmacological actions of the drug.

THE CHRONIC ADMINISTRATION OF COCAINE

The central stimulant action of cocaine is the basis of its chronic use, which is almost invariably illicit. The classical description of the cocaine user indicates a variety of bodily changes, including digestive disorders, loss of appetite, increased salivation, emaciation, and a sallow complexion, which together with hepatomegaly may be due to jaundice.[12] It has been thought that there is a degeneration of the CNS with tremor, sleeplessness, hallucination, and delirium, and a psychosis may occur.[13] The intravenous injection of cocaine gives the user "an ecstatic sensation of extreme physical and mental power,"[12] and there is a marked psychomotor stimulation, abolition of fatigue, and suppression of hunger. These effects of cocaine are but short-lasting in the chronic user, and frequent injections (every 10 to 15 min) are required to maintain the desired drug effects.[12] As repeated doses are administered, many signs of neurological toxicity, both central and autonomic, become apparent.[4] CNS signs include tremor, twitching, muscle spasm, and increases in deep tendon reflexes, and there may be convulsions. The blood pressure is raised, tachycardia occurs,

the respiratory rate is increased, there is mydriasis, exophthalmia, and sweating.

Cocaine is frequently taken by the habitué as a snuff, since it is very rapidly absorbed from the mucous membranes of the nose, and this practice leads to damage to the nasal septum. The mucous membranes become ulcerated and the underlying cartilage of the septum may perforate. There is crusting and epistaxis, resulting in a characteristic whistling on breathing. Surgery is possible to clean up such damage, and if the practice is stopped, the epithelia will heal to cover the perforation.[30]

One common observation in cocaine users is a sallow complexion, and this has been noted in the coca chewers of the High Andes.[10] Indeed, these latter show a definite hepatomegaly and these signs have been attributed to a mild jaundice. A number of studies have shown that cocaine produces considerable liver damage in animals, which could be the basis of the mild jaundice. Ehrlich[31] dosed mice with cocaine chronically and noted that this caused enlargement of the liver with fatty infiltration of the cells. Later work by McLachlan and Hodge[32] showed that when mice received cocaine orally for 60 days, there was a dose related liver enlargement with an increase in cell size, fatty infiltration, and vacuolar degeneration. Neutral fat and cholesterol were increased in proportion to the degree of liver damage, but the phospholipid content was unaltered, as was the ratio of phospholipids to nonlipid material. Similar alterations were seen in the livers of dogs and rats given cocaine on a chronic basis.

Marks and Chapple[33] have studied liver function in a group of 89 heroin and cocaine addicts and found abnormalities in 80% of the group, which were attributable to their drug intake. Although only 6 of the 89 were jaundiced, 69% had abnormal SGPT levels, 61% abnormal SGOT, and alkaline phosphatase was abnormal in 28%. In 26%, the serum protein was elevated.

It has been stated earlier that cocaine stimulates the cerebral cortex, elevating mood and increasing metabolic activity, and it is this which gives cocaine users the increased resistance to fatigue which has been claimed.[10] These phenomena have been extensively studied in the coca chewers of the High Andes, and it has been claimed that, along with increases in the basal metabolic rate, 50% of regular coca chewers show an actual temporary increase in muscular strength.[10] However, it has been shown that there is no difference between the responses of coca chewers with or without coca to cold stress.[34] Hanna[35] has studied the influence of coca chewing on cardiovascular responses to exercise in Peruvian Indians. In a submaximal work test, coca users showed lower exercise and recovery heart rates and higher blood pressures than nonchewers. On this basis, it cannot be concluded that coca provides an advantage to its users, but when these results were projected into maximal working conditions, a slight advantage was suggested.[35]

It has often been observed that drug abusers can be detected by the large numbers of injection marks to be found on the body, but this by itself does not indicate the nature of the drug(s) which have been injected. However, cocaine has been noted to cause characteristic bluish atrophic scarring at old injection sites, and these scars have been noted on the thighs, buttocks, back, upper arms, and shoulders.[36]

TOLERANCE TO COCAINE – DOES IT OCCUR?

The problem of whether or not tolerance to cocaine occurs has been debated for many years. Modern authorities comment on the very marked tolerance to cocaine seen in man, which permits the consumption of doses 10 to 50 times greater than normal.[37] Glatt[38] notes that doses of up to 2 g daily can be taken when combined with heroin. However, there is no universal agreement that tolerance does occur (see Reference 39), and when earlier work is consulted, it is apparent that there is a real controversy as to whether or not tolerance does develop to cocaine on chronic administration.

It was a very early observation that cocaine habitués could stop self-administration of the drug for long periods, but were able to resume use of the drug at doses many times higher than those normally considered to be toxic; this led some authors (see Reference 40) to suggest that the ability of such people to use very large doses of cocaine was due to their innate resistance to the drug rather than to an acquired tolerance. Tatum and Seevers[40] reviewed the literature up to that date, and they showed that there was no evidence to support the development of tolerance in a number of studies of the chronic administration of cocaine to animals. Indeed, it appeared that there

was a sensitization to the drug, which was retained even though drug administration was stopped periodically. This was seen in guinea pigs, rabbits, cats, and dogs.

Tatum and Seevers[40] have examined the effects of very prolonged daily administration of cocaine to dogs and rhesus monkeys. They chose a dose (30 mg) which gave only slight effects in the dog, and initially the animals showed only small increases in bodily activity and showed signs of apprehension. Within a week of commencing the daily administration of this dose, it was apparent that the stimulant action of cocaine had increased, and after 1 month, a group of new effects had become apparent. Some 5 min after injection, there were signs of pupillary dilatation, restlessness, and licking of the chops. These intensified, and 15 min after injection signs of cocaine poisoning were seen, with lateral spasmodic head movements, purposeless jumping back and forward which was seen even when free running was permitted, salivation, marked mydriasis, opisthotonus, and very rapid respiration with the tongue protruded. The body temperature rose between 3 and 3.5°C during this period. The great excitement seen in dogs before the expected injection of cocaine is accompanied by intense panting and tachycardia, but these symptoms disappear as soon as the cocaine is given, and the tachycardia may even be replaced by a bradycardia. In nonaddicted dogs, these changes in heart rate are never seen. After the preinjection excitement is dulled by cocaine, the characteristic pharmacological effects are then seen as previously described. These signs of anticipation can be relieved transiently by saline injections, which produce a short burst of motor activity; but when this is over, the expectant signs recur. No complete physiological record of the animals was kept, but during the treatment period, considerable weight loss was observed. It is interesting to note that the signs of extreme stimulation produced in these dogs by cocaine could be quieted by gentle handling of the animals, and this was accompanied by a reduction in the hyperthermia, since the maximum temperature rise in handled animals was only 1 to 1.5°C.

During the latter part of the phase of stimulation produced by cocaine, female dogs were receptive to the male, allowing copulation, but at other times no ardor was apparent. Male dogs showed priapism during the excitement prior to, and immediately after, injection. However, when placed with a female, the males made no attempt at copulation during the period of drug action.

Similar experiments were carried out using rhesus monkeys[40] and a similar pattern of increasing sensitivity to the drug was seen, which developed even more rapidly than in the dog. The hypersensitivity was not influenced by breaks in the continuity of dosing, and no signs of sexual excitement were seen.

Downs and Eddy[41] administered cocaine to dogs and found that there was an increase in the duration and intensity of the motor stimulant effect during the first 2 weeks of chronic administration, which then reached a plateau. The dogs showed a great craving for the drug, which was not satisfied by placebo injections of saline. The physical condition of the dogs was unaffected, weight gain being maintained throughout the experiment, and no withdrawal signs were evident at the end of the period of drug administration. In similar experiments in rats, Downs and Eddy[42] showed that the increased sensitivity to the motor stimulant effect of cocaine seen on chronic administration also occurs in this species. It is interesting to note that they found that this increased sensitivity is even more marked in the male than in the female.

Regrettably, there does not appear to be any study extant of the changes of the physiological effects of cocaine throughout a period of chronic administration to animals or to man (see chapter by M. Matsuzaki). However, it is apparent that cocaine habitués regularly consume doses which are markedly in excess of those normally considered to be toxic,[43] even though many bizarre neurological signs are apparent. It must therefore be concluded that tolerance does occur to some effects, so as to allow the intake of these very large doses, but not to the CNS effects, to which sensitization occurs as described. It is necessary to speculate about the causes for the sensitization occurring to some effects of cocaine on chronic administration. This sensitization is limited to the CNS effects of the drug, giving rise to a form of stereotyped behavior in animals, and it is obvious that no tolerance is seen to CNS effects in man since a psychosis may ensue after repeated doses.[37] At this point, it is interesting to note what may be a parallel between amphetamine and cocaine, which are both psychic energizers, and which both give rise to a psychosis in man. We have made a careful study of a number of the effects of amphetamine during chronic administration to rats and guinea pigs, and it appears that while tolerance develops readily to such actions as hyperthermia and anorexia, the stereotyped behavior induced by the drug increased markedly during the period of chronic administration. It may be that as cocaine and amphetamine have a number of features in common with respect to mode of action and effects, cocaine is like amphetamine in the unequal development of tolerance and in there being a hyperresponse to some effects on repeated dosage.[44,45] This perhaps provides an interpretation of the early reports of sensitization, since the early workers only dealt with the behavioral responses to the drug.

That tolerance does develop to some of the effects of cocaine is suggested by the considerable tachyphylaxis which develops to this drug in a number of animal systems.[46] Thus, tachyphylaxis has been noted to the pressor effect of cocaine in the spinal cat and to its contractile effect on rabbit aortic strips. In both these cases, the tachyphylaxis was reversed by the infusion of noradrenaline. However, cocaine had no effect on aortic strips from reserpinized animals, and the tachyphylaxis was not reversed by indirect-acting sympathomimetics, such as amphetamine. Washing and resting the aortic strips reversed the tachyphylaxis, but this reversal was prevented when a variety of noradrenaline synthesis inhibitors were incorporated in the bath fluid. It appears that the tachyphylaxis results from depletion of the neuronal stores of the transmitter, due to inhibition of reuptake. This would explain the inability of indirect-acting sympathomimetic amines to reverse the tachyphylaxis, since there is no transmitter available for them to release, and the reversibility of the tachyphylaxis by exogenous noradrenaline, the action of which would be potentiated due to the inhibition of uptake by cocaine. Resting serves to replenish stores of noradrenaline by the *de novo* synthesis of this amine. (For further discussion and data see chapter by M. Matsuzahi.)

WITHDRAWAL

It is a widely held view that the phenomenon of physical dependence to drugs, as defined by their ability to produce a well-defined withdrawal syndrome when their administration is stopped, is restricted to those CNS depressants which are abused, notably the narcotic analgesics, barbiturates and other sedative-hypnotics, and beverage alcohol, and that no abstinence signs occur when the administration of CNS stimulants, such as the amphetamines and cocaine, is stopped.

Cocaine usage is marked by an exceedingly great craving for the repeated administration of the drug, but as indicated above, there is no distinctive withdrawal syndrome when its use is stopped.[39] Early work on the experimental addiction of animals to cocaine notes the absence of such phenomena (q.v.), but Jaffé[47] states that the only effects seen in man when cocaine is withdrawn are a continued craving for the drug, fatigue, lassitude, sleep, hunger, and depression. No gross physiological disruptions occur, but Jaffé[47] suggests that the problem of whether or not an abstinence syndrome occurs must be reconsidered. The lassitude, fatigue, and depression which occur are hard to attribute to previous sleep loss due to the drug alone, and may constitute a type of withdrawal syndrome. It is interesting to note that although cessation of amphetamine use, like cocaine, does not give any withdrawal phenomena, it has been observed to cause very marked disturbances in certain EEG patterns during sleep, with prolonged periods of paradoxical (REM) sleep during withdrawal; these disturbances can be reversed by further doses of the drug.[48] It is thus likely that there is a withdrawal syndrome produced by the stimulant amines of this type, and although this is less severe than with the depressant drugs which cause addiction, it nevertheless must be considered when such drugs are withdrawn from habitués.

ACKNOWLEDGMENTS

The author wishes to thank Dr. P. A. Nasmyth for his helpful comments, and Mr. N. D. Palmer and the staff of the Library, St. Mary's Hospital Medical School, for their help in obtaining references.

REFERENCES

1. **Taylor, R. E.,** Effect of procaine on electrical properties of squid axon membrane, *Am. J. Physiol.,* 196, 1071, 1959.
2. **Bishop, G. H.,** Action of nerve depressants on potential, *J. Cell. Comp. Physiol.,* 1, 177, 1932.
3. **Blaustein, M. P. and Goldman, D. E.,** Competitive action of calcium and procaine on lobster axon, *J. Gen. Physiol.,* 49, 1043, 1966.
4. **Ritchie, J. M., Cohen, P. J., and Dripps, R. D.,** Cocaine; procaine and other synthetic local anesthetics, in *Pharmacological Basis of Therapeutics,* 4th ed., Goodman, L. S. and Gilman, A., Eds., Macmillan, New York, 1971, chap. 20.
5. **Shanes, A. M.,** Drug and ion effects in frog muscle, *J. Gen. Physiol.,* 33, 729, 1950.
6. **Gasser, H. S. and Erlanger, J.,** The role of fibre size in the establishment of a nerve block by pressure or cocaine, *Am. J. Physiol.,* 88, 581, 1929.
7. **Adriani, J.,** The clinical pharmacology of local anesthetics, *Clin. Pharmacol. Ther.,* 1, 645, 1960.
8. **Ritchie, J. M. and Greengard, P.,** On the mode of action of local anesthetics, *Ann. Rev. Pharmacol.,* 6, 405, 1966.
9. **Frank, G. B. and Sanders, H. B.,** A proposed common mechanism of action for general and local anaesthetics in the central nervous system, *Br. J. Pharmacol.,* 21, 1, 1963.
10. **Guttierez-Noriega, C. and von Hagen, V. W.,** The strange case of the coca leaf, *Sci. Mon.* (New York), 70, 81, 1950.
11. **Tanaka, K.,** Anticonvulsant properties of procaine, cocaine, adiphenine and related structures, *Proc. Soc. Exp. Biol. Med.,* 90, 192, 1955.
12. **Grollman, A.,** *Pharmacology and Therapeutics,* 5th ed., Henry Kimpton, London, 1962, 436.
13. **Cushny, A. R.,** *Pharmacology and Therapeutics,* 12th ed., Edmunds, C. W. and Gunn, J. A., Eds., Churchill, London, 1941, 442.
14. **Barbour, H. G. and Marshall, H. T.,** Heat regulation and water exchange. XII. The underlying mechanism of fever as illustrated by cocaine poisoned rabbits, *J. Pharmacol. Exp. Ther.,* 43, 147, 1931.

15. Eggleston, C. and Hatcher, R. A., A further contribution to the pharmacology of local anaesthetics, *J. Pharmacol. Exp. Ther.*, 13, 433, 1919.

16. Adriani, J. and Campbell, D., Fatalities following topical application of local anesthetics to mucous membranes, *JAMA*, 162, 1527, 1956.

17. Moe, G. K. and Abildskov, J. A., Antiarrhythmic drugs, in *Pharmacological Basis of Therapeutics*, 4th ed., Goodman, L. S. and Gilman, A., Eds., Macmillan, New York, 1971, chap. 32.

18. Salant, W. and Parkins, W. M., The response of the isolated intestine to cocaine and novocaine at different pH levels, *J. Pharmacol. Exp. Ther.*, 46, 435, 1932.

19. Crohn, N., Olson, W. H., and Necheles, H., The local effect of anaesthetic drugs on the motility of the gastrointestinal tract of the human and the dog, *Surg. Gynecol. Obstet.*, 70, 41, 1944.

20. Matsui, T. and Kuriaki, K., Effect of denervation and cocainization on activity of creatine synthesizing enzymes and phosphorylase in skeletal muscle, *Am. J. Physiol.*, 196, 461, 1959.

21. Iversen, L. L., *The Uptake and Storage of Noradrenaline*, Cambridge University Press, London, 1967.

22. Trendelenberg, U., The supersensitivity caused by cocaine, *J. Pharmacol. Exp. Ther.*, 125, 55, 1959.

23. Graham, M. H., Abboud, F. M., and Eckstein, J. W., Effect of cocaine on cardiovascular responses in intact dogs, *J. Pharmacol. Exp. Ther.*, 150, 46, 1965.

24. Lundholm, L. and Mohme-Lundholm, E., The effect of cocaine and adrenaline on blood lactic acid and oxygen consumption in rabbits, *Acta Pharmacol. Toxicol.*, 15, 257, 1959.

25. *Martindale-Extra Pharmacopoiea*, 26th ed., Pharmaceutical Press, London, 1972, pp. 1029–1033.

26. Luduena, F. P., Toxicity and irritancy of local anesthetics, in *International Encyclopedia of Pharmacology and Therapeutics*, Vol. 8, part 1, Pergamon, Oxford, 1971, chap. 9, p. 319.

27. Tatum, A. L., Atkinson, A. J., and Collins, K. H., Acute cocaine poisoning, its prophylaxis and treatment in laboratory animals, *J. Pharmacol. Exp. Ther.*, 26, 325, 1925.

28. Steinhaus, J. E. and Tatum, A. L., An experimental study of cocaine intoxication and its treatment, *J. Pharmacol. Exp. Ther.*, 100, 351, 1950.

29. Vourc'h, G., Incidents and accidents induced by local anaesthetics in their various clinical applications, in *International Encyclopedia of Pharmacology and Therapeutics*, Vol. 8, part 1, Pergamon, Oxford, 1971, chap. 10, p. 343.

30. Miles Foxen, E. H., *Lecture Notes of Diseases of the Ear, Nose, and Throat*, 3rd ed., Blackwell, Oxford, 1972, 108.

31. Ehrlich, P., Cocainreh, *Dtsch. Med. Wochenschr.*, pp. 717–719, 1890.

32. McLachlan, P. L. and Hodge, H. C., The influence of cocaine feeding on the liver lipids of the white mouse, *J. Biol. Chem.*, 127, 721, 1939.

33. Marks, V. and Chapple, P. A. L., Hepatic dysfunction in heroin and cocaine users, *Br. J. Addict.*, 62, 189, 1967.

34. Elsner, R. W. and Bolstad, A., Thermal and Metabolic Responses to Cold Exposure of Andean Indians at High Altitude, Technical Report AAL-TOR 62–64, Arctic Aeromedical Lab, Ladd AFB, Alaska, 1963.

35. Hanna, J. M., The effects of coca chewing on exercise in the Quecha of Peru, *Hum. Biol.*, 42, 1, 1970.

36. Yaffee, H. S., Dermatologic manifestations of cocaine addiction, *Cutis* (New York), 4, 286, 1968.

37. Snyder, S. H., CNS stimulants and hallucinogens, in *Chemical and Biological Aspects of Drug Dependence*, Mulé, S. J. and Brill, H., Eds., CRC Press, Cleveland, 1972, 55.

38. Glatt, M. M., *A Guide to Addiction and Its Treatment*, MTP Press, Lancaster, 1974, 143.

39. Isbell, H. and White, W. M., Clinical characteristics of addictions, *Am. J. Med.*, 14, 558, 1953.

40. Tatum, A. L. and Seevers, M. H., Experimental cocaine addiction, *J. Pharmacol. Exp. Ther.*, 36, 401, 1929.

41. Downs, A. W. and Eddy, N. B., The effect of repeated doses of cocaine on the dog, *J. Pharmacol. Exp. Ther.*, 46, 195, 1932.

42. Downs, A. W. and Eddy, N. B., The effect of repeated doses of cocaine on the rat, *J. Pharmacol. Exp. Ther.*, 46, 199, 1932.

43. Caldwell, J. and Sever, P. S., The biochemical pharmacology of abused drugs. I. Amphetamine, cocaine, and LSD, *Clin. Pharmacol. Ther.*, 16, 625, 1974.

44. Sever, P. S. and Caldwell, J., Species differences in amphetamine tolerance, *J. Pharmacol.* (Paris), 5(2), 91, 1974.

45. Sever, P. S., Caldwell, J., and Williams, R. T., Tolerance to amphetamine in two species (rat and guinea pig) which metabolize it differently, *Psychol. Med.*, 6, 35, 1976.

46. Maengwyn-Davies, G. D. and Koppanyi, T., Cocaine tachyphylaxis and effects on indirect-acting sympathomimetic drugs in the rabbit aortic strip and in splenic tissue, *J. Pharmacol. Exp. Ther.*, 154, 481, 1966.

47. Jaffé, J., Drug addiction and drug abuse, in *Pharmacological Basis of Therapeutics*, 4th ed., Goodman, L. S. and Gilman, A., Eds., Macmillan, New York, 1971, chap. 16.

48. Oswald, I. and Thacore, V. R., Amphetamine and phenmetrazine addiction. Physiological abnormalities in the abstinence syndrome, *Br. Med. J.*, 2, 427, 1963.

Clinical Aspects

*Clinical Aspects of Cocaine: Assessment of Acute
and Chronic Effects in Animals and Man*

CLINICAL ASPECTS OF COCAINE: ASSESSMENT OF ACUTE AND CHRONIC EFFECTS IN ANIMALS AND MAN*

Robert M. Post

TABLE OF CONTENTS

INTRODUCTION

This chapter will focus on the several different clinical effects of cocaine as they relate to both the dose and the duration of cocaine administration. Particular attention will be paid to the evolution of the cocaine effects with chronic administration and to the evidence that many parameters demonstrate sensitization or reverse tolerance following repeated doses. The effects of chronic cocaine in animals will be reviewed in an attempt to elucidate the mechanisms involved and how they might be relevant as models of psychotic behavior.

EFFECTS ON MOOD (EUPHORIA-DYSPHORIA) AND PHYSIOLOGY

Over several centuries, cocaine has been reported to be a potent euphoriant and psychomotor stimulant with the potential for producing mood elevation, alertness, increased capacity for work, and a variety of other effects closely paralleling those of amphetamine.[1-3] Until recently, however, there have been relatively few systematic studies of its effects in controlled conditions.[4,5]

Indians in the high Andes mountains have routinely chewed coca leaves producing an increased subjective sense of well-being, stamina, and decreased hunger. Their cocaine habit is to some extent related to environmental conditions, as they are able to give up cocaine when they return to lower altitudes, apparently without suffering any major withdrawal phenomenon or associated depression.[6] Freud and many other European and American physicians at the turn of the century became impressed with cocaine's effects on mood and widely prescribed the drug for their own and their patients' depressed moods.[7] Freud was particularly enthusiastic about its mood elevating

*This chapter is written under the auspices of and funded by the Federal Government and is not subject to copyright.

properties, initially not recognizing its potential for psychic habituation. He writes of the cocaine user:

After a short time (10 – 20 minutes), he feels as though he had been raised to the full height of intellectual and bodily vigor, in a state of euphoria, which is distinguished from the euphoria after consumption of alcohol by the absence of any feeling of alteration . . . . one can perform mental and physical work with great endurance, and the otherwise urgent needs of rest, food, and sleep are thrust aside, as it were. During the first hours after cocaine, it is even impossible to fall asleep. This effect of the alkaloid gradually fades away after the aforesaid time, and is not followed by any depression . . . . I could not fail to note, however, that the individual disposition plays a major role in the effects of cocaine, perhaps a more important role than with other alkaloids. The subjective phenomena after ingestion of coca differ from person to person, and only few persons experience, like myself, a pure euphoria without alteration. Others already experience slight intoxication. hyperkinesia, and talkativeness after the same amount of cocaine, while still others have no subjective symptoms of the effects of coca at all . . . .
Sigmund Freud (1854)[8]

Reports of cocaine's prominent euphorogenic properties continue to come from the drug subculture where abusers indicate that it is the drug of choice for producing exquisite effects on mood.[9] These subjective reports of cocaine's special properties and superiority as a euphoriant stand in contradiction to the evidence that cocaine is not easily discriminated from other stimulants[10,11] and that other stimulants are mistakenly identified as cocaine.[12]

Clinical Trial in Depression

In light of the similarity of cocaine's effects in blocking reuptake of norepinephrine, dopamine, and serotonin to many routinely useful antidepressants, its widely accepted effects as a euphoriant, and the possibility that it might have a rapid onset of action, a clinical trial was undertaken in moderately to severely depressed patients at the National Institutes of Health.[13] Cocaine was initially administered orally in doses similar to those reported effective by Freud and others, but prominent antidepressant effects were not observed. Ten patients received 12 double blind trials of oral cocaine for an average of 10 days. Initial doses of 5 to 50 mg/day were gradually increased to a final dose of 30 to 200 mg/day. Drug was given at 9:00 a.m. and 10:00 p.m. so that effects on mood during the day, as well as sleep, could be studied.[13,14]

The potential hazard of psychic dependence on cocaine was minimized in several ways. Patients were excluded from the study if they had a history of drug dependence. Cocaine was administered on a double-blind basis within the context of a therapeutic milieu that included group and individual therapy. Routine antidepressant medications were substituted at the end of the cocaine protocol. Prior to and during a patient's voluntary hospitalization, a number of experimental drugs (including cocaine) that might be administered during the course of hospitalization were discussed with patients and relatives. Thus, while patients were able to discuss the possible hazards of cocaine as well as other experimental drugs and give informed consent, they were unaware of when they were receiving cocaine during the hospitalization. The experimental trials were of short duration, and when clear effects on mood became evident, cocaine administration was discontinued and placebo substituted. Obviously, the drug was not self-administered, a condition most closely associated with the development of drug dependence.[3]

Oral Cocaine: Effects on Mood and Sleep

The results are summarized in Table 1. Only one patient appeared to have improved during oral cocaine administration; she also had two periods of rated hypomania at the highest doses. Three patients had equivocal response of small magnitude unassociated with a rebound in depression upon placebo substitution, and five patients showed no change. One patient, receiving the highest dose of cocaine during a second trial (after lower doses were unsuccessful in a first trial), showed an exacerbation of his depression, characterized by increasing agitation, verbal blocking, and the development of paranoid ideation.

TABLE 1

Effects of Oral Cocaine in Ten Depressed Patients

Number of patients	Effect on depression
1	Worse
5	No change
3	Equivocal response
1	Improved

Adapted from Post, R. M., Kotin, J., and .Goodwin, F. K., *Am. J. Psychiatry,* 131, 511, 1974.

No definitive conclusions should be drawn regarding the effects of oral cocaine in depression since cocaine is rapidly hydrolyzed in the gastrointestinal tract and absorption would be highly variable. However, Woods et al.[15] reported measurable levels of plasma cocaine in the dog after oral administration, and levels of cocaine in our patients (1/2 to 2 hr after a dose) were measurable in the nanogram range by mass fragmentography (in collaboration with Richard L. Hawks). Although oral cocaine did not significantly affect pulse, blood pressure, or ratings of mood, it did produce statistically significant effects on sleep,[14] suggesting that some cocaine or metabolite was being absorbed by the oral route and was physiologically active. The effects of cocaine on sleep are summarized in Figure 1 and indicate a significant reduction in both total and rapid eye movement (REM) sleep.[14] Other parameters were affected in the direction of producing a general impairment and disruption of sleep, but were not statistically significant. As the dose of cocaine was increased, there was greater REM suppression (p < .01) and a REM rebound was observed following discontinuation of the drug and placebo substitution.

Intravenous Cocaine

A clinical trial of intravenous cocaine in depressed patients was conducted in an attempt to avoid the ambiguities of dose and absorption inherent in the oral administration of cocaine. In contrast to the insubstantial effects of oral cocaine in most depressed patients, the intravenous route was associated with more clear effects on both mood and vital signs.[13] Twelve patients received a total of 57 cocaine and 15 placebo infusions in the context of a tape-recorded interview with a non-blind psychiatrist; a blind observer also rated patients following selected placebo and drug infusions. The interview was unstructured and nondirective. A low dose of cocaine or a placebo was administered during the first interviews so that baseline clinical observations could be made. After the patients' pulse and blood pressure achieved a stable baseline during an interview, the infusion was administered and pulse and blood pressure were measured at approximately 5-min intervals for a half hour or until vital signs returned to normal. After examining normal fluctuations within interviews when a placebo was administered, it was arbitrarily decided that less than a ten-point change in diastolic or systolic blood

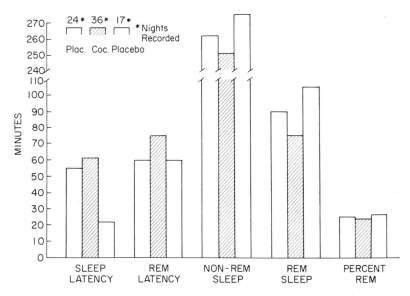

FIGURE 1. Six clinical trials were carried out in a placebo-cocaine-placebo design. For statistical analysis of a given sleep parameter, a mean for placebo, cocaine, and placebo nights for each patient was calculated, ranked, and compared with the Friedmann Two-Way Analysis of Variance. Cocaine significantly suppressed rapid eye movement sleep (p < 0.002) and total sleep (p < 0.03). (Adapted from Post, R. M., Gillin, J. C., Wyatt, R. J., and Goodwin, F. K., *Psychopharmacologica,* 37, 59, 1974.)

pressure or pulse would be categorized no change, increase of ten or more points a moderate change, and more than 15 points a marked change. Psychological changes were defined as absent, moderate, or marked according to the degree of mood change assessed from the patients' interview material and the observer's reports. Self-ratings were obtained a half hour after the infusion, in addition to the two-hourly ratings.

The starting doses of intravenous cocaine ranged from 2.5 mg to 8 mg; while the highest doses reached for each of the 12 patients ranged from 5 mg to 25 mg. Cocaine was infused over intervals of 1 to 3 min for the first several patients and then a duration of 1.5 min was adopted.

Physiology and Dose-response Effects on Mood

Effects on pulse and blood pressure varied in a systematic fashion according to the dose of cocaine administered.[13] Although there was wide individual variation in the dose of cocaine that produced a ten-point increase in pulse and blood pressure (2.5 to 16 mg), within a given individual and across all subjects, a relatively consistent dose-response relationship was evident (Figure 2). The average dose of intravenous cocaine associated

with no, moderate, or marked changes in vital signs as defined above was 6.2 mg, 9.5 mg, and 12.4 mg respectively. A close relationship was observed between the effects on vital signs and those on mood. Patients with little physiological change (even to a moderate dose of cocaine) showed few subjective or objective changes, while those with clear effects on pulse and blood pressure had clear effects on mood.

The type of mood and behavior change also tended to be closely related to physiological effects.[13] Infusions which produced mild to moderate increases in vital signs were more likely to be associated with positive affects and a sense of calmness and well-being, while higher doses of cocaine associated with more marked physiological changes produced intense mobilization of affect and sudden onset of tearfulness or a mixed euphoric-dysphoric picture with a predominance of dysphoria (Table 2). This pattern is illustrated in one patient (Figure 3) in whom a dissociation of objective and subjective reports was noted. At peak physiological effect as measured by her pulse, she suddenly began to cry and appeared markedly anxious, distraught, and depressed to blind observers, but reported an internal sense of

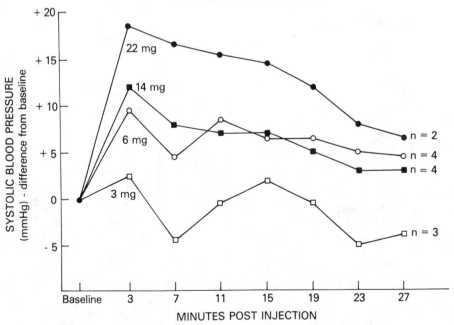

EFFECTS OF INTRAVENOUS COCAINE ON SYSTOLIC BLOOD PRESSURE
IN DEPRESSED PATIENTS

FIGURE 2. While some patients demonstrated greater reactivity than others to a given dose of cocaine, an overall dose-response relationship was manifest; higher doses were associated with larger increases in blood pressure. (Post, R. M., Kotin, J., and Goodwin, F. K., unpublished observation, 1974.)

TABLE 2

Type of Affective Response in Relation to Degree of Physiological Change

Predominant response	Physiological change	
	Moderate (>10 points)	Marked (>15 points)
Marked affective release and tearfulness	1	4
Dysphoria	3	*
Mixed affect	4	2
Calmness, well-being	7	1
No change	8	1
Total # of infusions	23	8

*Three of four patients experienced the marked affective release as dysphoric.

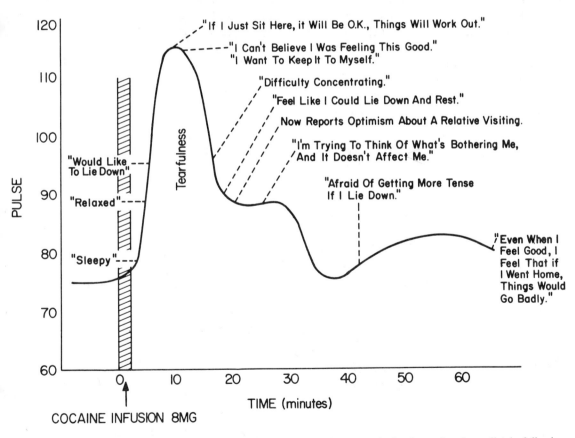

CORRELATION BETWEEN PHYSIOLOGICAL AND PSYCHOLOGICAL CHANGE AFTER INTRAVENOUS COCAINE

FIGURE 3. This patient was a 54-year-old female with moderate to severe unipolar depression. Immediately following intravenous injection of 8 mg of cocaine, she reported a sense of sleepiness and relaxation, but appeared tense and depressed and suddenly began to cry. During this time she continued to report a subjective sense of decreased depression, anxiety, and sadness. Forty minutes after the infusion, as pulse was returning to baseline levels, her reports of depression returned. This patient, atypically, showed a dissociation of her positive subjective feeling and her behavior, including the marked tearfulness that she experienced during peak increases in pulse and blood pressure. (Post, R. M., Kotin, J., and Goodwin. F. K., unpublished observation, 1974.)

relaxation and mood elevation accompanying these changes. As her pulse returned toward baseline, her depressive thoughts returned. Other patients reported the sudden onset of affective flooding as distinctly unpleasant, and all said that they would not want to repeat that experience even though they felt they benefited from the catharsis. Again, infusions of lower doses of cocaine, producing less marked physiological effects, were more likely to be reported as positive experiences, including the only patient who experienced a relatively pure euphoria. In these depressed patients in this experimental context, it was difficult to reach and maintain the end point of a positive effect on mood, as higher doses would tend to produce more dysphoria.[13] Figure 4 presents a schema summarizing some of the dose and time-course relationships (see below).

Relationship to Other Patient Populations

The physiological data in these depressed patients and, to some extent, the effects on mood have been closely replicated by the work of Resnick et al.[16] and Fischman and Schuster[11] in addict volunteers. As also reported in this volume, they demonstrated dose-related increases in pulse and blood pressure following cocaine which closely paralleled the time course of the subjective reports of the high. In addition, Resnick reported, as in our depressed patients, that higher doses (25 mg) were associated with more reports of dysphoric effects. These data are also consistent with the observations of Martin et al.[12] that the largest doses of a variety of sympathomimetic amines increased scores on a dysphoria scale.

The apparent inability of cocaine to produce consistent mood elevation without dysphoria in our depressed patients (even with gradually increasing doses which should have maximized the likelihood of reaching and not exceeding an optimal response), in contrast to the characteristic reports of mood elevation in addict volunteers in similar dose ranges, requires further exploration and clarification in relation to other or "normal" control populations. Apparent differences between groups may disappear in controlled studies of different populations under the same conditions; it is also possible that addicts may be more sensitive to the euphoric effects of cocaine (see below) or depressed patients more resistant. A demonstration of the depressed patient's reduced capacity for stimulant-induced euphoria would have obvious theoretical import. Such an investigation would be complicated by the difficulty of

INTERACTION OF DOSE, DURATION, AND ROUTE OF ADMINISTRATION
ON COCAINE-INDUCED PSYCHOPATHOLOGY

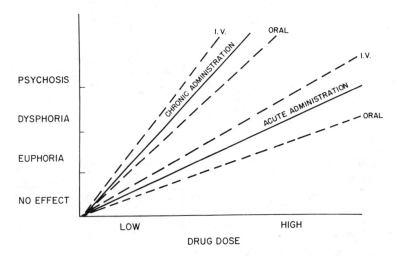

FIGURE 4. This figure represents a hypothetical schema for the interaction of drug administration variables and behavioral changes induced by cocaine. The continuum aspects of cocaine's effects are emphasized on the ordinant where, with increasing drug effect, euphoria is followed by dysphoria and paranoid psychosis. These latter effects appear to be more readily achieved with intravenous administration of higher doses over longer periods of time.

ethically studying a suitable "normal" control group and by the inherent problems of equating set and setting[17] for depressed compared to other control populations. A further question is to what extent does an infusion of cocaine nonspecifically activate ongoing motivational, cognitive, and affective states as distinct from a more specific effect on "euphorogenic" systems. Another thorny conceptual issue which current data are inadequate to answer is whether the failure to produce consistent euphoria in depressed patients with i.v. cocaine in our paradigm can be considered evidence against a bipolar theory of affective illness in which "high" and "low" are considered opposite ends of the spectrum. The data in depressed patients[13] and addict volunteers[12,16] suggest that some dysphoria may occur following a more intense drug effect.[18] To what extent the dysphoria occurring with high doses[12,13,16] or more chronic administration of cocaine or amphetamine[19,20] is relevant to various functional depressive syndromes or is merely a transitional phase between euphoria and early psychotogenic effects of the stimulants remains for further study. The dysphoria of high dose or chronic stimulant administration does, however, suggest a hyperaroused or overstimulated clinical state, in contrast to the dysphoria of the more classical retarded depression following stimulant withdrawal with either amphetamine,[21] or as occasionally reported, with cocaine.[1,2]

PSYCHOTOGENETIC EFFECTS

While anecdotal reports of cocaine psychoses are numerous, no controlled study of cocaine psychosis has been conducted like those with amphetamine.[19,20,22,23] Moreover, while case descriptions of cocaine psychoses have been provided by a number of sources, these have been largely based on the older literature,[24-26] and few current workers in the field (Robert Byck, personal communication, based on an informal survey at a recent symposium on cocaine) have seen a substantial number of cases of cocaine psychosis. The reasons for this may include the following aspects: current abuse patterns, drug availability, and cost are not conducive to the production of psychotogenic effects; such patients do not readily come to medical attention; or less

likely, the possibility may exist that cocaine is a more benign drug than previously thought.

Several psychotic syndromes have been reported which appear to depend both on dose and duration of administration. An acute overdose may produce a rapidly evolving picture of initial elation; increased irritability, anxiety, and agitation; a toxic-confusional psychosis with typical features of an organic brain syndrome; and may proceed to convulsions, cardiovascular and respiratory arrest, and death.[1,3,9,26,27] The toxic-confusional psychosis is of less theoretical interest than the other syndromes which appear to develop with more chronic cocaine administration and, in parallel with amphetamine psychoses, may not be associated with a clouded sensorium or a preponderance of visual hallucinations. These syndromes may be useful as models for manic-like and schizophreniform psychoses.[18,27] A grandiose-delusional psychosis associated with hyperactivity, pressure of speech, insomnia, and hypersexuality has been described[9,24,26] which appears to share many characteristics with a fulminant manic episode.

It was when I got back into that familiar snow feeling that I began to want to talk. Cocaine produces, for those who sniff its powdery white crystals, an illusion of supreme well-being, and a soaring over-confidence in both physical and mental ability. You think that you could whip the heavyweight champion; and that you are smarter than everybody.

Malcolm X (1945) as cited in Reference 9

When you shoot coke in the mainline there is a rush of pure pleasure to the head. Ten minutes later you want another shot. Intravenous C is electricity through the brain, activating cocaine pleasure connections. There is no withdrawal syndrome with C. It is a need of the brain alone.

William Burroughs (1966) as cited in Reference 9

Borne on the wings of two coca leaves, I flew about in the spaces of 77,438 worlds, one more splendid than another. I prefer a life of ten years with coca to one of a hundred thousand without it. It seemed to me that I was separated from the whole world, and I beheld the strangest images most beautiful in color and in form than can be imagined.

Paolo Mantegazza (1859) as cited in Reference 9

A paranoid psychosis has also been frequently reported, apparently highly similar to that reported with chronic amphetamine administration.[24-28]

Mental weakness, accompanied by irritability, erroneous

conclusions, suspicion, bitterness towards his environment, a false interpretation of things, groundless jealousy, etc., bring about in the individual, now suffering from insomnia, illusions of the senses while fully conscious. Hallucinations of vision, hearing, smell and taste, disturbances in the sexual sphere and the general condition master those who are severely affected. In many cocainomaniacs confusional insanity preceded by general mental disorders, vacancy of mind as in delirium tremens, extreme alarm due to false impressions, set in. A cocainist who had snuffed 3.25 gr. cocaine armed himself for protection against imaginary enemies; another in an attack of acute mania jumped overboard into the water; another broke the furniture and crockery into pieces and attacked a friend.

Louis Lewin (1931)[24]

I imagined every one was looking at me and watching me; even when locked in my own room, I could not persuade myself there were not watchers outside, with my eyes glued to imaginary peepholes. If I ventured into the street I thought I was followed and that the passers-by made remarks about me; I thought my vice was known to all, and on all sides I could hear the widespread word 'Cocaine . . . '. It is curious that directly after the effect of cocaine had passed away all the suspicions and delusions vanished instantly. I could see the absurdity and impossibility of the idea that a whole town was watching and talking about one obscure individual. I realized the folly of thinking that spies were in the room above, watching me through holes pierced in the ceiling. Yet, the overpowering desire to repeat the dose would overtake me, and almost instantly after taking it all delusions would return in full force, and no reasoning would banish them.

Wilson (1955) as cited in Reference 28

A late developing phase characterized by an amotivational state, ahedonia, and mental deterioration has been less well documented[9,24-26] and may be partially confounded by effects of malnutrition, withdrawal effects, and other drugs. Some authors highlight the differences between the cocaine syndromes and the functional psychoses,[24,25] especially the lack of systemization of delusions, the absence of a total "ensemble" typical of schizophrenia, and the low but reported incidence of delusions of parasitosis.

Abnormal sensations in the peripheral nerves cause the patient to believe there are animals under his skin. The result is frequently self-mutilation, and by a false application of subjective impressions, the mutilation of members of his family, in order to remove the foreign substance from the body. A woman injured herself with needles in order to kill the 'cocaine bugs'. A man who suffered from twinges and pains in the arms and feet thought he was being forcibly electrocuted. He thought he could see electric wires leading to his body.

Louis Lewin (1931)[24]

Whether the late developing cocaine syndromes are close models for some manic or schizophrenic syndromes or not, the effects of chronic cocaine on behavior may represent a valuable conceptual strategy and research tool for the study of the evolution of a spectrum of psychotic states related to an initial, identifiable biological insult. Even if the parallelism of the cocaine syndromes with spontaneous or endogenously produced psychopathology is not exact, some of the biological processes involved may overlap and the elucidation of mechanisms may be important to the understanding of both processes. It may be that to some extent, pharmacopathogenic processes recapitulate the psychopathogenic, and that careful study of multiple variables thought to influence the clinical manifestation of cocaine's effects may help clarify the interaction of similar variables in response to psychological stresses and other endogenous precipitants of psychopathology.

ACUTE AND CHRONIC EFFECTS OF COCAINE IN ANIMALS

In an attempt to more systematically understand the dose-response and time-course relationships of cocaine administration to behavior and biology, we have administered cocaine acutely and chronically to rats and monkeys. Under conditions of once or twice daily intraperitoneal administration, both moderate and high doses of cocaine produce increasing effects on selected behavioral and neurological indices.[29-31] This apparent sensitization or reverse tolerance to repeated doses of cocaine stands in contradiction to its effects in some administration paradigms where tolerance to some effects appears to be produced.[11] Definitive studies have not been carried out to differentiate the conditions required to produce tolerance versus reverse tolerance for a given parameter, but the interval between injections may be a critical variable. Extraordinarily high doses of cocaine have been tolerated when it has been administered in rapid, repeated sequences in dogs[32] or man.[3] Schuster[33] reported that an individual survived self-administration of 20 g of cocaine in 24 hr, which is consistent with the reports in addicts that large total doses can be tolerated when taken in frequently repeated applications; tachyphylaxis[34] to cocaine's toxic effects may occur in these circumstances. Doses of cocaine as small as 20 mg have been reported to produce serious side effects in individual patients.[9] Adriani[35] reported that overzealous application of cocaine solution to the nasopharynx by anesthesiologists was associated with a small yearly incidence of convulsions and deaths in his hospital experience. Usually tolerated intraperitoneal doses of cocaine (14 mg/kg) have also been associated with convulsions and death in some rhesus monkeys (unpublished observations). Eidelberg and collaborators reported that different groups of similar age, weight, and strain rats would have very different convulsive thresholds to cocaine.[36]*

Pharmacological Kindling?

There is increasing evidence that repetitive once or twice daily injections of cocaine can be associated with progressive sensitization or lowering of the threshold to convulsions with chronic cocaine administration. In 1932, Downs and Eddy[37] reviewed the literature up to that point and presented evidence that repeated administration of cocaine (75 mg/kg i.p.) would produce seizures after an average of 5.6 injections and death after 14.2 injections in male rats. We have replicated these findings with 60 mg/kg i.p., showing that six of eight animals had their first seizure after 20 ± 7 injections and died after an average of 21 injections;[38] two animals survived for an average of 80 injections without any evidence of convulsions. Similarly, repetitive administration of the same dose of cocaine intraperitoneally to rhesus monkeys (average dose = 14 mg/kg) resulted in the progressive development of convulsions to a previously subthreshold dose.[30] Once the animal had its first seizure at a given dose, it continued to seize with increasing frequency with repetitive administration. A similar increase in susceptibility to seizures has been documented with lidocaine in rats (60 mg/kg i.p.), which showed no convulsions after an average of the first 16 injections, but thereafter developed seizures with increasing frequency in 13 out of 21 animals.[39]

The development of seizures to a dose of cocaine which was previously subthreshold was reminiscent of the phenomenon of electrical kindling suggested originally by Goddard and collaborators[40] and further studied in many other laboratories.[41-43] In this paradigm, structures in the limbic system, particularly the amygdala, are stimulated in a repetitive fashion until the animals eventually develop seizures to the parameters of stimulation which were clearly subthreshold. We have proposed that the local anesthetic and psychomotor stimulant drugs may be "pharmacologically kindling" the limbic system by mechanisms potentially related to those of electrical kindling.[29,30,39,44] In addition to similar time-course characteristics, the seizures induced by lidocaine[39] are qualitatively similar to those produced by electrical stimulation of the amygdala and classified as typical "limbic seizures" by Goddard et al.[40] Animals, especially following more chronic seizure induction, rear up on their haunches supported by their tail and manifest intermittent clonic convulsions of the forepaws, head, and trunk (this particular seizure pattern is not seen during cocaine-induced convulsions, however.) Ellinwood and co-workers[45,46] also report behavioral and electrophysiological effects of cocaine which are consistent with a kindling mechanism.

In addition to the increased susceptibility to convulsions manifest during chronic repetitive cocaine administration in rats and monkeys, several behavioral parameters appear to also increase in intensity. Repetitive administrations of cocaine (10 mg/kg i.p.) in the rat are associated with increases in hyperactivity and stereotypy.[31] These results are highly similar to those reported by Segal and Mandell[47] and Klawans and Margolin[48] with amphetamine administration. Rebec et al.[49] have also documented that single units in the striatum and reticular formation become increasingly sensitized to amphetamine or apomorphine injections after chronic amphetamine pretreatment.

In the rhesus monkey, after a period of hyperactivity and stereotypy during the first 8 weeks of cocaine administration, animals show increasing amounts of inhibitory behavior characterized by catalepsy, staring, and visual tracking behavior (Table 3). Some rhesus monkeys enter the inhibitory phase initially without showing an initial hyperactive and stereotypic pattern.[30] With prolonged cocaine administration, some animals remain immobilized as long as 1 hr after the cocaine injection. After 8 to 10 weeks of repetitive cocaine administration on a twice-daily basis with 2 drug-free days per week, 4 of 13 animals

---

*Editor's note: Our laboratory experience indicates that acute intravenous doses of 1 mg/kg of cocaine have caused death. Doses of 3 to 5 mg/kg consistently cause convulsions and some deaths.

TABLE 3

Time Course of Cocaine Effects in a Subgroup of Seven Rhesus Monkeys

	Acute (1-8 weeks)	Chronic (>8 weeks)
Hyperactivity	+	
Stereotypy	+	
Scattering of attention (checking)	+	+
Anorexia	+	+
Motor inhibition		+
Catalepsy		+
Slow visual tracking		+
Staring		+
Oral-buccal-lingual dyskinesias		+

developed progressively increasing severity of oral-buccal- lingual dyskinesias. During both the acute excitatory phases and the more chronic inhibitory phases, animals showed significant increases in baseline levels of the dopamine metabolite HVA in cisternal CSF, with a similar trend for increases in probenecid-induced accumulations with HVA.[30] These and other data in this volume link many of the effects of acute and chronic cocaine administration to alterations in catecholamine pathways.

Progressive Effects of Lidocaine

A different set of behaviors was associated with the repetitive administration of lidocaine in the rat.[39] Here, there was not evidence of psychomotor stimulation, and instead, the animals developed an increased frequency of omniphagic activity, particularly coprophagia. Saline controls and experimental animals initially demonstrated no coprophagia after the first several injections of lidocaine, but eventually 80% of the animals developed this eating response. The chronic lidocaine-treated animals also showed an increased incidence of eating pieces of gauze and straw compared to saline-treated controls. Recent studies from our laboratory[50] have demonstrated that bilateral lesions of the amygdala block both the onset and the development of this progressive coprophagic behavior with chronic lidocaine administration.

Mechanisms of the Sensitization with Cocaine and Lidocaine

Thus, it appears that repetitive administrations of psychomotor stimulant and nonpsychomotor stimulant local anesthetics are capable of producing not only an increased susceptibility to

seizures, but increased severity of other behavioral pathology. The local anesthetics are known to have a prominent limbic focus for the convulsions[36,51-53] and the amygdala may be involved in some of the behavioral end points. Although further studies are required, alterations in blood and cerebrospinal fluid levels of cocaine with chronic administration do not appear to account for the chronic effects.[53,54] In addition to the pharmacological kindling hypothesis, multiple biochemical explanations may also be invoked for this apparent reverse tolerance effect. As reviewed elsewhere,[38] one might invoke alterations in postsynaptic receptor sensitivity or presynaptic uptake mechanisms,[55] as well as a change in the relative activation of the two kinds of dopamine receptors that have been postulated by Cools et al.[56] and Costall and Naylor,[57] or changes in agonist-antagonist dopamine receptor confirmation as postulated by Creese et al.[58] Cocaine also appears to potentiate catecholamine effects by direct receptor mechanisms that do not depend on the blockade of amine reuptake.[59-64] Gunne and Jonsson[65] report that repeated cocaine injections (100 mg/kg) once daily for 14 days produce increasing effects on urinary, but not brain, epinephrine and norepinephrine; these data may suggest the contribution of peripheral mechanisms.[65] Conditioning phenomena,[66] while they may play a role in the increasing effects to cocaine in some paradigms, do not appear to be an adequate explanation for all the results. Seizures and dyskinesias, as well as a variety of new behaviors which developed in these animals *de novo*, make a pure conditioning explanation, as suggested by Tilson and Reich,[66] highly unlikely.

The precise relationship of the progressive

development of pathological behaviors with chronic drug administration in animals to the development of the grandiose and paranoid psychoses in man associated with chronic cocaine administration remains to be elucidated. While there are only rough analogies between the behavior in man and animals receiving chronic cocaine administration, similar pharmacological and physiological mechanisms may nevertheless underlie the development of these species-specific behaviors. It is tempting to speculate that the ultimate mechanism involved in the sensitization or pharmacological kindling associated with chronic psychomotor stimulant administration may also be active in the development of the stimulant-induced paranoid psychosis in man. We have speculated elsewhere[44] that the capacity for increased response to a variety of stimuli, as uncovered by the cocaine-kindling model, may represent a basic mechanism in the central nervous system worthy of further study because of its potential relationship to the development of behavioral pathology in the functional psychoses.

REFERENCES

1. **Kosman, M. E. and Unna, K. R.,** Effects of chronic administration of the amphetamine and other stimulants on behavior, *Clin. Pharmacol. Ther.,* 9, 240, 1968.
2. **Bejerot, N.,** A comparison of the effects of cocaine and synthetic central stimulants, *Br. J. Addict.,* 65, 35, 1970.
3. **Richie, J. M. and Cohen, P. J.,** Cocaine; procaine and other synthetic local anesthetics, in *The Pharmacological Basis of Therapeutics,* 5th ed., Goodman, L. S. and Gilman, A. G., Eds., Macmillan, New York, 1975, 379.
4. **Zapata-Ortiz, V.,** Accion de la cocaina en sujetos no habituados, *Rev. Med. Exp.,* 3, 307, 1944.
5. **Zapata-Ortiz, V.,** Modificaciones psicologicas y fisiologicas producidas por la coca y la cocaina en los coqueros, *Rev. de Med. Exp.,* 3, 132, 1944.
6. **Zapata-Ortiz, V.,** The chewing of coca leaves in Peru, *Int. J. Addict.,* 5, 287, 1970.
7. **Jones, E.,** The cocaine episode, in *The Life and Work of Sigmund Freud,* Trilling, L. and Marcus, S., Eds., Basic Books, New York, 1953, 52.
8. **Freud, S.,** On the general effects of cocaine, *Drug Dependence,* 5, 15, 1970.
9. **Gay, G. R., Sheppard, C. W., Inaba, D. S., and Newmeyer, J. A.,** Cocaine in perspective: "Gift From The Sun God" to "The Rich Man's Drug", *Drug Forum,* 2, 409, 1973.
10. **Griffith, J.,** Structure-activity relationships of several amphetamine analogues in man, in *Symposium on Contemporary Issues in Stimulant Research,* Ellinwood, E., Ed., Plenum Press, New York, 1976.
11. **Fischman, M., Schuster, C., and Krasnegor, N.,** Cocaine: Cardiovascular and behavioral effects in man, in *Symposium on Contemporary Issues in Stimulant Research,* Ellinwood, E., Ed., Plenum Press, New York, 1976.
12. **Martin, W. R., Sloan, J. W., Sapira, J. D., and Jasinska, D. R.,** Physiologic, subjective, and behavioral effects of amphetamine, methamphetamine, ephedrine, phenmetrazine, and methylphenidate in man, *Clin. Pharmacol. Ther.,* 12, 245, 1971.
13. **Post, R. M., Kotin, J., and Goodwin, F. K.,** The effects of cocaine on depressed patients, *Am. J. Psychiatry,* 131, 511, 1974.
14. **Post, R. M., Gillin, J. C., Wyatt, R. J., and Goodwin, F. K.,** The effect of orally administered cocaine on sleep of depressed patients, *Psychopharmacologia,* 37, 59, 1974.
15. **Woods, L. A., McMahon, F. G., and Seevers, M. H.,** Distribution and metabolism of cocaine in the dog and rabbit, *J. Pharm. Exp. Ther.,* 101, 200, 1951.
16. **Resnick, R., Kestenbaum, R., and Schwartz, L.,** Acute systemic effects of cocaine in man: A controlled study by intranasal and intravenous routes of administration, in *Symposium on Contemporary Issues in Stimulant Research,* Ellinwood, E., Ed., Plenum Press, New York, 1976.
17. **Schacter, W. and Wheeler, L.,** Epinephrine, chlorpromazine, and amusement, *J. Abnorm. Soc. Psychol.,* 65, 121, 1962.
18. **Post, R. M.,** Cocaine psychoses: A continuum model, *Am. J. Psychiatry,* 132, 225, 1975.
19. **Angrist, B. and Gershon, S.,** The phenomenology of experimentally-induced amphetamine psychosis—preliminary observations, *Biol. Psychiatry,* 2, 95, 1970.
20. **Griffith, J. D., Cavanaugh, J. H., Held, J., and Oates, J. A.,** Experimental psychosis induced by the administration of d-amphetamine, in *Amphetamines and Related Compounds,* Costa, E., and Garattini, S., Eds., Raven Press, New York, 1970, 897.

21. **Watson, R., Hartmann, E., and Schildkraut, J. J.,** Amphetamine withdrawal: Affective state, sleep patterns, and MHPG excretion, *Am. J. Psychiatry,* 129, 263, 1972.
22. **Anggard, E., Jonsson, L. E., Hogmark, A. L., and Gunne, L.-M.,** Amphetamine metabolism in amphetamine psychosis, *Clin. Pharm. Ther.,* 14, 870, 1973.
23. **Bell, D. S.,** The experimental reproduction of amphetamine psychosis, *Arch. Gen. Psychiatry,* 29, 35, 1975.
24. **Lewin, L.,** *Phantastica: Narcotic and Stimulating Drugs,* E. P. Dutton, New York, 1931, 75.
25. **Gordon, A.,** Insanities caused by acute and chronic intoxications with opium and cocaine, *JAMA,* 51, 97, 1908.
26. **Owens, W. D.,** Signs and symptoms presented by those addicted to cocaine, *JAMA,* 58, 329, 1912.
27. **Ellinwood, E. H.,** Amphetamine psychosis: Individuals, settings, and sequences, in *Current Concepts on Amphetamine Abuse,* National Institute of Mental Health Publication HSM 72-9085, U.S. Government Printing Office, Washington, D. C., 1972, 143.
28. **Woods, J. H. and Downs, D. A.,** *Drug Use in America: Problem in Perspectives,* Technical papers of the Second Report of the National Commission on Marihuana and Drug Abuse, Appendix, Vol. 1, Patterns and Consequences of Drug Use, U.S. Government Printing Office, Washington, D. C., 1973, 116.
29. **Post, R. M. and Kopanda, R. T.,** Cocaine, kindling, and reverse tolerance, *Lancet,* 1, 409, 1975.
30. **Post, R. M., Kopanda, R. T., and Black, K. E.,** Progressive effects of cocaine on behavior and central amine metabolism in rhesus monkeys, *Biol. Psychiatry,* in press, 1976.
31. **Post, R. M. and Rose, H.,** Increasing effects of repetitive cocaine administration in the rat, *Nature,* 260, 731, 1976.
32. **Gutierrez-Noriega, C. and Zapata, Ortiz, V.,** Cocanismo experimental. 1. Toxicologia general acostumbramiento y sensibilizacion, *Rev. Med. Exp.,* 3, 279, 1944.
33. **Schuster, C. R., Fischman, M., and Krasnegor, N.,** Comparative Cocaine Dose-response and Time-action Curves in Man, presented at the 14th Annual Meeting of the American College of Neuropsychopharmacology, Demember 16–19, 1975, San Juan, Puerto Rico.
34. **Teeters, W. R., Koppanyi, T., and Cowan, F. F.,** Cocaine tachyphylaxis, *Life Sci.,* 7, 509, 1963.
35. **Adriani, J.,** Cocaine: Clinical observations, presented at the 14th Annual Meeting of the American College of Neuropsychopharmacology, December 16–19, 1975, San Juan, Puerto Rico.
36. **Eidelberg, E., Lesse, H., and Gault, F. P.,** An experimental model of temporal lobe epilepsy: Studies of the convulsant properties of cocaine, in *EEG and Behavior,* Glaser, G. H., Ed., Basic Books, New York, 1963, 272.
37. **Downs, A. W. and Eddy, N. B.,** The effect of repeated doses of cocaine on the rat, *J. Pharm. Exp. Ther.,* 46, 199, 1932.
38. **Post, R. M.,** Progressive effects of repetitive cocaine administration on behavior and seizures, in *Symposium on Contemporary Issues in Stimulant Research,* Ellinwood, E., Ed., Plenum Press, New York, 1976.
39. **Post, R. M., Kopanda, R. T., and Lee, A.,** Progressive behavioral changes during chronic lidocaine administration: Relationship to kindling, *Life Sci.,* 17, 943, 1975.
40. **Goodard, G. V., McIntyre, D. C., and Leech, C. K.,** A permanent change in brain function resulting from daily electrical stimulation, *Exp. Neurol.,* 25, 295, 1969.
41. **Racine, R. J.,** Modification of seizure activity by electrical stimulation. II. Motor seizure, *Electroencephalogr. Clin. Neurophysiol.,* 32, 281, 1972.
42. **Wada, J. A. and Sata, M. S.,** Generalized convulsive seizures induced by daily electrical stimulation of the amygdala in cats, *Neurology,* 24, 565, 1974.
43. **Pinel, J. P. J. and Van Oot, P. H.,** Generality of the kindling phenomenon: Some clinical implications, *Can. J. Neurosciences,* 2, 467, 1976.
44. **Post, R. M. and Kopanda, R. T.,** Cocaine, kindling, and psychosis, *Am. J. Psychiatry,* 133, 627, 1976.
45. **Stripling, J. and Ellinwood, E.,** Sensitization to cocaine following chronic administration in rats, in *Symposium on Contemporary Issues in Stimulant Research,* Ellinwood, E., Ed., Plenum Press, New York, 1976.
46. **Ellinwood, E., Kilbey, M., Castellani, S., and Khoury, C.,** Behavioral and electrophysiological effects of cocaine, in *Symposium on Contemporary Issues in Stimulant Research,* Ellinwood, E. Ed., Plenum Press, New York, 1976.
47. **Segal, D. S. and Mandell, A. J.,** Long-term administration of d-amphetamine: Progressive augmentation of motor activity and stereotypy, *Pharmacol Biochem. Behav.,* 2, 249, 1974.
48. **Klawans, H. L. and Margolin, D. I.,** Amphetamine-induced dopaminergic sensitivity in guinea pigs, *Arch. Gen. Psychiatry,* 32, 725, 1975.
49. **Rebec, G. and Groves, P.,** Changes in neuronal activity in the neostriatum and reticular formation following acute or long-term amphetamine administration, in *Symposium on Contemporary Issues in Stimulant Research,* Ellinwood, E., Ed., Plenum Press, New York, 1976.
50. **Pert, A., Squillace, K., and Post, R. M.,** Effects of bilateral amygdala lesion on lidocaine-induced omniphagia, unpublished manuscript.
51. **Wagman, I. H., DeJong, R. H., and Prince, D. A.,** Effects of lidocaine on spontaneous cortical and subcortical electrical activity, *Arch. Neurol.* (Chicago), 18, 277, 1968.
52. **Riblet, L. A. and Tuttle, W. W.,** Investigation of the amygdaloid and olfactory electrographic response in the cat after toxic dosage of lidocaine, *Electroencephalogr. Clin. Neurophysiol.,* 28, 601, 1970.
53. **Hawks, R. L., Squillace, K., and Post, R. M.,** unpublished observations.
54. **Mulé, S. J.,** Pharmacokinetics and Metabolism of Cocaine, presented at the 14th Annual Meeting of the American College of Neuropsychopharmacology, December 16–19, 1975, San Juan, Puerto Rico.

55. **Trendelenberg, U. and Graefc, K.-H.,** Supersensitivity to catecholamines after impairment of extraneuronal uptake or catechol-0-methyl transferase, *Fed. Proc.,* 34, 1971, 1975.

56. **Cools, A.,** Heterogenous neuropharmacology of the caudate-raphe connection in animals and man, in *Symposium on Contemporary Issues in Stimulant Research,* Ellinwood, E., Ed., Plenum Press, New York, 1976.

57. **Costall, B. and Naylor, R. J.,** The behavioral effects of dopamine applied intracerebrally to areas of the mesolimbic system, *Eur. J. Pharmacol.,* 32, 87, 1975.

58. **Creese, I., Burt, D. R., and Snyder, S. H.,** Dopamine receptor binding: Differentiation of agonist and antagonist state with ^{3}H-dopamine and ^{3}H-haloperidol, *Life Sci.,* 17, 993, 1975.

59. **Nakatsu, K. and Reiffenstein, R. J.,** Increased receptor utilization: Mechanism of cocaine potentiation, *Nature,* 217, 1277, 1968.

60. **Maxwell, R. A., Wastila, W. B., and Eckhardt, S. B.,** Some factors determining the response of rabbit aortic strips to dl-norepinephrine-7-^{3}H hydrochloride and the influence of cocaine, guanethidine and methylphenidate on these factors, *J. Pharm. Exp. Ther.,* 151, 253, 1966.

61. **Bevan, J. A. and Verity, M. A.,** Sympathetic nerve-free vascular muscle, *J. Pharm. Exp. Ther.,* 157, 117, 1967.

62. **Reiffenstein, R. J.,** Effect of cocaine on the rate of concentration to noradrenaline in the cat spleen strip: Mode of action of cocaine, *Br. J. Pharmacol. Chemother.,* 32, 591, 1968.

63. **Kalsner, S. and Nickerson, M.,** Mechanism of cocaine potentiation of responses to amines, *Br. J. Pharmacol.,* 35, 432, 1969.

64. **Davidson, W. J. and Innes, I. R.,** Dissociation of potentiation of isoprenalin by cocaine by inhibition of uptake in the cat spleen, *Br. J. Pharmacol.,* 39, 175, 1970.

65. **Gunne, L.-M. and Jonsson, J.,** Effects of cocaine administration on brain, adrenal, and urinary adrenaline and noradrenaline in rats, *Psychopharmacologia,* 6, 125, 1964.

66. **Tilson, H. A. and Reich, R. H.,** Conditioned drug effects and absence of tolerance to d-amphetamine-induced motor activity, *Pharmacol. Biochem. Behav.,* 1, 149, 1973.

Clinical Aspects

*Clinical Aspects of Cocaine: Assessment of
Cocaine Abuse Behavior in Man*

CLINICAL ASPECTS OF COCAINE:
ASSESSMENT OF COCAINE ABUSE BEHAVIOR IN MAN*

Richard B. Resnick and Elaine Schuyten-Resnick

TABLE OF CONTENTS

INTRODUCTION

Cocaine use has increased tremendously in the past decade. The psychedelic Sixties are over and many believe that we are now in the cocaine Seventies. As one writer expressed it: "A blizzard of cocaine is blowing over us."[1] Since the early 1970s, cocaine use has been moving steadily from the ghetto to the middle and upper classes and has changed from a little-known and infrequently used drug into the recreational drug of choice among people in many social and economic groups. This increase in cocaine use is especially intriguing, since the drug is not only illegal, it is very, very expensive.[2,3]

Awareness of this phenomenon is reflected by recent press[4-6] and television[7] coverage of cocaine use. Newspaper and magazine articles assert that cocaine snuffing has become commonplace at social gatherings of both the rich and the poor. Symbolic of the drug's appeal among users are the various nicknames it has endearingly been given, such as "king," "queen," and the "champagne of drugs."

Accurate estimates of cocaine usage are very difficult to obtain. In a 1971 survey of 56,745 students in the seventh through twelfth grades in Dallas, Texas, 2,108 or 4% reported having used cocaine, with 1,250 acknowledging that they had used it at least one time during the week the questionnaire was given.[8] In 1973 the National Commission on Marihuana and Drug Abuse estimated that nationwide cocaine use was 3.2% for adults and 1.5% for youth.[9] A recent national survey estimates that the cocaine use among youths 12 to 17 years old doubled between 1972 and 1974.[10] The same survey found that 17% of those who live in cities with populations of a million or more reported using cocaine within the preceding year.[10a]

Despite this widespread and increasing nonmedical use of cocaine, until very recently there were no controlled studies of the subjective, behavioral, or physiologic effects of the drug in man. We have reviewed the medical literature through 1973 and found that systematic assessment of cocaine abuse behavior in man was notably absent. It has been argued, for example,

*Supported by a grant from the National Institute on Drug Abuse and a contract with the New York State Office of Drug Abuse Services.

that cocaine shares many of the behavioral properties of the amphetamines,[11] but there is no experimental evidence of the effects that cocaine has on human performance. The need for studies is further emphasized by unconfirmed and contradictory reports in the literature regarding cocaine effects.

In 1974 investigators at New York Medical College began a series of controlled studies with cocaine. Seventy-five individuals, referred to us for their "regular use" of cocaine, were clinically interviewed regarding their patterns of cocaine use and its subjective effects. An additional source of information came from four individuals seen in private individual psychotherapy; they had been using between $200 and $1,000 worth of cocaine a week. Another group of over 300 individuals who were applying for treatment of opiate abuse in our clinic was surveyed regarding the patterns and effects of its cocaine use. This group is a known subgroup of cocaine abusers.[12-14] We elicited information from these individuals using structured clinical interviews and recording the data on Cocaine Use Questionnaires. Laboratory data were obtained on approximately 50 of the non-opiate-abusing group, who were studied to assess their physiological, subjective, and behavioral responses to measured doses of intranasal and intravenous cocaine.

CLINICAL INTERVIEWS

One group of individuals who were clinically interviewed to learn about their "regular use" of cocaine was predominantly middle to upper class, white, and highly educated. The group of opiate users were Black, White and Puerto Rican, from all levels of society, with the majority being lower middle class or poor.

We found that patterns of cocaine-using behavior resemble those patterns generally associated with other commonly used recreational drugs, such as marijuana and alcohol. Types of users, grouped by their characteristic patterns of cocaine use, fall into the five patterns established by the National Commission on Marihuana and Drug Abuse that cover the entire spectrum of drug-using behavior.[9] Each pattern is intended to reflect distinct meanings that the drug use has for the users within each group.

Some cocaine use can be regarded as *experimental* and is motivated by curiosity or a desire to experience an altered mood state. This type of use is short-term and nonpatterned. Some individuals in this group found the drug effects primarily dysphoric and said they will not use it again.

The pattern that best describes the majority of cocaine users we have interviewed is called *recreational*. They use the drug in social settings among friends in order to share a pleasurable experience. This type of use tends not to escalate in frequency or amount, and the reinforcement for continued use is strengthened by nonpharmacologic factors. They report that they will usually accept cocaine when it is offered to them in a social situation, but they do not seek to obtain supplies of the drug. Most of these individuals genuinely like to use cocaine, but they have an attitude of "I can take it or leave it."

A pattern of drug use that has grown significantly in the past decade, according to the National Commission, is *circumstantial* drug use. This type of use is motivated by the user's perceived need or desire to achieve an anticipated effect in order to cope with a specific problem, situation, or condition of a personal or vocational nature. For example, we have found this pattern of cocaine use to be prevalent among professional musicians and others in the music business, who say they will refuse to perform at a recording session or concert unless they have taken cocaine, since they feel that without it they will not be as creative.

A smaller group of users may escalate from recreational or circumstantial use into *intensified* drug-using behavior. The Commission defines this group as using at least daily and motivated by an individual's perceived need to achieve relief from a persistent problem or stressful situation, or his desire to maintain a certain self-prescribed level of performance. We have found that daily users of cocaine tend to space each dose of the drug, as if trying to achieve a sustained rather than an intense effect. Most individuals of this group snort the cocaine from three to twenty times a day, each individual having a dose schedule from which he rarely deviates, so long as supplies of the drug are available. Some use as often as every hour, others only three times a day.

The pattern that the Commission called the "most disturbing," but which encompasses the smallest number of users, is *compulsive* use. This type of drug-using behavior is patterned, at a high frequency and high level of intensity, and characterized by a high degree of psychological dependence. The most striking feature of this pattern is that the drug use dominates the individual's life and precludes other social functioning. We found that the cocaine users in this category use the drug for episodic or sporatic binges to get "high." These can occur from once a week to once or twice a year and can last from hours to days. These binges are very similar to alcohol binges; they use large quantities of cocaine for days until the supply or their money runs out.

One behavioral effect of cocaine that some individuals in each of these groups experience is an often overwhelming compulsion or craving to take more, as soon as the acute effects have subsided. Individuals who are not compulsive users of the drug often comment on this effect. For this reason, although cocaine is known to be nonaddicting (it does not produce physical dependence), many individuals develop a strong psychological dependence on it. Laboratory experiments with animals have demonstrated beyond dispute that cocaine is the most powerful reinforcer of all psychoactive substances.[9] In our interviews, certain individuals reported that at times the drug must be made unavailable to them in order to break a cycle of compulsive use. In a dramatic example of this problem, one individual in our clinic asked the doctor to lock up his bank book so he wouldn't be able to buy more cocaine. He explained that he had already used most of his savings and knew that, if it were available, all his money would be spent on cocaine in a matter of days. Another compulsive user reported having spent $24,000 in insurance money over a 3-month period, all on supplies of cocaine.

For many other users of the drug, however, there is no such liability. In fact, some users report the contrary; they prefer using cocaine to many other drugs because it is short-acting and they regard it as being relatively safe. Some people feel they can use cocaine, knowing that its effects will be gone in a short time, get a profound "high," and then go on with whatever they plan to do with their time. Unlike psychedelics or other long-acting drugs, they don't have to set aside whole days to accommodate their drug use.

One of cocaine's most sought-after effects is its reputed aphrodisiac quality. For many it is considered the choice drug to enhance sexuality. Users report that it produces more intense sensual feelings, particularly tactile sensations, and that it prolongs sex due to delaying of orgasm. Some individuals say that it increases their ability to fantasize and that they are able to talk about or act-out their sexual fantasies, which they would have felt too disinterested in or too inhibited to permit without cocaine. Although some individuals say that when cocaine is applied to the penis it increases erections, it is more commonly reported that cocaine inhibits erections in men.

Reports in the medical literature suggest that cocaine administered chronically (i.e., every day) may produce reverse tolerance or sensitization.[15-17] We were, therefore, interested in investigating whether this effect was reported or observed by people who have used cocaine daily. We asked individuals how long they had used it without skipping a single day and whether they found that they needed more, less, or the same amount of cocaine on the last day as on the first if they wanted to achieve the same effect. Many individuals reported having had periods of daily use ranging from 30 to 90 days, but not one of them reported having experienced a difference in subjective effects from the first to the last day of use, when they have used cocaine of uniform potency. We suspect that the difference between the reports of sensitization in animals and the lack of this effect in the groups of people we interviewed may be explained by a cumulative drug effect in the animal studies, where doses used far exceed doses taken by humans. This explanation is supported by animal studies that report sensitization after cocaine is given chronically in high doses, but not when it is given in low doses.[18] For most individuals the cost of cocaine precludes their using extremely high doses. Even those who engage in high-dose compulsive patterns of use do not use it chronically in quantities as high as those found in the animal studies.

Psychotic reactions to cocaine are another commonly reported phenomenon in the medical[19,20] and nonmedical literature. In searching for the scientific basis for the assertions regarding cocaine-induced psychosis, we found that the reports in the medical literature are anecdotal and usually limited to the self-reports of a few individuals. There is a striking absence of information on the individual's pre-morbid personality or the circumstances or set in which the drug was taken. In our experience, paranoid ideation is often associated with the set in which cocaine is taken, rather than being a specific pharmacologic effect of the drug. Individuals who have experienced paranoid feelings when self-administering cocaine have been struck by the absence of this effect when they received it in our laboratory. Nevertheless, the possibility that cocaine can induce hallucinations and paranoid ideation is suggested by one experiment at the Addiction Research Center.[21] In this experiment, which was recorded on film,[22] a subject was given repeated intravenous injections of cocaine at short intervals, beginning with 20 mg every 30 min and increasing to 50 mg at 5- to 10-min intervals. Over a 12-hr period, he received more than 2,000 mg of cocaine, at which time he began to show evidence of visual hallucinations (seeing insects) and had delusions that consisted of thoughts that he was being watched by detectives. Even in this controlled situation, however, one can speculate that the experimental set (being filmed and being watched) may have contributed to his paranoid feelings.

We elicited no reports of cocaine psychosis in any of the people we interviewed, nor was anyone able to recall having seen someone who had such a reaction. We also inquired among attending and resident physicians who work in emergency rooms of major New York City hospitals, where there were frequent reports of amphetamine psychosis some years ago. Not one of them reported having seen a case of psychosis associated with cocaine. As Woods and Downs[2] suggest, the conditions under which cocaine is taken today are very different from those that many early observers found when they described the psychotic behaviors presumed to be cocaine-induced. Since the set may be a critical factor in influencing paranoid responses to cocaine, today's more relaxed attitudes toward illicit drugs may be contributing to the recent lack of reports of psychotic reactions to the drug.

COCAINE USE QUESTIONNAIRES

As part of our routine intake process all individuals applying for treatment of opiate abuse were asked about their use of cocaine. Interviews were conducted by professional staff, using openended questions and recording the information on a standardized form. The Cocaine Use Questionnaires were designed to get detailed histories of past and present cocaine use and to elucidate information on why this group uses cocaine, how it makes them feel, and in what way they believe it

affects their behavior and their lives. A study sample of 212 questionnaires was used for data analysis.[23]

The population was predominantly male, ranging in age from 18 to 56, with a mean age of 27. Subjects came from various socioeconomic backgrounds with an ethnic distribution of 38% Puerto Rican, 38% Black, and 24% White. One hundred ninety-nine of the 212 individuals interviewed (94% of the sample) acknowledged having used cocaine at least one time. Sixty-eight percent of those who had tried it reported having used cocaine during the 6 months preceding their intake interview. Twenty-eight percent said they had used it during the week of the interview. Average cocaine use during the week and 6 months prior to being interviewed is shown in Tables 1 and 2.

The age at which cocaine was first tried ranged from 12 years to 40 years, with the mean age of first use being 20 (Figure 1). Thirty-four percent said they had used it for the first time at 12 to 17 years of age. Route of administration for first use was reported as 38% intravenous and 62% intranasal. Opiate users are the only major group of cocaine users who regularly self-inject the drug, and most who do so mix the cocaine with heroin, a combination referred to as a "speedball."

All subjects were asked whether they considered themselves to have ever been a "regular user"

TABLE 1

Frequency and Amount of Cocaine Used by a Sample of 199 Opiate-dependent Patients During the 7 Days Prior to Being Interviewed (N = 56)

Frequency (days/week)		Amount (dollars/day)	
1–2 Days	71%	Less than $10	25%
3–4 Days	16%	$11–$49	54%
5–7 Days	12%	$50–$100	16%
		$100 or more	5%

TABLE 2

Frequency of Amount of Cocaine Used by a Sample of 199 Opiate-dependent Patients During the 6 Months Prior to Being Interviewed (N = 130)

Frequency (days/week)		Amount (dollars/day)	
Less than 1 day	56%	Less than $10	25%
1–2 Days	23%	$10–$50	54%
3 Days or more	21%	$50 or more	21%

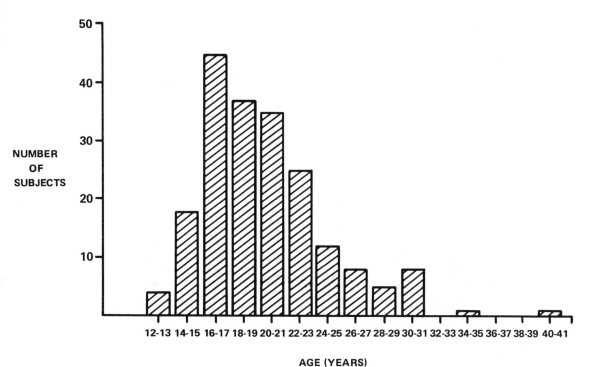

FIGURE 1.   Distribution of ages that subjects first tried cocaine (N = 199).

of cocaine. Forty-four percent of the sample defined themselves as having been a "regular user" of the drug at some time. For three fourths of this group, regular use was defined as being $10 to $50 of cocaine during each day of use and using 3 to 7 days a week for periods ranging from weeks to months (Table 3).

Following the first exposure to cocaine, 23% of the sample had used it again by the next day and another 23% used it by the end of the same month. By the end of the year in which they first tried cocaine, a total of 75.4% had used it at least one more time. Only 2% stated that they never used the drug again. The group who were self-defined regular users tended to use cocaine a second time much sooner than those who were not regular users (Figure 2).

Since we were interested in finding out about peoples' subjective experiences when they took cocaine, all subjects were asked to report the effects they got from the drug and to rate these effects as "good" or "bad." They were instructed to report all effects spontaneously and were not given categories within which to fit their perceptions. Those "good effects" most frequently reported were related to the stimulant properties of

TABLE 3

Average Frequency and Amount of Cocaine Used by a Group of 88 Self-defined "Regular Users" (N = 88)

Frequency (days/week)		Amount (dollars/day)	
Less than 1 day	2%	Less than $10	1%
1–2 Days	24%	$10–$49	61%
3–4 Days	18%	$50–$99	19%
5–7 Days	56%	$100 or more	14%
		No response	5%

cocaine, as shown in Table 4. More than half the sample (51%) reported that they never had "bad effects" from cocaine. Those individuals who did experience "bad effects" reported a range of effects but most frequently noted feeling nervous and shaky, fear or paranoia, irritable or depressed, nausea and rapid heartbeat (Table 5).

Forty-eight percent of users reported a biphasic effect from cocaine that consisted of primarily euphoric acute effects, followed by dysphoric effects as the acute effects subsided. This dysphoria is referred to as "post-coke blues" or "crashing" and is characterized by feelings of fear and paranoia, depression, tiredness, wanting more cocaine, and being nervous (Table 6). Inter-

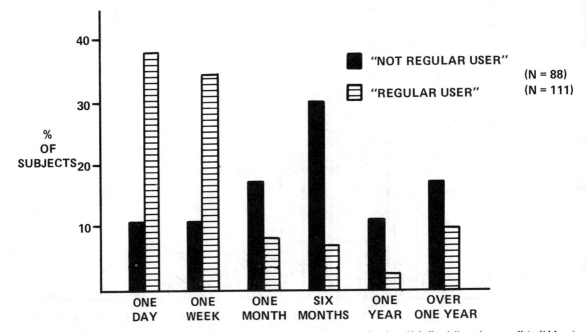

FIGURE 2. Comparison of intervals between first and second use of cocaine in self-defined "regular users" (solid bars) and those who were not "regular users" (striped bars).

<table>

| TABLE 4 |
</table>

TABLE 4

"Good Effects" from Cocaine Most Frequently Reported by 199 Opiate-dependent Subjects

Effects	Number of subjects reporting
Alert/energetic	61
Up	48
High	36
Talkative/sociable	36
Sexually stimulated	30
Rush	29
Pleasurable	21
Confident	9
Forget my troubles	5
More relaxed	5

TABLE 5

"Bad Effects" from Cocaine Most Frequently Reported by 97 Opiate-dependent Subjects*

Effects	Number of subjects reporting
Nervous/shaky	30
Fear/paranoia	23
Irritable/depressed	20
Nausea/vomiting	18
Rapid heartbeat	16
Violent	3

*In the sample of 199 subjects, 102 reported never experiencing "bad effects."

estingly, many of these "crash" effects are similar to those reported as "bad effects" of cocaine; apparently many individuals do not distinguish between the effects of the drug and the effects of the drug wearing off.

Cocaine is most frequently used in social situations rather than being taken by individuals when they are alone. Asked in what setting they first took cocaine, 61% reported using it in a private setting (i.e., their apartment, a friend's home, motel room); 33% said they had used it in a public place such as school, a park, the street, or in a bar.

Ten percent of the sample believed that they had a "problem" with cocaine, three fourths of whom stated they would elect to seek treatment for the problem, if such treatment were available. For the remainder of the group, cocaine was only seen as a problem in terms of its expense. As many of them put it: "It keeps me broke."

TABLE 6

Percent of Subjects Who Experience "Crashing" and "Crash Effects" Most Frequently Reported

Do you "crash" after cocaine?		What effects do you get when you crash?	
		Effects	Number of subjects reporting
Yes	48%	Fear/paranoia	29
No	47%	Depression	28
No response	5%	Tired	27
		Want more	26
		Nervous	24
		Sweating/chills	13
		Insomnia	8
		Nausea/vomiting	8

LABORATORY DATA

This part of our studies was undertaken to assess physiologic and subjective effects, over a 30-min observation period, of acute doses of 10 mg and 25 mg cocaine administered by intranasal and intravenous routes[24] and of 50 mg and 100 mg administered intranasally only. Intranasal cocaine was given by drops; intravenous doses were given over a 90-sec period. Physiologic parameters measured were heart rate, blood pressure, respiratory rate, oral temperature, and hand-grip strength. We assessed subjective effects by ratings of "high," pleasantness, speeding, hunger, strength, and number of statements rated true on a 36-item Addiction Research Center Inventory for acute amphetamine effects.[25]

The results showed that by the intranasal route, 10 mg of cocaine produced no changes different from placebo and the 25-mg dose produced minimal changes, but only in systolic blood pressure and feelings of "high." When administered intravenously, however, both doses of cocaine produced significant dose-related physiologic and subjective responses (Figure 3). The onset of effects occurred within 2 min of cocaine administration and in most instances peaked within 10 min. As Figure 3 shows, some effects persisted beyond the 30-min observation period, particularly at the higher dose. There were no significant changes in respiratory rate, oral temperature, or hand-grip strength following either dose. As can be seen in the graphs, there is a concordance in the shape of the curves showing changes in physiologic and subjective effects. This relationship, however, was not consistently found in each subject. Some

individuals, particularly more experienced cocaine users, rated subjective effects lower than other subjects, who had equally large physiologic changes. The effects of 50 mg intranasally were barely distinguishable from the effects of 25 mg. Effects of 100 mg, however, were comparable to those produced by an intravenous dose of 25 mg.

The four items that were most frequently rated true on the Acute Effects Scale following cocaine administration are listed in Table 7. Nine items that were the best dose-related indicators of cocaine effects and that also discriminated between the two routes of administration are listed in Table 8. The tenth item on this table, "I feel more relaxed," was the most frequent spontaneous report of subjects regarding an effect they experienced from the cocaine.

After the 25-mg intravenous dose, one of the subjects had a marked affective response (crying) together with a strong "high." We later learned that this individual had entered the experimental session feeling depressed. The dysphoric reaction following cocaine that this subject experienced is consistent with a report on the effects of cocaine in depressed patients.[26]

Although mean ratings of pleasantness were higher after the larger dose of intravenous cocaine, the reverse was true for occasional subjects. The seven statements on the Acute Effects Scale that were more frequently rated "true" after the lower intravenous doses (Table 9) are items that reflect an increased interpersonal awareness and general pleasantness.

Half the subjects reported that they felt uncomfortable from symptoms of anxiety and depression beginning 20 to 40 min after use of cocaine. These

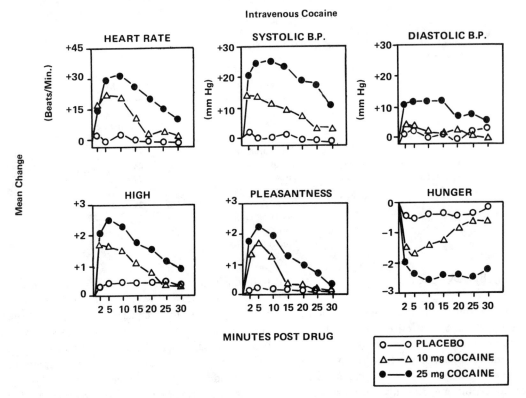

FIGURE 3. Time course over a 30-min observation period for physiologic and subjective effects of placebo and 10 mg and 25 mg cocaine administered intravenously.

TABLE 7

Statements on the Acute Effects Scale That Were Rated "True" Most Frequently After Administration of Cocaine

1. I feel as if something pleasant had just happened to me.
2. I am in the mood to talk about the feeling I have.
3. A thrill has gone through me one or more times since I started the test.
4. I feel like joking with someone.

effects persisted beyond the period of observation, and the subjects stated that they were characteristic of "crashing."

SUMMARY

Our clinical and laboratory studies have begun to elucidate some physiologic, behavioral, and subjective effects of cocaine in man. We have described five profiles of typical cocaine-using behavior, based on the patterns of drug use established by the National Commission on Marihuana and Drug Abuse. We have described some

TABLE 8

Items 1 Through 9 are the Best Dose-related Acute Effects Indicators of Cocaine Effects Which Also Discriminated Between Intravenous and Intranasal Administration. Item 10 was the Most Frequent Spontaneous Report of Subjects

1. I have a pleasant feeling in my stomach.
2. My thoughts come more easily than usual.
3. I feel less discouraged than usual.
4. My memory seems sharper to me than usual.
5. I fear that I will lose the contentment that I have now.
6. I have a weird feeling.
7. Right now I feel as if all my needs are satisfied.
8. I feel an increasing awareness of bodily sensations.
9. I have a floating feeling.
10. I feel more relaxed.

demographic characteristics of a subgroup of cocaine users who also use opiates and subjective cocaine effects experienced by this subgroup. A ten-item true/false scale that can be used to assess acute effects of intravenous and intranasal cocaine is presented. Our data provide information that

TABLE 9

Statements on the Acute Effects Scale That Were More Frequently Rated "True" Following 10 mg Than 25 mg Intravenous Cocaine

1. I feel as if something pleasant had just happened to me.
2. I am in the mood to talk about the feeling I have.
3. I can completely appreciate what others are saying when I am in this mood.
4. I feel a very pleasant emptiness.
5. I feel so good that I know other people can tell it.
6. I feel like joking with someone.
7. I would be happy all the time if I felt as I feel now.

helps to affirm certain prevalent beliefs about cocaine and to dispel others.

One of the major liabilities of cocaine use is the strong reinforcing property which in some individuals leads to an overwhelming compulsion for the drug and to serious social and psychological consequences. For other individuals cocaine use may be chronic, but does not escalate in frequency or amount and apparently carries little or no serious risk.

The onset, intensity, and duration of subjective effects coincide very closely with changes in cardiovascular measures, particularly systolic blood pressure. Subjective and physiologic changes from 100 mg intranasally are comparable to those produced by 25 mg administered intravenously. Surprisingly, the most frequent spontaneously reported effect following a single dose of cocaine in the laboratory was "I feel more relaxed." Roughly half the users experience a biphasic effect that consists of pleasant sensations followed by a dysphoric state that is commonly referred to as "post-coke blues" or "crashing." We found no evidence to support the view that cocaine taken every day will produce either sensitization or tolerance to its effects. We also found no evidence of psychotic reactions to cocaine. Paranoid ideation associated with use of cocaine appears to be related more to the psychological set under which it is taken than to a specific pharmacologic effect.

REFERENCES

1. Rhodes, R., A very expensive high, *Playboy*, Vol. 22, No. 1, January 1975, 131.
2. Woods, J. H. and Downs, D. A., The psychopharmacology of cocaine, in *Drug Use in America: Problem in Perspective*, technical paper of the 2nd Report of the National Commission on Marihuana and Drug Abuse, Vol. 1, U.S. Government Printing Office, Washington, D.C., 1973.
3. Gay, G. R., Inaba, D. S., Sheppard, C. W., and Newmeyer, J. A., Cocaine: History, epidemiology, human pharmacology, and treatment. A perspective on a new debut for an old girl, *Clin. Toxicol.*, 8(2), 149, 1975.
4. Plate, T., The politics of dope, *New York Magazine*, May 20, 1974, 8.
5. Schmeck, H. M., Cocaine is re-emerging as a major problem, while marijuana remains popular, *The New York Times*, November 15, 1972, 82.
6. Anon., Life and leisure: It's the real thing, *Newsweek*, September 27, 1971, 124.
7. The David Suskind Show, WNEW-TV, METRO-MEDIA, March 14, 1975.
8. Gossett, J. T., Lewis, J. M., and Phillips, V. A., Extent and prevalence of illicit drug use as reported by 56,745 students, *JAMA*, 216, 1464, 1971.
9. Wood, J. H. and Downs, D. A., Defining the issues, in *Drug Use In America: Problem in Perspective*, 2nd Report of the National Commission on Marihuana and Drug Abuse, Washington, D.C., March 1973.
10. Abelson, H. I. and Atkinson, R. B., Public Experience with Psychoactive Substances: A Nationwide Study Among Adults and Youth, Response Analysis Corporation, Princeton, New Jersey, August 1975.
10a. O'Donnell, J. A., Voss, H. L., Clayton, R. B., Slatin, G. T., and Room, R. G. W., Young Men and Drugs – A Nationwide Survey, NIDA Research Monograph 5, National Institute on Drug Abuse, Rockville, Maryland, February 1976.
11. Ray, O. S., *Drugs, Society and Behavior*, C. V. Mosby, St. Louis, 1972.
12. Chambers, C. D., Taylor, M. J. R., and Moffet, A. D., The incidence of cocaine abuse among methadone maintenance patients, *Int. J. Addict.*, 7, 427, 1972.
13. Edmundson, W. T., Davies, J. E., Acker, J. D., and Myer, B., Patterns of drug abuse epidemiology in prisoners, *Ind. Med. Surg.*, 41, 15, 1972.

14. Sheppard, C. W., Gay, G. R., and Smith, D. E., The changing face of heroin addiction in the Haight-Ashbury, *Int. J. Addict.*, 7, 109, 1972.
15. Downs, A. W. and Eddy, N. B., The effects of repeated doses of cocaine in the dog, *J. Pharmacol. Exp. Ther.*, 46, 195, 1932.
16. Tatum, A. L. and Seevers, M. H., Experimental cocaine addiction, *J. Pharmacol. Exp. Ther.*, 36, 401, 1929.
17. Post, R. and Kopanda, R. T., Cocaine, kindling, and reverse tolerance, *Lancet*, 1, 409, 1975.
18. Ellinwood, E. and Stripling, J. S., Behavioral Electrophysiological Effects of Chronic Cocaine Intoxication, presented at the ACNP annual meeting, San Juan, Puerto Rico, December 16—19, 1975.
19. Post, R. M., Cocaine psychoses: A continuum model, *Am. J. Psychiatry*, 132(3), 225, March 1975.
20. Goodman, L. S. and Gilman, A., *The Pharmacological Basis of Therapeutics*, 3rd ed., Macmillan, New York, 1965.
21. Wikler, A., personal communication, April 24, 1975.
22. Isbell, H., Clinical Manifestations of Drug Addiction (film), made at the Addiction Research Center, Lexington, Kentucky, 1953.
23. Schuyten-Resnick, E., Resnick, R. B., Pribyl, S., Kestenbaum, R. S., and Freedman, A. M., Patterns and Effects of Cocaine Use, presented at the Collegium Internationale Neuro-Psychopharmacologicum, 10th Congress, Quebec, Canada, July 4—9, 1976.
24. Resnick, R. B., Kestenbaum, R. S., and Schwartz, L. K., Acute Systemic Effects of Cocaine in Man: A Controlled Study By Intranasal and Intravenous Routes of Administration, presented at the National Drug Abuse Conference, New Orleans, April 6, 1975; the Committee on Problems of Drug Dependence in Washington, D.C., May 20, 1975; and Annual Meeting of ACNP, December 1975.
25. Hill, E. H., Haertzen, C. A., Wolbach, A. B., and Miner, E. J., The addiction research center inventory: Appendix, *Psychopharmacologia*, 4, 184, 1963.
26. Post, R. M., Kotin, J., and Goodwin, F. K., The effects of cocaine on depressed patients, *Am. J. Psychiatry*, 131, 511, 1974.

Sociological, Treatment and Rehabilitation Aspects

Sociological Aspects of Cocaine Use and Abuse

SOCIOLOGICAL ASPECTS OF COCAINE USE AND ABUSE*

Jöel L. Phillips and Ronald D. Wynne

TABLE OF CONTENTS

*The work upon which the chapter is based was performed in large part under Contract ADM-45-74-144 with the National Institute on Drug Abuse, of the Alcohol, Drug Abuse and Mental Health Administration, Department of Health, Education and Welfare.

INTRODUCTION

Cocaine has had a long and romantic history, especially in America. During the late 1800s, it enjoyed great popularity as the active ingredient in hundreds of patent medicines and soft drinks. Adherents claimed it possessed near-magical powers, both curative and preventative. By the first decades of the 1900s, however, cocaine was seen as a key factor in the "depravity" of blacks, a spur to crime, and a deadly vice. The growing reactions to cocaine and the other "drugs of abuse" led to an outpouring of state and Federal regulatory activity, starting well before World War I, and culminating in the 1914 Harrison Act. Other than for increasingly limited medical application, the use of cocaine went "underground" following 1914, where it remained for many years.

This chapter discusses aspects of contemporary use and abuse of cocaine, following on the drug's resurgence of popularity in the last few years. The materials are largely drawn from the final report of our project for the National Institute on Drug Abuse — *Cocaine: The Facts and Myths.*[1] That volume includes a comprehensive summary of historical and scientific information on cocaine and coca, statistical data concerning the use and abuse of cocaine, an overview of pertinent Federal and state laws, and the results of a limited field study of current cocaine street myths and rituals. The field effort included interviews with a variety of users, dealers, and law enforcement officials and the solicitation of letters concerning their experiences from other users.

THE "NEW" POPULARITY OF COCAINE

Our analysis of the 20th Century cocaine literature shows a relative dearth of published articles between 1935 to 1960, and a sudden increase in the early 1960s, due predominantly to an upsurge of scientific interest in psychoactive drugs of all kinds.[2]

It seems clear that the current popularization of cocaine is the result of no single social, legal, or cultural factor. Rather, the etiology of its use is rooted in a complex series of forces that came together in the late 1960s, and resulted both in a desire for, and a supply of, cocaine:

● With increasing police emphasis in the late 1960s on "cracking down heavily on the amphetamine black market," cocaine smuggling and use enjoyed a renaissance.[3]

● "Some narcotics experts trace the current cocaine popularity back to Dr. Timothy Leary, the professor turned drug cultist who expounded the virtues of the conscious-expanding drugs . . . like LSD, DMT and Methedrine or 'speed'."[4]

● King suggests that the revival of cocaine use is a direct result of the channeling of heroin addicts into methadone programs in the early 1970s.[5] Methadone patients might seek out cocaine to get the euphoric feeling that they used to get (or were hopeful of getting) with heroin. Such euphoria clearly does not result from orally administered methadone.

● During the late 1960s, there was an increased general interest in and use of illicit drugs. Reflective of these social changes were many drug-related songs, movies, books, and articles in popular magazines. For instance, a 1971 *Newsweek* article noted that cocaine was "abundant," with all the "pot heads" on the scene trying it at "least once."[6] A prominent disc jockey, both on the radio and in the *Realist* magazine, talked about cocaine as the "thinking man's Dristan®."

EXTENT OF CURRENT USE

Although no one study or survey has been designed specifically to examine either cocaine use or its users, relevant items are typically included in questionnaires on illegal drug use.

The most popular test population has been high school students. The National Commission on Marihuana and Drug Abuse reviewed all available survey data from before 1972 based on student populations, and reported that cocaine had been used by:

● 1.2% of junior high students
● 2.6% of senior high students
● 10.4% of college students

The Marihuana Commission sponsored its own national probability sample survey of drug use, which showed that 1.5% of the youth (ages 12 to 17) and 3.2% of the adults (18 and older) reported using cocaine. Further, 1.6% of the adults and 1.1% of the youth had used cocaine in the previous 6 months. However, as the Commission's final report indicated, this "sample did not include the transient 'street' population among whom use of heroin and cocaine is presumably high."[7] A number of high school studies, compiled by Glenn, demonstrate an increasing awareness and use of cocaine among junior high and high school students.[8]

Other studies demonstrated that socioeconomic level, ethnic group, and size of community are related to self-reported cocaine use. Thirty-five thousand students in nineteen senior and six junior high schools in the East, Midwest, South, and Far West, representing various social and ethnic backgrounds, were polled as to their drug-taking behavior.[9] The percentage of students who had tried cocaine ranged from 13.8% (of 1,324 students polled in a high school located in a large West Coast city, ethnically mixed) to a low of 1.5% (of 486 junior high school students located in an East Coast city).

A more localized but still broad-based survey estimated that 6,000 individuals (0.1% of the population) used cocaine six or more times per month in the State of New York.[10] However, it was also estimated that an *additional* 95,000 individuals also used cocaine, but *less* than six times a month.

CHARACTERISTICS OF COCAINE USERS

"Cocaine is the drug of choice, not only among whites but, ever increasingly, among affluent black drug users as well. Cocaine has traditionally been the status drug among black athletes, show business personalities, and underworld figures (whose drug usage is very limited and distinctly snobbish: black mob leaders condescendingly regard heroin addicts — black or white — as trash). It now seems to be attracting an even broader black clientele. Among Latin Americans in New York, cocaine is often the preferred drug of entertainers, expensive prostitutes, very successful businessmen, and certain religious sects for whom cocaine use is literally an act of faith. And among white drug users, cocaine is especially popular with rock stars, writers, younger actors and actresses, and stockbrokers and other Wall Street types. The main thing these otherwise varied people have in common is an income that can support the luxury of cocaine."[11]

While this quotation neatly sums up the popular beliefs, there is little empirical knowledge about the characteristics of cocaine users, professionally, ethnically, or socially. What little information there is comes from the Federal Government's DAWN and CODAP systems, concerns cocaine users who have come to the attention of the drug abuse authorities (not necessarily for their use of cocaine, however), and largely seems to ignore the kinds of people listed above. As background to interpret this data, a brief description of these information systems follows.

The CODAP and DAWN Drug Abuse Reporting Systems

DAWN (Drug Abuse Warning Network) is a data collection system funded jointly by the National Institute on Drug Abuse (NIDA) and the Drug Enforcement Administration (DEA). The system receives information on "drug abuse incidents" — adverse drug effects that have led abusers to appear in a crisis information center or a hospital emergency room, or to become the subject of a medical examiner's report (autopsies, etc.). Pre-1975, incident data were also collected from hospital in-patient facilities. Preselected reporting sources are now located in the 24 Standard Metropolitan Statistical Areas (SMSAs).

CODAP (Client-Oriented Data Acquisition Process) is a data collection and reporting system operated by NIDA. The CODAP files date back to April 1, 1973, when specifically designed forms on patients admitted to Federally funded drug treatment agencies were first collected. Data, collected during admission to a program, concern demographic characteristics, drug use history, and treatment background. These data are reported to NIDA, via the cognizant state drug abuse agencies, for all clients who are considered "admitted" to programs. Quarterly updates are also provided to NIDA concerning all clients still in treatment at the end of the quarter.

DAWN Findings

Table 1 provides information on the characteristics of 3,069 cocaine users as reported via the DAWN system between April 1974 and April 1975.[12] As Table 1 shows, the reported cocaine users are predominantly white, male, and under 30, and obtained the drug "on the street." Note that 13% of the users were reportedly housewives. The data reinforce, not surprisingly, the belief that most users (61%) use cocaine for its psychic effects. What is surprising is the proportion of the cases (30%) reporting the motivating factor as dependency on cocaine.

Data from 1973 to 1974 concerning frequency of use are shown in Table 2. Since the frequency of use was reported for only half the cases, it proved very difficult for DEA to interpret the

TABLE 1

Characteristics in Users in 3,069 Cases
Involving Cocaine (1974–1975)

	%
Sex	
Male	64
Female	36
Race	
White	58
Black	27
Other	3
Unknown/No response	12
Age	
Under 9	*
10–19	21
20–29	53
30–39	10
40–49	3
50 and over	1
Unknown/No response	12
Employment Status	
Working	24
Unemployed	30
Student	2
Housewife	13
Retired	*
Unknown/No response	*
Motivation for use	
Psychic effects	61
Dependency	30
Suicide attempt	2
Unwilling/Unknowing/Other	*
Unknown/No response	8
Source of the drug	
Legal prescription	*
Forged prescription	*
Stolen	1
Street buy	74
All others	5
Unknown/No response	20

*Less than 0.5%

From Drug Abuse Warning Network
(Project DAWN) Files, IMS America,
Inc., Ambler, Pennsylvania (see Refer-
ence 12).

findings, and the item was dropped from later
reporting forms.[13] (Additional data on frequency
of use [from CODAP reports] are shown in Table
4.)

TABLE 2

Frequency of Cocaine Use Based on
2,319 Cases Involving the Use of Cocaine
(July 1973–April 1974)

Frequency of use	N	%
Daily	468	20.6
Weekly	460	20.3
Monthly	177	7.8
One time	173	7.6
Unknown	991	43.7
Total	2,269*	100.0

*Data incomplete because this informa-
tion is not collected from one data
source – Medical Examiners

From Drug Abuse Warning Network
(Project DAWN) Files, IMS America,
Inc., Ambler, Pennsylvania.

CODAP Findings

The most recent CODAP data useful for this
analysis are from 1973. As shown in Table 3,
during the first 9 months of 1973 only 1% of the
clients who entered drug treatment programs that
report through this system reported cocaine as
their primary drug of choice. And only about 10%
reported any cocaine-related "problems" (e.g.,
admitted during the course of an intake interview
that they use or have used cocaine).

An analysis done by NIDA of the characteristics of 730 clients who reported their primary
drug of abuse as cocaine is shown in Table 4, in
comparison with all other clients in CODAP-
reporting programs. The key distinction between
the cocaine clients in this system and all other
clients is that cocaine users are relatively younger
males who use their drug of choice relatively less
frequently.

While both the CODAP and DAWN findings
indicate the predominant user group to be white
males under 30, the CODAP reportees, compared
to the DAWN reportees, are older, include more
males and blacks, and are more frequent users of
cocaine.

HOW COCAINE IS USED

Routes of Administration
Inhalation
    Inhalation (referred to as "snorting,"

TABLE 3

Proportion of Cocaine Users Among Clients Admitted to Drug Treatment Programs (April–December 1973)

	Quarter 1 4/73–6/73		Quarter 2 7/73–9/73		Quarter 3 10/73–12/73	
CODAP admissions	N	%	N	%	N	%
Total admissions	18,515	100.0	21,347	100	26,069	100.0
Primary cocaine	182	1.0	207	1.0	280	1.1
Secondary cocaine	1,422	7.7	1,760	8.2	2,078	8.0
Other cocaine	435	2.3	392	1.8	472	1.8
Total cocaine	2,039	11.0	2,359	11.0	2,830	10.9

Adapted from Client Oriented Data Acquisition Process (CODAP) Files/Division of Scientific and Program Information, NIDA.

Note: The numbers in this table do not add to the totals for all CODAP admissions cited in other tables due to missing information regarding date of admission and because of reports received for pre-April 1, 1973 admissions.

TABLE 4

Characteristics of 730 Primary Cocaine Users and 70,602 Other Drug Users: Sex, Race, Age, Extent of Use

Variable	Primary cocaine users	Other drug users
Sex		
Male	79.2	72.9
Female	20.5	24.8
No data	0.3	2.2
Race		
White	54.0	54.4
Black	41.5	37.2
Other	3.0	5.4
No data	1.5	3.1
Age		
Mean	24.6	26.9
Median	22.7	23.8
Extent of use		
Daily	33.3	54.8
Several times/wk	15.2	10.7
Once/wk	6.3	4.5
Less than once/wk	27.7	17.3
No use at admission	12.1	6.4
No use in last 30 days	5.5	6.4

Adapted from Client Oriented Data Acquisition Process (CODAP) Files/Division of Scientific and Program Information, NIDA.

"tooting," or taking a "snort" or a "toot") is the most common route of administration. Table 5 indicates that over 60% of the cocaine cases reported through the DAWN system "snorted." Elaborate rituals involving a variety of paraphernalia have been developed for snorting. The most common procedure is to line up a small pile of cocaine powder (a "line" or "rail") on a hard, smooth surface, and then to snort the whole pile in one long and continuous inhalation. One nostril is pinched while the other is used for snorting, and vice versa. The effects (if cocaine is present) are usually apparent to the inhaler within a few minutes.

Other Ways to Take Cocaine

The other route of administration commonly employed by cocaine users is by intravenous (i.v.) injection. In addition, cocaine can be, and is, taken orally. A popular area for direct application of cocaine is on the genital region, in order to prolong the sex act. Cocaine is also reportedly used, again sexually, in enema solutions.

Reasons for Preference of Inhalation Over Injection

The main reason cited by users we interviewed for the preference of inhalation over injection was the relatively short duration ("often less than 15 minutes") of cocaine effects when used intravenously. Many users expressed a fear of using syringes. A number also mentioned the relative costs. Given the shorter duration of the i.v. effects (in comparison with the admittedly less intense inhalation effects), more cocaine, and thus more money, is likely to be involved in using the drug in this manner.

Use of Cocaine and Other Drugs
Heroin

A series of surveys have demonstrated a relationship between the use of cocaine and other drugs, most notably heroin. Kestenbaum et al. cite a study by the New York State Narcotic Commission which found that nearly 82% of 180 randomly selected (and certified) narcotics addicts reported using cocaine during 1969 to 1970. They also cite a study conducted at the Clinical Research Center, Lexington, Kentucky, in which it was found that "of 1,096 opiate addicts, 72.9 percent reported cocaine abuse during 1968-69."[14]

TABLE 5

Route of Administration in 2,319 Cases Involving the Use of Cocaine (July 1973–April 1974)

Method	No.	%
Oral	92	4.0
Injection i.v.	291	12.5
Injection other	48	2.1
Injection unspecified	252	10.9
Snorted	1.421	61.3
Other	46	2.0
Unknown	169	7.2
Total	2.319	100.0

Adapted from Drug Abuse Warning Network (Project DAWN) Files, IMS America, Inc., Ambler, Pennsylvania.

But not all of the figures have been this high. Gay et al., for instance, analyzed clinical records at one treatment center and found that during any one data collection period, only 20% of their addicts, at most, reported using cocaine (while treatment was underway.)[15]

Use of Drugs Other Than Heroin

Cocaine users, for a number of reasons, tend to be multiple (or "polydrug") users, often using cocaine in combination with other drugs. One of our interviewees said:

"I like coke and smoking pot, coke and downs, coke ... and anything and everything. It's hard to say ... The combination is whatever's available and that's that."

Many of our subjects preferred depressant combinations:

"I love [cocaine with] downers, barbiturates. They seem to have a nice mixture. Whereas cocaine after a while will act like an amphetamine, the downer will mellow you out. Quaaludes®, as the downer, seem to mix well. Drinking and coke goes well, too."

What seems to us a reasonable explanation for this use of depressants is that they may reduce the "jittery" or anxious state that reportedly, for many users, follows upon dissipation of cocaine's euphoric effects.

On the other hand, for some of the users, cocaine's relative expense and unique euphoric effect preclude their mixing drugs:

"It's a treat; you just don't want to take away from a cocaine high. It's definitely a treat to most people."

Factors Restricting Frequency/Amount of Use

Woods and Downs[16] speculated that, at least for "occasional" users, the setting was the key determinant in regulating the frequency with which they used cocaine. Our interviewees provided support for this speculation:

"You go to a party where there's a lot of coke, it's a status trip . . . so you do it.

"Cocaine is above all a social drug, and if you have some, you share it with your friends."

It has been reported that many users believe that extensive use has psychotoxic results (e.g., they would "freak out" or overdose).[16] Another barrier to a very extensive use of cocaine might be the heavy abuse of other drugs, especially heroin. And a final barrier is likely to be the price: current U. S. street prices, ca. mid 1975, range from $55 to over $100 per gram.

Rituals of Use

Paraphernalia

Local "head shops" (stores specializing in drug use-related paraphernalia) typically stock some of the many devices currently used in connection with the ritual of "snorting" cocaine. These include spoons, ranging from cheap metal ones (resembling small salt spoons) to exquisitely designed, very expensive gold and silver ones that hold enough for a single "snort." Head shops also carry curved glass tubes, often termed "tooters" or "snorters" and used in lieu of straws or rolled up bills to inhale the cocaine.

The smaller end fits in the nose, and the larger end is placed over a "line" of cocaine. The powder is typically scraped into thin lines on a table top, mirror, or any other smooth surface. Such fancy glass tubes or straws are in common use. Most of the users we interviewed continue to use rolled-up dollar bills, however.

Some drug speciality stores sell complete cocaine kits including glass snorters, razor blades, a mirror, and different size vials in which to carry the cocaine. The entire contents fit into small leather cases resembling miniaturized versions of shaving kits. The razor blade is used to chop the cocaine into a fine consistency. The crushed and cut-up powder is then placed on a mirror (or any

uniformly flat and smooth surface) and is usually divided into either one large or two small piles or "lines." The amount in each pile varies among users, is rarely measured precisely, and is determined by habit or individual preference. Several interviewees familiar with the subject said that this approach differed from the use of heroin, in which the amounts used are much more closely measured. A typical "line" of cocaine is about the thickness of a felt-tip pen mark and at least several inches long.

Side Effects of Inhalation: Nose Problems

There are several current practices among cocaine users to prevent the build-up of cocaine particles in the nasal passages:

- Cutting or grinding the cocaine into a fine powder.
- Snorting water into the nose. (Some of our interview subjects use wine.)
- Using nose drops and nasal sprays. A doctor in the Los Angeles area, commenting on the number of patients coming to his office with complaints that nasal sprays were not helping their congestion, said, "Sales of these sprays and drops have rocketed . . . and I directly attribute that increase to the widely extended use of cocaine."[17]

Settings and Reasons for Use

General Pleasure

Among the users we interviewed, the most frequently offered explanation for cocaine's popularity was its extremely pleasurable and euphoric properties. Other frequently given explanations are

- It enhances parties and social situations and is often taken in group settings.
- There has been almost no "bad" publicity concerning cocaine and its effects.
- It's profitable, and many users also buy and sell the drug.

Sports

The use of cocaine by athletes is not a new phenomenon.

"Some years ago the members of the Toronto Lacrosse club experimented with coca, and during that season when the club held the championship of the world, coca was used in all its important matches. The Toronto club was composed of men accustomed to sedentary work, while some of the opposing players were sturdy men accustomed to out-of-door exercise. The games were all severely contested, and some were played in the hottest weather of one summer ... The more stalwart appearing men, however, were so far used up before the match was completed that they could hardly be encouraged to finish the game, while the coca chewers were as elastic and as free from fatigue as at the commencement of the play."[18]

The extent to which cocaine is used by athletes as a performance aid is unknown, but it has clearly relevant physiological effects. However, because of its acute toxic effects when used in large doses, the conventional medical view is that "cocaine should never be used in connection with athletics."[19]

There seems to be a widespread belief that professional athletes use cocaine extensively. We were told a number of anecdotes about the use of cocaine — both socially and as a performance aid — by well-known professional football and basketball players by several reliable (law enforcement) sources.

While few of our subjects reported using cocaine for any athletic events, a number reported using it for the perhaps equally strenuous activities of housecleaning and sexual intercourse.

Sex

Of all the drugs of abuse, cocaine has been most strongly identified as possessing aphrodisiac qualities. This has historical precedence with coca's use as an aphrodisiac by some South American Indians. Cocaine can have paradoxical sexual effects. On the one hand, as a sensory stimulant, it increases the intensity of orgasm. On the other hand, it can both inhibit and retard the climax, in both males and females. Applied directly to the genital areas, it causes a "tingling" sensation (it is a local anesthetic) and a prolongation of the period of intercourse.[20]

It may be that some part of the aphrodisiac role attributed to cocaine results from the expectations of users who have heard that cocaine has strong sexual properties. As noted by Goode, this has likely been the case for marijuana.[21] Thus, if a user expects to be "turned on sexually" by cocaine, this may often happen. One of the cocaine users we interviewed for this study said:

"... Everybody says that it's an aphrodisiac. Again, I think some people say it because it's supposed to be ... I

think that it's just peer group identification. I remember when I first started doing coke, I remember everybody would be sitting around saying, 'Oh, I just got to get laid.' I said it a couple of times, but I never felt that way. I was more content to sit there and enjoy it."

In spite of some scientists' views that cocaine has no true aphrodisiac qualities,[22] cocaine's reputation as a sexual stimulant is still strong among users and nonusers alike. Clearly, more research needs to be done in this area before any conclusive statements can be made.

TRAFFICKING IN COCAINE

The South American Connection

In all likelihood, the cocaine inhaled by a user anywhere in the United States had its beginnings as bundled coca on the backs of llamas, being led out of the Andean highlands of Bolivia or Peru to laboratories run by brokers with contacts in organized crime in the major Latin countries. The brokers process the coca leaves into a paste that is usually sold in two-kilogram lots for the equivalent of a few hundred dollars. The paste is then smuggled mainly into Brazil and Chile, where it is refined at more sophisticated laboratories into cocaine HC1 and then made ready for wholesale exportation.[23] Large quantities of leaves are needed for the process: 1 kilo of leaves yields 7 g of paste (a ratio of 143:1) and 100 g of paste yield 81 g of cocaine HC1.

According to the Drug Enforcement Administration, there are several routes by which cocaine enters the United States:

- One route originates in Peru, then travels through Ecuador and Panama to Mexico, from where it enters the United States via air, land, or sea. Texas port cities such as Houston and Galveston are the destination.
- A second route starts in Chile and extends through other Latin American countries to various ports on the U. S. Pacific Coast, probably most often in California.
- A third route starts in Bolivia, on to the West Indies, and then the United States, with Miami and New York City being the major ports of entry.

The profits along this cocaine trail are extraordinary and are, by all accounts, going up, indicative of the increasing demand. According to

Ashley, in 1971 a pure "gram" of Bolivian flake, the best illicit cocaine available, ". . . could be had for from $40–$50 . . . A quarter ounce (seven grams) went for $200-$225, and an ounce brought $600-$700."[25] A look at the prices reported in the 1975 *Pharm Chem Newsletter* reveals price increases across the board: up to $100 for a gram; $425 for one quarter of an ounce; and ounces ranging between $1,100 to $2,000. The majority of the ounce prices were $1,500 and up.

Fooner quotes the price of cocaine as being $1,600 to $1,800 per pound in Bogota or Guayaquil, and about $6,500 per pound, or approximately $1,300 a kilo, when it is delivered to a wholesaler.[26] Two years earlier in 1971, the *New York Times* reported that a kilo (2.2 lb) sold for about $900 in Chile.[27]

Control of the Market

Over the last 10 years, there has been a realignment in the cocaine smuggling setup — in particular, a shift of the traffic center. According to Fooner:

"In the 1950s, Miami became the center because it was easy for Spanish-speaking smugglers to use the Cuban community as a cover. Miami-based Cuban traffickers serviced New York and other markets around the country. Now the center seems to have shifted to New York, with Colombian smugglers in the ascendancy."[28]

According to Federal experts, the Chileans, possessing a source of cocaine in their mountains, moved into the trade about 4 years ago. Two years ago, apparently the Chilean dealers stopped selling cocaine "directly to U. S. recipients and started working through Colombian criminal groups, using Colombian rather than Chilean couriers."[29]

However, the cocaine trade does not seem to be the prerogative of any one organized crime syndicate, unlike the situation that has traditionally characterized the heroin network.

Adulterants

With the increase in street demand for cocaine, the quality or purity of cocaine has decreased in the last several years.[30] The potential street buyer of cocaine is usually confronted with cocaine that has either been diluted or adulterated.

Cocaine (as well as heroin) is often adulterated by many substances not chemically classified as drugs. Sugars in the form of lactose and, to a lesser degree, inositol and mannitol are often used. Although these sugars are regularly used in pharmaceutical preparations and, therefore, are considered to be relatively safe, "medical knowledge of these substances is based on oral use."[31]

A more dangerous cut, involving nondrug substances, uses cornstarch, talcum powder, and oven flour. The source quoted just above reports that there have been numerous cases of people injecting heroin or cocaine cut with talc and cornstarch, resulting in emboli in the lungs and eyes, which can lead to respiratory failure and blindness.

Pharm Chem statistics for both 1973 and 1974 indicate that cocaine is most often cut with other local anesthetics such as procaine (Novocaine®) and lidocaine (Xylocaine®). The other local anesthetics, benzocaine and tetracaine, are used less frequently. With the addition of some of these adulterants, it is very possible that "street" cocaine will be far more lethal than if the substance were pure cocaine.[32]

Costs and Purity of "Street" Cocaine

There is a definite relationship among purity levels, cost, and the amount of cocaine purchased, based on our own analysis of data provided us by the DEA. Table 6 clearly shows that purchasers on the wholesale level (defined by the DEA as any purchase of cocaine that is at least 14% pure or a minimum weight of 14 g) obtain a purer sample than do small-time dealers on the retail level. The wholesale cocaine is less expensive overall, considerably more pure, and thus, considerably cheaper per gram of pure cocaine. Overall, the undercover agents purchased more cocaine, and a

TABLE 6

Cocaine Prices and Purity Information (DEA Statistics Fiscal Year 1974)

	Wholesale	Retail
Gross g purchased	2188.06	293.35
Total cost	$82,505	$12,355
Cost/gross g	$37.70	$42.10
Average purity	40.8%	9.6%
Net g of pure cocaine	892.04	28.19
Cost/net g	$90.00	$440.00
Number of data points*	55	47

*Data point = a purchase by an undercover agent.

better quality of cocaine, at the wholesale than at the retail level. These findings are also bolstered by the results of analyses of street samples conducted by Pharm Chem Laboratories in Palo Alto.[33]

Conclusion

The final monopolistic control of the cocaine trade has not been resolved. It may never be. But, as Ianni suggested in his book, *Black Mafia,* the new route of drugs from South America "should" have an important impact on the American drug scene:

"The most important effect will be the continued displacement of Italian-American syndicates from the international drug traffic as this new section replaces the older one which came through Europe. The street implications are enormous. It not only means that new patterns of wholesaling will be established, changing the ethnic balance of power in organized crime; it also means that cocaine may very well displace heroin as the 'street drug'."[34]

REFERENCES

1. **Phillips, J. L. (edited and with introduction by Wynne, R. D.),** *Cocaine: The Facts and Myths,* Final report to Natl. Inst. on Drug Abuse, Contract No. ADM-45-74-144, Wynne Associates, Washington, D.C., July, 1975.

2. **Phillips, J. L. and Wynne, R. D.,** *A Cocaine Bibliography — Nonannotated,* DHEW Publ. No. (ADM) 75-203, Natl. Inst. on Drug Abuse, Rockville, Maryland, 1975.

3. **Brecher, E.,** *Licit and Illicit Drugs,* Little, Brown & Co., New York, 1972.

4. **Ottenberg, M.,** Cocaine: The new no. 1 drug, *Washington Star,* August 5, 1974, A1.

5. **King, R.,** *Drug Hang-up: America's Fifty-Year Folly,* Norton, New York, 1972.

6. Anon., Life and leisure: It's the real thing, *Newsweek,* September 27, 1971, 124.

7. National Commission on Marihuana and Drug Abuse, *Drug Use in America: Problem in Perspective,* U.S. Govt. Printing Office, Washington, D.C., 1973.

8. **Glenn, W. A.,** *A Compendium of Recent Studies of Illegal Drug Use,* unpublished report prepared for Natl. Inst. on Drug Abuse under Contract No. HSM-42-72-169, Research Triangle Institute, Raleigh, North Carolina, March 1973.

9. **Elinson, J.,** *A Study of Teen-age Drug Behavior,* Summary progress report for the period 9/1/71 through 6/30/72 under Natl. Inst. of Mental Health grant No. MH-17589-03, Columbia University College of Physicians and Surgeons, New York, June, 1972.

10. **Chambers, C. and Inciardi, J.,** *An Assessment of Drug Use in the General Population,* Special Report No. 2, N.Y. State Narcotic Addiction Control Commission, Albany, 1971.

11. **Plate, T.,** Coke: The big new easy-entry business, *New York Magazine,* November 5, 1973, 63.

12. The data in Table 1 are from a special unpublished analysis of cocaine users provided to us by Betty O'Brien of IMS America, Inc., Ambler, Pennsylvania, the DAWN contractor.

13. Cocaine Policy Task Force Report, Drug Enforcement Administration, Washington, D.C., July, 1974.

14. **Kestenbaum, R. S., Resnick, R. B., and Schwartz, L. K.,** Acute System Effects of Cocaine in Man: A Controlled Study by Intranasal and Intravenous Routes of Administration, Division of Drug Abuse Research and Treatment, Dept. of Psychiatry, New York Medical College, 1975.

15. **Gay, G. R., Sheppard, C. W., Inaba, D. S., and Newmeyer, J. A.,** An old girl: Flyin' low, dyin' slow, blinded by snow: Cocaine in perspective, *Int. J. Addict.,* 8, 1027, 1973.

16. **Woods, J. H. and Downs, D. A.,** The psychopharmacology of cocaine, in *Drug Use in America: Problem in Perspective,* U.S. Govt. Printing Office, Washington, D.C., 1973.

17. **Hopkins, J.,** Cocaine: A flash in the pan, a pain in the nose, *Rolling Stone,* Vol. 81, April 9, 1971, pp. 1, 6.

18. **Mortimer, W. G.,** *Peru History of Coca, the Divine Plant of the Incas,* J. H. Vail and Co., 1901. Reprinted as *History of Coca,* And/Or Press, San Francisco, 1974.

19. Methods used for improving athletic performance, *JAMA,* 115, 1281, 1940.

20. **Gay, G. R., Sheppard, C. W., Inaba, D. S., and Newmeyer, J. A.,** An old girl: Flyin' low, dyin' slow, blinded by snow: Cocaine in perspective, *Int. J. Addict.,* 8, 1027, 1973.

21. **Goode, E.,** Marijuana and sex, *Evergreen Review,* Vol. 66, 1969, 19.

22. **Gallant, D. M.,** The effect of alcohol and drug abuse on sexual behavior, *Med. Aspects of Hum. Sexuality,* Vol. 11, 1968, 30.

23. **Plate, T.,** Coke: The big new easy-entry business, *New York Magazine,* November 5, 1973, 63.

24. Drug Traffic in South America, Drug Enforcement Administration, Washington, D.C., 1970.

25. **Ashley, R.,** *Cocaine: Its History, Uses and Effects,* St. Martin's Press, New York, 1975.

26. **Fooner, M.,** Cocaine: The South American connection, *World,* Vol 2, 1973, 22.

27. U.S. agents try, but fail, to stop the flow of cocaine from Latin countries, *New York Times,* January 25, 1971.

28. **Fooner, M.,** Cocaine: The South American connection, *World,* Vol. 2, 1973, 22.

29. **Ottenberg, M.,** Cocaine: The no. 1 drug, *Washington Star,* August 5, 1974, A1.

30. **Malone, M. H.,** It's the real zing, *Pacific Information Service on Street Drugs,* Vol 2, 1973, 24.

31. **Perry, D. C.,** Heroin and Cocaine adulteration, *Pharm. Chem. Newsletter,* 3, 1, 1974.

32. **Malone, M. H.,** It's the real zing, *Pacific Information Service on Street Drugs,* Vol. 2, 1973, 24.

33. *Pharm Chem Newsletter,* Vol. 3, 1974; Vol. 5, 1975. Includes analyses of 1180 street drug samples purported to be cocaine.

34. **Ianni, F. A.,** *Black Mafia: Ethnic Succession in Organized Crime,* Simon and Schuster, 1974.

Sociological, Treatment and Rehabilitation Aspects

Acute and Chronic Toxicology of Cocaine Abuse:
Current Sociology, Treatment, and Rehabilitation

ACUTE AND CHRONIC TOXICOLOGY OF COCAINE ABUSE: CURRENT SOCIOLOGY, TREATMENT, AND REHABILITATION

George R. Gay and Darryl S. Inaba

TABLE OF CONTENTS

INTRODUCTION

Cocaine, at various times also known as "snow," "flake," "girl," "her," "coke," "lady," "blow," "toot," "she," "jam," "happy trails," "rock," "nose candy" or "candy," "the star spangled powder," "la dama blanca" (the white lady), "the gift of the sun god," "heaven-leaf," "the rich man's drug," and "the pimp's drug,"[1-4] has certainly held moments of high drama on the historical stage during the ten centuries of its recorded use.

A thorough understanding of the chemistry, pharmacology, and neuropharmacology of this substance is needed for the intervention and treatment of the chronic cocaine abuser as well as the acute toxicity or "caine" reaction. Though previously presented in other chapters, it is relevant here to underscore some of the more important clinical characteristics of cocaine abuse.

CURRENT SOCIOLOGY AND EPIDEMIOLOGY

In the current drug subculture, cocaine has become the "champagne of drugs" with probably the greatest potential for an explosive growth in popularity. The cocaine-using population looks down on other drug types and indeed represents the "upper" class of drug abusers.[5,6] Truly the "rich man's drug" may be purchased illicitly, ranging in price from $500 to $1500 an ounce,[3,7] which is usually diluted or "stepped on" by the street dealer. The most commonly sold unit of cocaine available on the illicit drug market is a gram or "spoon" of coke. Sold at prices ranging from $50 to $75 a gram, the average good "line" or "snort" of coke (60 to 200 mg) would cost $5 to $10. This is about three times the cost for a reasonably effective dose of liquor and about ten times the cost of a fairly effective dose of marijuana. This high price of illicit cocaine (pure, legal cocaine wholesales for about $20 an ounce [30 gm]) may be the only obstacle preventing current widespread use of this substance.

The recent influx of cocaine abuse amongst Hollywood elite, popular musicians, and other upper economic classes has revived the practice of "snorting" or "horning" (in which a "line" of cocaine is inhaled into a nostril, often through a specially rolled high denomination bill) and has to some extent supplanted intravenous use. Hugh Romney, or "Wavy Gravy" of "The Hog Farm" (which distributed food at Woodstock), has called cocaine "The Thinking Man's Dristan."[3] One of the complications seen as a result of this practice, however, is alleged perforation of the nasal septum from necrosis secondary to the vasoconstricting effects of cocaine. "Sniffers," "snorters," or "snarfers" are also prone to infections of the mucous membranes and entire respiratory system. In addition, a "reactive hyperemia" (or clogging of nasal airways by engorged membranes) occurs as the vasoconstriction wears off. Thus the items carried by chronic cocaine sniffers include: (a) the paraphernalia (spoon, snuffbox, etc.) and (b) the nose drops.

Cocaine is the drug of "special occasions," both social and sexual; hoarded and then doled out like champagne or rare old brandy.[8]

The pharmacologic properties which afford cocaine its high degree of desirability and expense are its stimulant effects on the CNS. Cocaine is the prototype of the stimulant drug that is capable of producing euphoric excitement and (in high dosage) hallucinatory experience. Coke is also venerated as the most suitable adjunct to sexual activity, especially the performance aspects of sexuality. These properties rank it high in the esteem of the experienced drug abuser and lead to the highest degree of psychic dependence[2,9,10]. Bearing witness to this is a passage written on the effects of cocaine by Paolo Mantegazza, a century before those written by Iceberg Slim and Malcolm X:

Borne on the wings of two coca leaves, I flew about in the spaces of 77,438 worlds, one more splendid than another. I prefer a life of ten years with coca to one of a hundred thousand without it. It seemed to me that I was separated from the whole world, and I beheld the strangest images most beautiful in color and in form than can be imagined.

Paolo Mantegazza (1859) as cited in Reference 11

I felt like the top of my skull had been crushed in. It was like I had been blown apart and all that was left was my eyes. Then tiny prickly feet of ecstasy started dancing through me. I heard melodious bells tolling softly inside my skull.

Iceberg Slim (1967) as cited in Reference 12

It was when I got back into that familiar snow feeling that I began to want to talk. Cocaine produces, for those who sniff its powdery white crystals, an illusion of supreme well-being, and a soaring over-confidence in both physical and mental ability. You think that you could whip the heavyweight champion and that you are smarter than everybody.

Malcolm X (1945) as cited in Reference 13

On a more clinical level, experiments have shown that rats taught to press a lever in order to obtain a drug would do so up to 250 consecutive times for caffeine, 4,000 times for heroin, and 10,000 times for cocaine.[2]

Intravenous cocaine is described as a "splash" or "orgasmic rush," in common with high-dose intravenous amphetamine abuse.[14-16]

When you shoot coke in the mainline there is a rush of pure pleasure to the head . . . . Ten minutes later you want another shot . . . intravenous C is electricity through the brain, activating cocaine pleasure connections . . . . There is no withdrawal syndrome with C. It is a need of the brain alone.

William Burroughs[29]

Many current "coke-heads" agree with Freud's description of cocaine as an aphrodisiac.

Orgasms go better with coke.[17]

Also, applied locally on the genital areas, tingling (partially due to local anesthetization) and prolongation of intercourse may be achieved. The chronic cocaine user comes much closer to fitting the picture of a "sex-crazed, depraved dope fiend" than do the narcotic addicts to whom this description is classically applied.[8]

In an evaluation of cocaine's role in sexuality, Newmeyer[18] studied the sexual and drug-taking habits of 95 clients of the Haight-Ashbury Free Medical Clinics in San Francisco from October 1972 to March 1975. Responding to an extensive (137-item) questionnaire about 11 different drugs, 75% (71) subjects described having used cocaine at least once during their lives and 44% (42) admitted present use (March 1975) of cocaine at least occasionally "to make sex better." Further pattern of responses clearly demonstrated "coke" to be the most esteemed of all drugs in regard to sexual enhancement. Cocaine ranked especially high in the "ego" or active, performance-enhancement aspects of sexuality, but ranked second to the psychedelics in the "id" or passive, fantasy-enhancement aspects of sexuality.

A retrospective study of the heroin-abusing clients seen at the Haight-Ashbury Free Medical Clinics demonstrated a striking rise in the incidence of cocaine use beginning in mid-1970.[19] Interview data of 741 heroin addicts who were first seen between March 1971 and April 1972 were reviewed. Among those clients seen between March to September 1971 (303), 10.0% reported moderate to heavy use of cocaine within the last 2 months. Of those clients seen between September 1971 and January 1972 (264), 13.6% reported moderate to heavy use within the last 2 months, and of those seen in February 1972 to April 1972

(147), the percentage reached 20.7%. Thus, it appears that the incidence of cocaine use rose rapidly during 1970 and the first half of 1971, then increased more slowly until mid-1972. Clients who were cocaine users tended to be significantly younger, less often Caucasian, more often Catholic, and more often single than their nonusing or rarely using counterparts. The data also showed that those clients who were recent users of cocaine were slightly more middle class in background, education, and employment. The cocaine users tended to have been significantly younger when they first used heroin and other drugs, and their use of all illegal drugs was more extensive, particularly prior to their use of heroin. There is inconclusive evidence to show that these cocaine users had less extensive arrest records, but more extensive participation in sexual activities outside of marriage.

An evaluation of illicit cocaine samples offered for anonymous analysis to Pharm Chem Laboratories in Palo Alto, California from October 1972 to March of 1975 also revealed a well-established and fairly "honest" (price and quality) cocaine market in the San Francisco Bay Area (see Table 1).[18] Assuming an average retail cost of $65 per gram, it was estimated that an aggregate *monthly* expenditure of $2,000,000 was spent by some 120,000 Bay Area "countercultural youth" cocaine users during the first few months of 1975.

On a national scale evidence is accumulating that cocaine use has undergone a similar rise as seen in the San Francisco Bay Area from mid-1970.[4,5] The Department of Justice reported that cocaine seized in the U.S. rose from 370 lb in 1969 to 751 lb by 1971, while arrests involving cocaine increased from 987 in 1969 to 1,284 in 1971. Further, agents of the U.S. Bureau of Narcotics and Dangerous Drugs (now the Drug Enforcement Agency) and officials of the Chilean government reported on August 13, 1971 that the flow of cocaine from Chile to the U.S. was at record levels. Little cocaine actually originates in Chile; most is produced in Peru, Bolivia, and Ecuador, sent to Chilean laboratories where it is refined and then shipped.

Today "body carriers" are mostly free lancers.... When a shipment is "hit" (by U.S. Agents) coming in through Central America, Mexico, or the Caribbean it averages 80, 90 or 100 lbs. That means organization.[20]

While none of these events "proves" that cocaine use is rising nationally (increased seizures could reflect increased vigilance or efforts devoted to cocaine), they do seem to bear out our local statistics regarding cocaine use.

In spite of this recent increase of cocaine abuse, it is only fair to state that *chronic* cocaine abuse is still a fairly rare occurence in the drug-taking subculture. This is most probably related to the tremendous financial cost that would be generated by a chronic pattern of abuse.

CLINICAL TOXICOLOGY AND TREATMENT

Intervention with the chronic cocaine abuser is often initiated by treatment of the early stimulation phase of a "caine" or acute toxic reaction. Though a complete caine reaction is rarely seen, it occurs frequently enough to warrant full review.

Cocaine is absorbed from *all* mucous mem-

TABLE 1

Analysis of Illicit Cocaine Samples: San Francisco Bay Area (October 1972 to March 1975)

Period	Median cost of grams	Median % purity of grams	Median cost of ounces	Median % purity of ounces
1. October 1972 – March 1973	$50	46%	$1,020	50%
2. October – December 1973	$53	64%	$1,190	59%
3. July – October 1974	$62	–*	$1,280	–*
4. October – December 1974	$66	–	$1,382	–
5. January – March 1975	$62	–	$1,444	–

"Cutters" – diluents and adulterants were also analyzed by Pharm Chem Laboratories. Twenty-five percent of the samples contained cocaine-like alkaloid adulterants, especially lidocaine (Xylocaine®), but also procaine and benzocaine. Sucrose, glucose, mannitol, and inositol were common diluents.

*Quantitative or % analyses were restricted by the DEA after December 1973.

branes. Absorption may even occur from the urinary bladder if inflammation is present.[21,22] However, the local vasoconstriction caused by cocaine limits the rate of its absorption. Despite this fact, its rate of absorption may easily exceed the rate of detoxification and excretion. This leads to cocaine's celebrated high toxicity. After absorption, cocaine is rapidly metabolized by the liver by a process of hydrolysis to benzoic acid and ecgonine (both of these products may be recovered from the urine)[23-25] and other metabolites (see chapter by A. L. Misra). *It has been estimated that the liver can detoxify one minimal lethal dose of cocaine an hour.* Taken in incremental intravenous doses, as much as 10 gm of cocaine can be detoxified in 1 day![22,24,26]

The fatal dose of cocaine (that dose which causes death 100% of the time) is stated to be 1.2 gm (1,200 mg) after oral ingestion. However, the LD_{50} (that dose which results in death 50% of the time) is approximately 500 mg after oral ingestion in a 150-lb man. But this can be very misleading in

that the fatal dose after application to *mucous membranes* may be as low as *30 mg*![14,23,24,26,27] Ingested cocaine is rapidly hydrolyzed in the stomach and is therefore much less toxic than by other routes of administration. The stated fatal doses are also misleading from the standpoint that there is a considerable individual variation (as emphasized by Freud)[28] in susceptibility to the drug. Anaphylactic sensitivity to cocaine and subsequent death have also occurred with its usage, even in small dosage.

Table 2 illustrates the biphasic nature of a "caine" reaction, and Table 3 outlines basic therapy employed at the Haight-Ashbury Free Medical Clinic in the management of acute cocaine toxicity.

Death from acute toxicity most often occurs within 2 to 3 min, but may be delayed as much as 30 min after symptoms develop. If a patient survives the first 3 hr after such an episode, he is likely to recover.[30] Psychological support to the recovering victim of overdose can also be of the

TABLE 2

The "Caine" Reaction

Phase	Central nervous system	Circulatory system	Respiratory system
I Early stimulative	Excitement, apprehension; other symptoms of emotional instability Sudden headache Nausea, vomiting "Twitchings" of small muscles, particularly of face, fingers	Pulse varies – probably will slow (Usual) elevation in blood pressure may occur Fall in blood pressure may occur Pallor of skin	Increased respiratory rate *and* depth
I-a Advanced stimulative	Convulsions (tonic and clonic) resemble Grand Mal seizure	Increase in both pulse rate *and* blood pressure	Cyanosis, dyspnea, rapid (gasping or irregular) respiration
II Depressive	Paralysis of muscles Loss of reflexes Unconsciousness Loss of vital functions Death	Circulatory failure No palpable pulse Death	Respiratory failure Ashen gray cyanosis Death

From Gay, G. R., Inaba, D. S., Sheppard, W., and Newmeyer, J. A., *Clin. Toxicol.,* 8(2), 149, 1975. With permission.

TABLE 3

Treatment of the "Caine" Reaction

1. Administration of Oxygen, by positive pressure and artifical respiration if necessary. First, be *assured* that an open airway is present.
2. Trendelenburg position (head down). Wrap arms and legs if necessary to increase central return of blood.
3. Inject *small amounts* of short-acting barbiturates (e.g., 25 to 50 mg sodium pentothal) *if* convulsions are *present*. May be repeated but *gently*. (Do *not* force general depressant effect to point of no return.) Recent work by Rappolt* indicates that 1.0 to 6.0 mg of the β-blocker propranolol (Inderal®) given i.v. in 1.0-mg increments terminate a "cocaine OD" within less than 3 min. Oral propranolol (40 mg) may be used, but onset usually coincides with the duration of action of cocaine, per se, some 40 min.
4. Keep patient cool and keep crowds away. (Keep cool yourself; crowd hysteria can "gang-panic" anyone.)
5. General muscle relaxants may be given to facilitate administration of positive pressure oxygen.
6. Continuously monitor vital signs.
7. Have some ice handy for hyperpyrexia.

The health professional must recognize the sociological reality that any true "acute" cocaine OD will (by all odds far-and-away) most likely be seen in medical settings, with physicians literally overwhelming their trusting and helpless patients by using cocaine as a local anesthetic for endoscopic procedures. One can only conclude ruefully (and a bit sardonically) that cocaine is perhaps most dangerous in the hands of an infant or of a physician.

*Rappolt, R. T., Ed. *Clinical Toxicology,* San Francisco, California.

utmost importance once vital life processes are assured. When recovery occurs, it may be complete in 1 to 3 hr; or there may be persisting headache or a feeling of listlessness for a day or longer. Cases associated with a marked circulatory collapse or respiratory failure of several minutes' duration show a high incidence of permanent cerebral damage secondary to hypoxia.

Chronic toxicity of cocaine ranges from the Andean leaf chewers[31-33] to the classic "burned-out," "over-amped" coke "freak" and polydrug abuser of the 1967 Haight-Ashbury "hippie era." Continued high-dose abuse of cocaine can lead to irrationality, paranoia, a proness to violence, and a true toxic psychosis similar in all clinical characteristics to chronic amphetamine or "speed" abuse.[9,34-37]

Driving that train
High on cocaine
Casey Jones . . . you'd better
Watch your speed
Trouble ahead
Trouble behind
And you know that notion
Just crossed my mind . . . .
And you know that notion
Just crossed my mind.

Grateful Dead from "Workingman's Dead"
Warner Bros. Records, Inc., #1869
(1970)

Beware the toxic paranoia of the
cranked-up speed-freak or coke-head —
they may bristle in steel.

Haight Street Omar (1971)

As use continues, initial ecstatic gratification may be replaced with an increased nervousness, depression, and insomnia. Intermittent and concomitant use of heroin or other "downers" is not uncommon to the chronic cocaine abuser.[38]

. . . sit up all night shooting cocaine at one minute intervals, alternating with shots of heroin, or cocaine and heroin mixed in the same injection to form a "speed ball.

William Burroughs[39]

Despite early psychic rewards, true physical dependence is not seen. Further, it is felt that tolerance, both to the pleasurable and the toxic effects of cocaine, is not seen. Indeed, some authors suggest a decreased tolerance (increased sensitivity), to the pleasurable effects.[9,16,24,40,41]*

Cocaine is a really great drug, it's a great way to feel good, and you can function and work clearly on it, like for 12 or 15 hours straight, without losing your perspective the way you do on uppers or speed. But it's not controllable. It's not that you have an increased need or tolerance, it's that it's so pleasant you can't control your use of it. And when you're heavily into it, it makes you cold toward people, in the sense that you're thinking of so many other things that you can't possibly accomplish them all, and you're thinking of how to do all the things and you don't think about all the people you're around . . . . Also, it can get you physically fucked up . . . .

Paul Kantner as cited in Reference 2

*See chapter by M. Matsuzaki for a detailed presentation of this controversial issue.

Treatment of the chronic cocaine abuser is symptomatic and supportive, recognizing that like chronic amphetamine abuse, three distinct phases are involved in the complete detoxification process. Originally outlined by Chambers[42] for amphetamine addiction, these phases are

1. Initial detoxification
2. Initial abstinence
3. Long-term aftercare

Modified for the cocaine abuser, initial detoxification consists of dealing with an initial drug-induced, paranoid psychotic state. As with traditional talk-down procedures for psychedelic drugs, the physically exhausted and potentially psychotic "coke-head" must be approached in a cautious, yet nonconfrontive manner. Gentle, quiet vocal reassurance along with a quiet environment (if possible) has reaped tremendous results in dealing with this initial phase of cocaine detoxification. Once credibility and rapport have been established, definitive therapy may be offered with the approval of the patient. (Often times a coke abuser will come in asking for some form of pharmacological relief.) At the Drug Detox Project of the Haight-Ashbury Free Medical Clinics the authors have had excellent results and greater patient compliance by using sedative-hypnotic drugs during the initial detox from cocaine. We do not recommend the general use of phenothiazine derivatives with their greater side effects and adverse reactions. Affording the patient some sleep (with 1 to 1.5 gm chloral hydrate or 30 to 60 mg flurazepam) and treating his agitated-depressive state with 20 to 40 mg/day diazepam or 30 to 60 mg/day chlordiazepoxide (also helpful for muscular cramps and spasms of withdrawal) are the important aspects of the first 3 to 10 days of initial detoxification.

The initial abstinence phase of treating chronic cocaine abuse involves a discontinuation (via tapering) of all sedative medications. A stronger counseling relationship is established with the patient and a more formalized psychosocial rehabilitative approach is initiated. Though generally accepted that cocaine addiction does not manifest a phsyical withdrawal syndrome, chronic abusers have been observed to enter into a depressive and apathetic state of consciousness sometimes accompanied by muscular cramps, headaches, and continued sleep disturbances during this second phase of treatment.

Come here mama . . . come here quick This old cocaine really got me sick Cocaine, . . . Cocaine running around my brain. Dave Von Ronk
Cocaine Blues

Though somewhat controversial, tricyclic antidepressants (doxepin or amitriptyline) in a mild therapeutic dose given once a day at bedtime have been effective in cases of severe refractive depression following chronic cocaine abuse. Tricyclic antidepressants should not be administered during the initial detoxification phase to avoid potentiation of an anticholinergic crisis sometimes seen with chronic abuse. In addition, it is best not to initiate their use while the patient is still receiving any sedative medications.

Although not our personal method, the regime of R. T. Rappolt, Sr.* should be mentioned here. This consists of treatment during the first 7 days of abstinence from cocaine with the butyrophenone haloperidol, Haldol®, in oral dosage of 10 to 25 mg the first day, and 25 mg per day the following 6 to 7 days. This treatment is found to effectively block the central euphoric and emetic properties of cocaine (postulated to be by competitive dopamine blockade).

Caveat: Because of the rather strikingly common extrapyramidol reactions following these high dosages, it is recommended to use concomitantly benztropine mesylate (Cogentin®) or diphenhydramine (Benadryl®) in usual anti-parkinsonian dosage. Further, haloperidol should not be used in conjunction with other CNS depressant drugs.

The duration of time spent in this initial phase of detoxification varies greatly with the individual needs of the patient and terminates when the patient is no longer in need of any continued pharmacologic support (may last for several months).

The long-term aftercare phase of detoxification is a prolonged process of contact and follow-up of the drug free ex-cocaine abuser. Recognizing his individual emotional, psychosocial needs and providing workable alternatives to drugs in meeting those needs are absolutely essential if rehabilitation in any true sense is to be achieved.

Though recidivism to chronic cocaine abuse is much lower than that of heroin or barbiturate

*Rappolt, R. T., Sr., personal communication.

abuse (probably because of economic limitations), continued sporadic use after treatment and retention of patients past the initial detoxification phase are the drawbacks with the above (idealistic and complete) detoxification approach. Invariably, the cocaine abusers completing the full detoxification approach outlined above at the Haight-Ashbury Free Medical Clinics were those who had established strong and ongoing counseling relationships with the project staff during the initial detoxification phase. Thus, it is important here to note that cocaine abuse, as with all forms of chronic compulsive drug-taking behavior, is not simply a pharmacologic-physiologic phenomenon but is comprised of a more complex interaction between psychological, emotional, and social variables, as well as chemical and physiologic parameters.

CONCLUSION

In its pharmacologic action, cocaine, perhaps more than any other of the recognized psychoactive drugs, reinforces and boosts what we recognize as the highest aspirations of American initiative, energy, frenetic achievement, and ebullient optimism (even in the face of great odds). On the coin's darker side of course are exhaustion, paranoia, and violence.

Cocaine, the truly American drug first used by the Andean Indians, is now restating the Yankee energy and vitality of free enterprise and even being incorporated into our leisure hours ("coke-time"). It is inevitable that cocaine, perhaps the most rapturously euphoric drug known to man,

would be rediscovered by the drug experimenters of the "Snorting Seventies."

The characteristics of drug dependence to cocaine can be summarized by a strong psychic dependency without the development of classical phsyical dependence and absence of a characteristic physiologic abstinence syndrome when the drug is withdrawn. Psychic dependence and a withdrawal depressive neuropsychiatric state with sleep disturbances may persist for several months after cessation of chronic high-dose cocaine abuse. Chronic cocaine abuse, still fairly rare but increasingly reported, can be treated via a three-phasic approach:

1. Initial detoxification — utilizing the traditional talk-down techniques along with sedative-hypnotic medication
2. Initial abstinence — increasing psychosocial counseling and rehabilitation with occasional employment of tricyclic antidepressants in cases of severe and continued depression
3. Long-term aftercare — prolonged follow-up with positive support therapy

Cocaine is probably the best example of a substance which induces deep psychic dependence without classical physical dependence that ultimately leads to a sporadic, profound type of drug abuse.

Whiffaree an' a whiffarye
Gonna keep on a-whiffin' until I die
An' ho, ho, baby, take a whiff on me.
Huddie Ledbetter ("Leadbelly")
"Take a Whiff on Me"
Electra Records EKL-301/2
(1933)

REFERENCES

1. **Gay, G. R., Inaba, D. S., Sheppard, C. W., and Newmeyer, J. A.,** Cocaine: History, epidemiology, human pharmacology, and treatment. A perspective on a new debut for an old girl, *Clin. Toxicol.,* 8(2), 149, 1975.
2. **Perry, C.,** The star-spangled powder, or through history with coke spoon and nasal spray, *Rolling Stone,* 115, August 1972.
3. **Hopkins, J.,** Cocaine: a flash in the pan, a pain in the nose, *Rolling Stone,* 81, April 29, 1971.
4. Cocaine is re-emerging as a major problem, *New York Times,* November 15, 1971.
5. Cocaine: The "Aristocrat" among dope, *San Francisco Examiner,* December 12, 1971.
6. Fifth Annual Report to the California State Legislature, Drug Abuse Information Project, San Francisco, December 1971.
7. **Anon.,** *The Gourmet Cokebook,* White Mountain Press, 1972.
8. **Gay, G. R. and Sheppard, C. W.,** Sex-crazed dope fiends — myth or reality, in *Proceedings of the National Academy of Science,* Committee on the Problems of Drug Dependence, Washington, D.C., May 1972.
9. **Eddy, N., Halbach, H., Harris, I., and Seevers, M.,** Drug dependence: Its significance and characteristics, *Psychoparmacol. Bull.,* 3, 1, 1966.
10. **Einstein, S.,** *The Use and Misuse of Drugs,* Wadsworth, Belmonth, California, 1970.
11. **Musto, D. F.,** A study in cocaine: Sherlock Holmes and Sigmund Freud, *JAMA,* 204(1), 125, 1968.
12. **Lengeman, R. R.,** *Drugs from A to Z: A Dictionary,* McGraw-Hill, New York, 1969.
13. **Malcolm X,** *The Autobiography of Malcolm X,* Haley, A., Ed., Grove Press, New York, 1964.
14. **Blum, R. H., Ed.,** A history of stimulants, in *Drugs I. Society and Drugs,* Jossey-Bass, San Francisco, 1969, 98.
15. **Bejerot, N.,** A comparison of the effects of cocaine and synthetic central stimulants, *Br. J. Addict.,* 65, 35, 1970.
16. Interim report of the commission of inquiry into the non-medical use of drugs, *Le Dain Commission,* Crown Copyrights, Ottawa, 1970.
17. **Rappolt, R.,** Practical treatment of drug abuse, *Semin. Drug Treat.,* 1(3), 207, 1971.
18. **Newmeyer, J. A.,** The Current Status of Cocaine Use in the San Francisco Bay Area, presented at the National Drug Abuse Conference, New Orleans, April 6, 1975.
19. **Smith, D. E. and Gay, G. R.,** *It's So Good, Don't Even Try It Once: Heroin In Perspective,* Prentice-Hall, Englewood Cliffs, New Jersey, 1972.
20. Chilean cocaine increases in U.S., *New York Times,* August 13, 1972.
21. **Lee, J. A. and Atkinson, R. S.,** *A Synopsis of Anaesthesia,* Williams and Wilkins, Baltimore, 1965.
22. **Wylie, W. D. and Churchill-Davidson, H. C.,** *A Practice of Anaesthesia,* Year Book Medical, Chicago, 1966.
23. **Adriani, J.,** *The Chemistry and Physics of Anesthesia,* 2nd ed., Charles C Thomas, Springfield, Illinois, 1962, 398.
24. **Krantz, J. C., Jr. and Carr, C. J.,** *Medical Pharmacology,* 6th ed., Williams and Wilkins, Baltimore, 1965.
25. **Fish, F. and Wilson, D. C.,** Excretion of cocaine and its metabolites in man, *J. Pharm. Pharmacol.,* 21 (suppl.), 135S, 1969.
26. **Peterson, D. I. et al.,** The effect of various environmental factors on cocaine and ephedrine toxicity, *J. Pharm. Pharmacol.,* 19, 810, 1967.
27. **Dreisbach, R. H.,** *Handbook of Poisons,* 6th ed., Lange, Los Altos, California, 1969, 231.
28. **Freud, S.,** *The Cocaine Papers,* Afghani Oil Press, San Francisco, 1974.
29. **Burroughs, W.,** *Naked Lunch,* Grove Press, New York, 1966.
30. **Brainerd, H., Krupp, M., Chatton, M., and Margen, S.,** *Current Diagnosis and Treatment 1970,* Lange, Los Altos, California, 1970, 808.
31. **Buck, A. A., Sasaki, T. T., Hewitt, J. J., and MacRae, A. A.,** Coca chewing and health. An epidemiologic study among residents of a Peruvian village, *Am. J. Epidemiol.,* 88, 159, 1968.
32. **Kosman, M. E. and Unna, K. R.,** Effects of chronic administration of the amphetamines and other stimulant drugs on behavior, *Clin. Pharmacol. Ther.,* 9, 240, 1968.
33. **Negrete, J. C. and Murphy, H. B. M.,** Psychological deficit in chewers of coca leaf, *Bull. Narc.,* 19, 11, 1967.
34. **Hekiman, L. J. et al.,** Characteristics of drug abuser admitted to a psychiatric hospital, *JAMA,* 205, 125, 1968.
35. **Kane, F. J. and Taylor, T. W.,** Mania associated with the use of I.N.H. and Cocaine, *Am. J. Psychiatry,* 119, 1098, 1963.
36. **Kramer, J. C., Fischman, V. S., and Littlefield, D. C.,** Amphetamine abuse: Pattern and effects of high doses taken intravenously, *JAMA,* 201, 89, 1967.
37. **Post, R. M.,** Cocaine psychoses: A continuum model, *Am. J. Psychiatry,* 132(3), 225, 1975.
38. **Sheppard, C. W., Gay, G. R., and Smith, D. E.,** The changing face of heroin addiction in Haight-Ashbury, *Int. J. Addict.,* 7, 109, 1972.
39. **Burroughs, W.,** *Junkie,* Ace Books, New York, 1953.
40. **Murphy, H. B., Rios, O., and Negrete, J. C.,** The effects of abstinence and of re-training on the chewer of the coca leaf, *Bull. Narc.,* 21, 41, 1969.
41. **Jaffe, J. H.,** Drug addiction and drug abuse, in *The Pharmacological Basis of Therapeutics,* 4th ed., Goodman, L. S. and Gilman, A., Eds., Macmillan, New York, 1970, 276.
42. **Chambers, C. D.,** Some considerations for the treatment of non-narcotic drug abusers, in *Major Modalities in the Treatment of Drug Abuse,* Brill, L. and Lieberman, L., Eds., Little, Brown & Co., Boston, 1970.

Indexes

AUTHOR INDEX

SUBJECT INDEX

A

Abuse, see also Use
  historical aspects, 3–10, 135–137, 251
  polydrug users, 236–237
    table, 235
  sociological aspects, 232–240
  tables, 247–249
  trafficking in cocaine, 238–240
  treatment, 193–194, 247–251
Acetaminophen, 45
Acetylcholine, 169
N-Acetylnorpseudoecgonine methyl ester, 22
Acquired sensitivity, see Sensitivity, acquired
Acute administration, see Administration, acute
Acute effects scale, 225–227
  tables, 226
Addiction Research Center, experiments at, 222, 225
Adiphenine
  Kovat values, table, 43
Administration, see also Use
  acute
    distribution, table, 85
    effects in animals, 210–213
    electrophysiological effects, 169–171
    pharmacokinetic studies, 83–84, 85–86
    physiologic effects, 225–227
    psychomotor effects, 168–169
    seizure susceptibility, 171–172
  characteristics of users, see Characteristics of users
  chronic, see also Dependence; Tolerance
    distribution, table, 85
    effects in animals, 210–213
    general implications, 86–88, 138–139, 143, 221
    pharmacokinetic studies, 83–84, 85–86
    pharmacological kindling, see Pharmacological
      kindling
    physiological effects, 139–141, 174–178, 195–196,
      206–208
  pharmacokinetic studies, 83–84, 85–86, 105–119
  routes
    inhalational, 234–237
    intravenous, 105–107, 205–206, 225–227, 236
    oral, 204–205, 237
    precava, 108–119
  self-injection studies in rats, 105–119
Adrenal cortex, hypertrophy, 176
Adrenergic responses potentiation of, 87–88, 161
Adulterants, 239
Aggression, see Behavior, effect on, aggression
Alcohol, 220
Alkaloids, medical, history of, 5–8, 16
Allococaine
  physical properties, table, 18
  spectral data, table, 20
  stereochemistry, 25–26
Allococaine picrate
  physical properties, table, 18
Alloecgonine, 26
Allopseudococaine
  physical properties, table, 18

spectral data, table, 20
  stereochemistry, 25–26
Allopseudococaine hydrochloride
  physical properties, table, 18
Allopseudococaine picrate
  physical properties, table, 18
Allopseudoecgonine, 25–26
Amines, biogenic, see Biogenic amines
Amitriptyline
  Kovat values, table, 43
  $R_f \times 100$ values, table, 52
Amphetamine
  anti-convulsant effects, 173
  biogenic amines, 93, 95, 97–99
  locomotor effects, 168–169, 175, 203
  mixed with cocaine, 46
  physiologic effects, 225
  psychotogenic effects, 209
  $R_f \times 100$ values, tables, 43, 52
  self-injection studies in monkeys and rats, 108
  use, 10
d-Amphetamine
  behavioral changes, 128, 131
    table, 130
  biogenic amine effects, 93, 97–99
    table, 98
  EEG effects, 138–139, 142–143
    figure, 140
  locomotor effects, 116
  3-MT concentrations, table, 96
  pimozide effects, table, 98
Amygdala, effects on, 150–154, 169–173, 177–178
Analysis, see Determination; Isolation
Anhydroecgonine, 16–19, 36
Antecedent-stimulus-produced attack, 124–126
Antifatigue action, 192
Aphrodisiac effects, 221, 238
Atropine
  Kovat values, table, 43
  psychomotor effects, 169
  structure, 16

B

Barbiturate self-injection studies in rats and monkeys, 108
Behavior, effect on
  aggression
    antecedent-stimulus-produced attack, 123–126
    comparison with other drugs, 128–129
    consequent-stimulus-produced attack, 124, 126–127
    figures, 125–130
    general discussion, 123–124, 129–131
    spontaneous attack, 127–128
    tables, 104, 105, 127
  characteristics of users, see Characteristics of users
  clinical aspects, 104, 105, 127, 203–213, 219–227
  conditioning, 177
  convulsant, see Convulsant effects
  dependence, see Dependence
  electrophysiological effects, 169–171

TITLES OF INTEREST

CRC PRESS HANDBOOKS AND MANUALS:

CRC HANDBOOK of CHEMISTRY and PHYSICS, 57th Edition
Edited by **Robert C. Weast, Ph.D.,** Consolidated Natural Gas Co., Inc.

CRC HANDBOOK SERIES in CLINICAL LABORATORY SCIENCE
Chief Executive Editor, **David Seligson, Sc.D., M.D.,** Yale University School of Medicine.

CRC HANDBOOK SERIES in MARINE SCIENCE. Compounds from Marine Organisms
Edited by **Joseph T. Baker, M.Sc., Ph.D., F.R.A.C.I.,** and **Vreni Murphy,** Roche Research Institute of Marine Pharmacology (Australia).

METHODOLOGY for ANALYTICAL TOXICOLOGY
Edited by **Irving Sunshine, Ph.D.,** Cuyahoga County Coroner's Office (Ohio).

CRC PRESS "UNISCIENCE"^{TM} TITLES:

ADVANCES in FORENSIC and CLINICAL TOXICOLOGY
By **A. S. Curry, Ph.D., F.R.I.C., F.R.C.,** Central Research Establishment (England).

DRUGS as TERATOGENS
By **James L. Schardein, B.A., M.S.,** Parke, Davis and Company.

IMMUNOASSAYS for DRUGS SUBJECT to ABUSE
Edited by **S. J. Mulé, Ph.D.,** New York State Narcotic Addiction Control Commission; **Irving Sunshine, Ph.D.,** Cuyahoga County Coroner's Office (Ohio); **M. Braudé, Ph.D.,** and **R. E. Willette, Ph.D.,** both with the National Institute on Drug Abuse.

CRC CRITICAL REVIEWS^{TM} JOURNALS:

CRC CRITICAL REVIEWS^{TM} in TOXICOLOGY
Edited by **Leon Golberg, M.D., B.Chir., D.Sc., D.Phil., F.R.C. Path.,** Chemical Industry Institute of Toxicology.

Direct all inquiries to CRC Press, Inc.

49.95
1.40
9-16
25.00